Andreas U. Bayer, M.D.

INHERITED RETINAL DISEASES
A Diagnostic Guide

INHERITED RETINAL DISEASES

A Diagnostic Guide

Juan M. Jiménez-Sierra, M.D.
Associate Professor of Ophthalmology
Universidad Nacional Autonoma de México
Ophthalmology Hospital
Association for the Prevention of Blindness in Mexico
(Hospital Asociación para Evitar la Ceguera en México)
Mexico City, México
Former Retinal Electrophysiology Fellow, Doheny Eye Institute
Los Angeles, California

Thomas E. Ogden, M.D., Ph.D.
Professor of Physiology and Biophysics
University of Southern California
School of Medicine
Director, Electrophysiology Laboratory
Doheny Eye Institute
Los Angeles, California

Gretchen B. Van Boemel, B.A.
Certified Ophthalmic Technician
Doheny Eye Institute
Los Angeles, California

with **499** *illustrations, including* **76** *in color*

THE C. V. MOSBY COMPANY
St. Louis • Baltimore • Philadelphia • Toronto • 1989

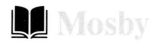

Editor: Eugenia A. Klein
Assistant Editor: Barbara S. Menczer
Project Manager: Mark Spann
Production Editor: Donna L. Walls
Book Designer: Susan E. Lane

Copyright © 1989 by The C.V. Mosby Company

All rights reserved. No part of this publication may be reproduced, stored in a retrieval system, or transmitted, in any form or by any means, electronic, mechanical, photocopying, recording, or otherwise, without prior written permission from the publisher.

Printed in the United States of America

The C.V. Mosby Company
11830 Westline Industrial Drive, St. Louis, Missouri 63146

Library of Congress Cataloging-in-Publication Data
Jiménez-Sierra, Juan M.
    Inherited retinal diseases : a diagnostic guide / Juan M. Jiménez-Sierra,
  Thomas E. Ogden, Gretchen B. Van Boemel.
      p. cm.
    Includes index.
    ISBN 0-8016-3944-1
     1. Retina—Diseases—Genetic aspects—Handbooks, manuals, etc.
  2. Retina—Diseases—Diagnosis—Handbooks, manuals, etc. I. Ogden,
  Thomas E. II. Van Boemel, Gretchen B. III. Title.
    [DNML: 1. Retinal Diseases—diagnosis. 2. Retinal Diseases—
genetics.   WW 270 J611]
RE661.G45J56 1989
617.7'3043—dc19
DNLM/DLC
for Library of Congress   89-2917
                                                                                            CIP

C/W/W 9 8 7 6 5 4 3 2 1

FOREWORD

Inherited retinal diseases, with the exception of retinitis pigmentosa, are rare. Most ophthalmologists encounter only a few of the 72 diseases discussed in this book during their careers. Although the diseases are studied during training, once in practice the distinctions are soon lost to memory. When an unusual retinal degeneration is seen, the first thought might be to refer the patient for diagnosis to someone specializing in retinal diseases. However, a retinal specialist may not be readily available. This guide will help the general ophthalmologist meet the ensuing diagnostic challenge. The unique format of this guide will suggest the category of disease and possible diagnosis and will provide useful information to impart to the patient.

The authors have successfully devised a logical approach to the diagnosis of retinal disease based on anatomic abnormality and electrophysiologic tests. They provide a brief summary of the cardinal findings, inheritance, and natural history of each disease in an easily assimilated format. The work is extensively illustrated, and references to the original descriptions of most of the diseases are provided. Because recognition of the inheritance pattern is basic to diagnosis of these conditions, a practical summary of patterns of inheritance is provided. This is a valuable addition to a book intended for the practitioner.

The authors have accomplished their aims; they have provided a very useful guide to diagnosis. The text, because of its brevity and clarity, should receive an enthusiastic welcome from those in training as well as from those in practice.

Stephen J. Ryan

Dedicated with affection to my parents,
Juan and Lola.

Juan M. Jiménez-Sierra

PREFACE

Every ophthalmologist occasionally sees a patient with an obscure retinal abnormality that seems inherited. The diagnosis may not be obvious, even to those who specialize in the retina and can summon from memory the 70 or so diseases that might be considered in the differential diagnosis. It is especially frustrating for the general ophthalmologist; many of these diseases are rarely seen, and the diagnostic possibilities swirl in dimly recalled memories from that period of cramming for board examinations. Only 15 to 20 of the more common of these diseases are even mentioned in general textbooks of ophthalmology, and those mentioned are given only as representatives of a class of diseases. The basic information is usually buried within the text of a large reference book, and developing a proper differential diagnosis requires time-consuming research.

Residents and fellows in ophthalmology have a similar problem. There is no convenient source for quick review of the salient features of the inherited retinal diseases. It is this void that this text seeks to fill. In many cases the original photographs of a condition are reproduced so that looking up the original articles describing the more rare diseases is unnecessary. Every disease is well illustrated; thus the text is also an atlas.

We hope that the general ophthalmologist will use this text to achieve a more definitive diagnosis for those patients with inherited retinal abnormalities, and we particularly hope the ophthalmologist will feel more comfortable in ordering the electrophysiology tests on which a final diagnosis may be based. There is also a more subtle motive for producing the text. Electrophysiology officially came of age in ophthalmology when the American Academy of Ophthalmology formally required all approved residency training programs to provide facilities for such tests. Laboratories for visual electrophysiology have become more common, and many practitioners have installed the equipment in their offices. Yet there is widespread confusion about the proper use of these tests for the diagnosis of inherited retinal diseases. These tests are reviewed in general terms in the appendices, and appropriate tests are clearly indicated for each of the diseases presented. We hope that this information will encourage more general use of the tests.

Treatment is not available for most of the inherited retinal diseases, but genetic and prognosis counseling may be very helpful to the patients and their families in coping with the disease. Such counseling depends entirely on accurate diagnosis and identification of inheritance patterns. The latter are fully explained and are an important feature of the text.

This manual was written by Dr. Jiménez-Sierra while he was a visiting scholar at the Doheny Eye Institute. He has a large practice in inherited retinal diseases in Mexico City, and most of the fundus photographs are of his patients' eyes. Dr. Ogden, who edited the manuscript and provided the appendix on electrophysiology, has been a visual electrophysiologist since 1962. His experience with clinical testing includes over 12,000 tests.

Ms. Van Boemel, who contributed the appendix on psychophysical testing, is a graduate student in psychology at the University of California, Irvine, and is an experienced electrophysiology and psychophysics technician.

For many of us, diagnosis of a rare and perhaps obscure condition in a patient is a cause for excitement and pleasure and perhaps for a feeling of pride. It can brighten an otherwise routine day. We hope this text will help the reader achieve some of these gratifying experiences.

Juan M. Jiménez-Sierra
Thomas E. Ogden
Gretchen B. Van Boemel

ACKNOWLEDGEMENTS

The authors gratefully acknowledge the support of the Hospital Asociación para Evitar la Ceguera en México and the Doheny Eye Institute. We are particularly grateful to Luis Sanchez-Bulnes, M.D., and Rafael Sanchez-Fontan, M.D., without whose encouragement this project could not have been completed.

The outstanding artwork represents the considerable talents of Patricia Chevez, M.D. We also wish to thank Ann Dawson for helpful suggestions and editorial assistance, as well as Eugenia A. Klein and Barbara S. Menczer of the C.V. Mosby Co. for their constant encouragement and support.

CONTENTS

Part I **INTRODUCTION**
Juan M. Jiménez-Sierra and Thomas E. Ogden

Classification of Disease, 2

Inheritance Patterns, 3

Genetic Counseling, 3

Anatomic Basis of Disease Classification, 7

Organization of the Manual, 9

Part II **REVIEW OF DISEASES**
Juan M. Jiménez-Sierra and Thomas E. Ogden

Abnormalities of Choroidal Vessels, 17
 Choroidal Atrophies, 18

Abnormalities of Bruch's Membrane, 45
 Bruch's Membrane Disorders, 47

Abnormalities of Retinal Pigment Epithelium (RPE), 59
 Macular Pattern RPE Dystrophies, 60
 Generalized RPE Dystrophy, 75
 Focal RPE Dystrophies, 83
 Congenital Pigmentary Anomalies, 100

Abnormalities of the RPE-Photoreceptor Complex, 111
 Flecked Retina Diseases, 112
 Rod-Cone Dystrophies (Retinitis Pigmentosa), 118
 Rod-Cone Dystrophies (RP-Associated Syndromes), 150
 Cone and Cone-Rod Degenerations, 166

Abnormalities of Photoreceptors, 175
 Rod System Disorders (Congenital Stationary Night Blindness [CSNB]), 176
 Cone System Disorders (Stationary Cone Disorders), 188

Abnormalities of the Inner Retina, 197
 Inner Retinal Diseases, 199

Vitreoretinal Abnormalities, 207
 Vitreoretinal Dystrophies, 208

Other Causes of Retinal Diseases, 229
 Congenital Infections, 230
 Toxic Retinopathies, 234
 Nutritional Disease, 240

Part III   **APPENDICES**

Review of Electrophysiologic Tests, 245
Thomas E. Ogden

Review of Psychophysical Tests, 255
Gretchen B. Van Boemel

INHERITED RETINAL DISEASES
A Diagnostic Guide

Part I INTRODUCTION

Classification of Disease
Inheritance Patterns
Genetic Counseling
Anatomic Basis of Disease Classification
Organization of the Manual

This manual was written with a very specific goal in mind. It is designed to help the general ophthalmologist arrive at diagnoses for patients with conditions rarely seen in the office, but for whom a correct diagnosis is vital if they are to understand the hereditary implications of their disease. Certain assumptions are made concerning the level of knowledge of the reader. It is assumed that there is familiarity with the basic ophthalmologic examination but lack of familiarity through disuse with quantitative methods of color vision testing, clinical electrophysiology, and dark adaptometry. It is also assumed that expressions common to the general practice of ophthalmology are familiar.

Most of the diseases presented in this manual are progressive, bilateral, and symmetric. It is likely that several listed as different are only different expressions of the same disease (macular pattern dystrophies). Some diseases (e.g., Leber's amaurosis) have a widely varying presentation and may actually represent several different but unidentified diseases. We use standard terminology for the diseases, but we group them by anatomic, clinical, and laboratory criteria in a way we hope will facilitate diagnosis. We have not generated a new classification.

Most of the diseases considered are properly referred to as dystrophies because they are hereditary, symmetric, and progressive; with onset after birth. Other nonhereditary, progressive diseases that are not always symmetric and bilateral are called degenerations. A third general category of stationary, bilateral, and symmetric diseases are present at birth (e.g., congenital stationary night blindness). We also present a small group of nonhereditary diseases (e.g., vitamin A deficiency) that may be mistaken for hereditary disorders.

CLASSIFICATION OF DISEASE

Classification of posterior pole diseases has been based on several different criteria. No classification is entirely satisfactory because the pathology of many of the diseases is incompletely understood. Previous classifications in the literature have been based largely on the following points, which are usually combined to arrive at a correct diagnosis:

Appearance of the predominant lesion. Many disease groups are recognized immediately from the appearance of the retina. These include the flecked retina diseases, the pigmentary retinopathies, and pattern dystrophies of the macula.

Topographic distribution of the disease in the posterior pole varies among diseases and may be localized (regional) or diffuse. The pattern of involvement provides important clues to the disease process.

Age at onset provides an additional basis for differentiation. Diseases may be present at birth (congenital), or they may develop during the first decade (infantile), during the second decade (juvenile), during or after the third decade (adult), or after the seventh decade (senile).

Progression is an important distinguishing characteristic among the degenerations that are progressive and, for instance, the stationary nyctalopias, which are present from birth but not progressive.

Symptoms are the basis of distinguishing the night-blinding disorders and color vision defects.

Inheritance pattern is the basis for separating a number of diseases whose clinical appearance may be virtually identical but whose progression and prognosis vary greatly according to inheritance pattern.

INHERITANCE PATTERNS

Most inherited retinal and choroidal diseases are not treatable. Once the diagnosis is established, the most important services an ophthalmologist can provide to the patient are genetic counseling and discussion of the probable prognosis for visual function. The disorders follow any of the Mendelian inheritance modes, depending on whether the involved genes are located on the autosomal or on the sex (X) chromosomes.

Autosomal Dominant Inheritance (AD)

Every generation is affected. Males and females are affected with equal frequency. The trait is transmitted only by an affected individual. Those without the trait do not transmit it. Autosomal dominant diseases are as a group more variable in expression, milder, and later in onset than recessive diseases. The risk to offspring of an affected parent is 50% because the defect involves one member of a chromosome pair and only one member of the pair is transmitted.

Conclusive evidence of autosomal dominant inheritance requires that there be affected individuals of both sexes in each of three successive generations.

Autosomal Recessive Inheritance (AR)

Only members of the same generation are affected. Usually the trait is only present in siblings, not parents. The trait is transmitted from asymptomatic carrier parents who each have one affected chromosome. Expression of the trait requires that both members of a chromosome pair be affected. The probability of receiving an affected chromosome from one parent is 50%, and the probability of disease from receiving two affected chromosomes, one from each parent, is 25%. Consanguinity is common in the families of patients with autosomal recessive diseases. Males and females are affected with equal frequency. These diseases are less variable in expression, are more severe, and begin at an earlier age than the dominantly inherited diseases. Every child of an affected person is a carrier of the trait. Obviously, if both parents are affected, all of their children will also be affected.

Sex-Linked Recessive Inheritance (X-L)

With this pattern of inheritance only males are affected. The father of an affected male is never affected; neither are the sons of an affected male. The trait is transmitted through the mother, who is normal but is a carrier, with the abnormal gene on one of her two X-chromosomes. The probability of transmission of the trait to her sons is 50% because males obtain their X-chromosomes from their mothers. The probability of transmission of the affected X-chromosome to a daughter from a carrier mother is also 50%. The affected male has only one X-chromosome and this is transmitted, along with the abnormal gene, to 100% of his daughters. Sex-linked recessive diseases are earlier in onset, show less variability in expression, and are more severe than diseases with AD inheritance.

The female carriers of X-L diseases often have mild fundus and electrophysiological abnormalities.

GENETIC COUNSELING

The goal of genetic counseling is to provide accurate information to a family concerning the prognosis of affected members and the probability that they will transmit the defect to their offspring. Because there is no treatment for most of these diseases, the only possibility for their control is through family planning.

Genetic counseling is based on an accurate diagnosis and a correctly analyzed pedigree. The diagnosis alone is insufficient because some of the diseases have more than one mode of inheritance. For example, retinitis pigmentosa occurs sporadically and can be inherited as an autosomal dominant, autosomal recessive, or sex-linked recessive trait. Careful family histories should be obtained from these patients to corroborate the diagnosis and to identify family members who may have the disease with incomplete expression or who may be carriers. Examination of the family is also essential to identify affected members and carriers. Diseases such as choroideremia (X-L) and Best's disease (AD) have only one mode of transmission, which is established with the diagnosis.

Particular attention should be paid to consanguinity when the history is taken. Consanguinity is common in small communities and suggests the possibility of autosomal recessive disease.

Diseases are sometimes referred to as genetically simplex or multiplex. Simplex inheritance implies that no other affected family members have been identified. The disease is assumed to represent a mutation of the affected gene. Multiplex inheritance implies that siblings of the affected patient are also affected, but no members of another generation have the trait. These terms are used when it is suspected that the disease has occurred for the first time in that generation. A subject with an inherited disorder born to normal parents, without family history or suggestions of consanguinity, may represent a gene mutation. The siblings are not at risk for the disease in this case. The children of the mutant may inherit the disease by any of the Mendelian modes of inheritance.

Successful recognition of different inheritance patterns is greatly facilitated by construction of an accurate pedigree chart. The diagrams on pages 5-7 show the symbols used to designate different familial status and typical pedigrees illustrating autosomal dominant, autosomal recessive, and X-linked recessive inheritance.

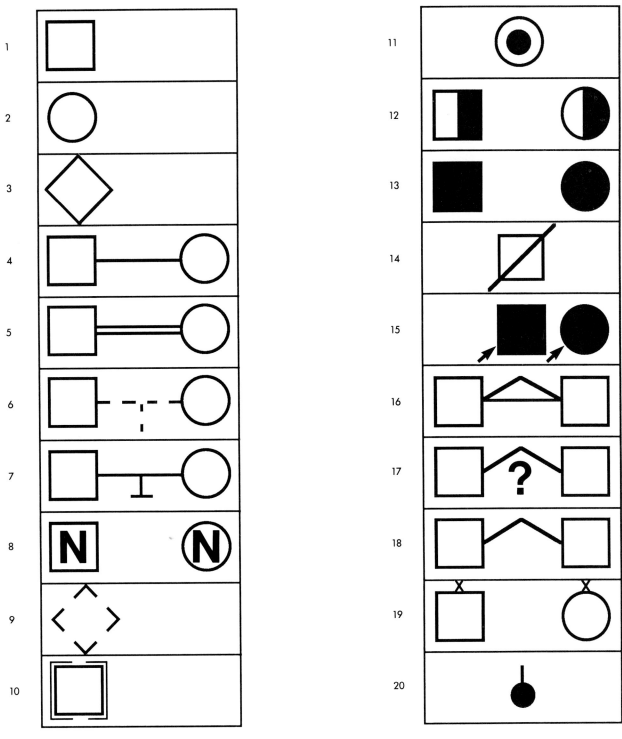

Pedigree symbols commonly used. 1, male; 2, female; 3, sex unknown; 4, marriage; 5, consanguineous marriage; 6, born out of wedlock; 7, childless marriage; 8, number of children (N) of sex indicated; 9, pregnancy; 10, adopted; 11, carrier of X-linked recessive trait; 12, heterozygotes for autosomal recessive trait; 13, affected individuals; 14, death; 15; propositus, proband or index case; usually the patient, male or female; 16, monozygotic or identical twins; 17, twins of unknown zygosity; 18, dizygotic or fraternal twins; 19, X indicates that the patient was examined; 20, abortion or stillborn, sex unknown.

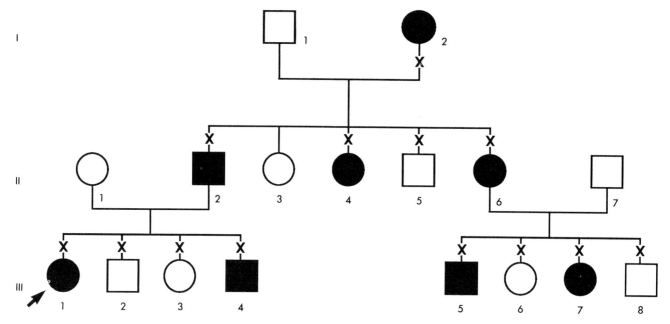

Autosomal Dominant Inheritance (AD)
I-2, II-4, II-6, III-7: Affected females; III-4, III-5: affected males; II-2: affected male (father of propositus); and III-1: affected female, propositus.

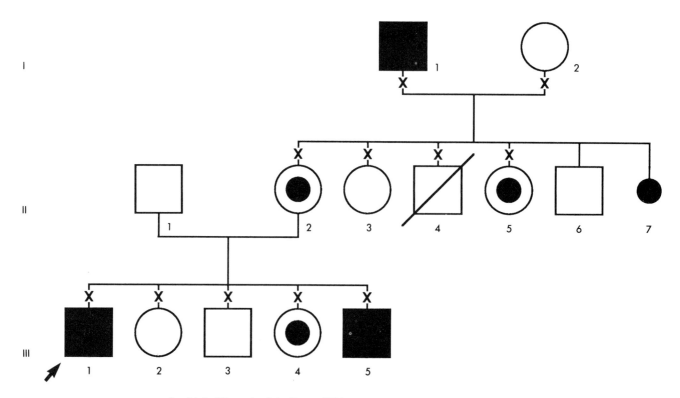

Sex-Linked Recessive Inheritance (X-L)
I-1: Affected male; II-2: female carrier, mother of propositus; II-4: Deceased male; II-5: female carrier (fundus abnormal); II-7: abortion; III-1: propositus, affected male; III-4: female carrier (fundus abnormal); and III-5: affected male.

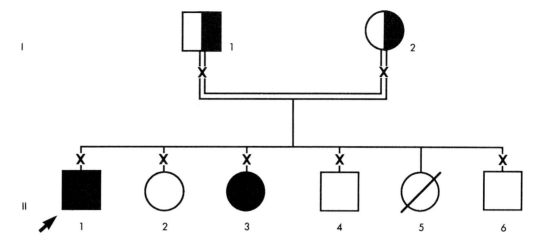

Autosomal Recessive Inheritance (AR)
I-1 and I-2: A consanguineous marriage of carriers; II-1: propositus; II-3: affected female; and II-5: deceased female.

ANATOMIC BASIS OF DISEASE CLASSIFICATION

Anatomic localization of the primary abnormality to a retinal layer or the choroid provides the best basis for classification, when this information is available. The inherited retinal and choroidal disorders presented in this book are grouped on the basis of retinal layer and area of the posterior pole primarily involved. The following section briefly reviews retinal anatomy and its clinical applications. Important terms are defined. Our definitions are, for the most part, standard but need to be stated to prevent misunderstanding.

Central retina is the retina of the posterior pole within about 3 mm of the fovea. The macula lutea is an area of yellow pigmentation extending about 1 mm laterally and 0.5 mm above and below the fovea. The macula is divided into the fovea or clinical macula (b), with its central foveola or pit (a), and a surrounding parafovea (c) that in turn is surrounded by the perifovea (d). The entire area within the outer circle is considered central retina. It should be recalled that the foveola and central fovea

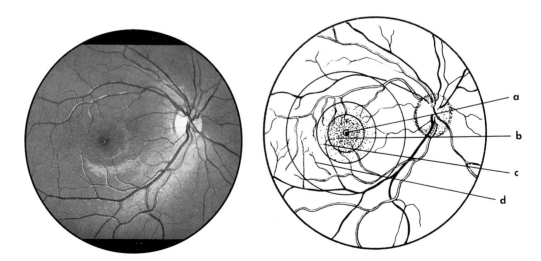

Normal fundus photograph. The central retina is well defined about the fovea (*b*), corresponding to the clinical macula, with its central foveola (*a*). The region surrounding the fovea is the parafovea (*c*). Surrounding the parafovea is the perifovea (*d*).

are rod free; the maximum density of rods, and therefore the greatest retinal sensitivity to light, occurs at an eccentricity of 18 to 20 degrees of visual angle.

Peripheral retina is divided into near periphery, midperiphery, and far periphery, together extending about 14 mm from the macula. Beyond the far periphery is the 2 mm wide ora serrata.

The **choroid** is a thin, highly vascular membrane that is the posterior extension of the uveal tract. All of the capillaries of the choroid are arranged in a single layer on its inner surface, the choriocapillaris. This location provides for efficient transfer of metabolites to and from the retina. The choriocapillaris vessels are unusual in being fenestrated; many small membrane covered holes occur on the membrane of the endothelial cells. The fenestrations are permeable to fluorescein dye, which freely leaves the vessels to account for the "choroidal flush" seen in the angiogram.

Bruch's membrane is a multilayered, noncellular basement membrane separating the choriocapillaris and the retinal pigment epithelium (RPE). It is freely permeable to metabolites passing into and out of the retina. It effectively separates the retina from the choroid. Breaks in Bruch's membrane occur in many disease processes and result in a breakdown of this separation and growth of choroidal vessels into the subretinal space, that is, subretinal neovascularization.

The **retinal pigment epithelium** (RPE) is a monolayer of epithelial cells that are the metabolic pathway and service facility for the receptors. The basal surface of the RPE is specialized for metabolite transfer, and the apical surface is adorned with microvilli in contact with the receptors. A major function of the RPE is phagocytosis of the ends of the photoreceptors, and abnormality of this function may be involved in some of the pigmentary retinopathies.

The **photoreceptor layer** consists of the outer segments of the receptors, in other words, the part of the cell containing the photopigments. Outer segments grow continuously during life but maintain a proper length by shedding their outer tips, which are phagocytosed by the RPE. In the absence of proper relations between the outer segments and the RPE, for instance, in retinal detachment, the outer segments are lost; they regenerate when proper conditions are restored.

The **external limiting membrane** and **outer nuclear layers** are specialized parts of the receptors without clinical significance. These and the receptor layer are avascular and dependent on the choriocapillaris for nourishment.

The **outer plexiform layer** contains synaptic processes of receptor, bipolar, and horizontal cells and the axons of foveal receptors that course laterally, forming Henle's layer in the macula. Henle's layer may be the site of schisis or splitting of layers.

The **inner retina** is considered that part of the retina nourished by the retinal circulation. It consists of the inner nuclear, inner plexiform, ganglion cell, and nerve fiber layers and the vitreoretinal interface.

The **inner nuclear layer** contains the cell bodies of the horizontal, bipolar, amacrine, and Müller cells. It is nourished by a capillary network of retinal origin.

The **inner plexiform layer** contains processes of the bipolar, amacrine, and ganglion cells, processes of Müller cells, and many microglial cells. It may be a site of retinal schisis.

The **ganglion cell layer** contains the cell bodies of the ganglion cells and displaced amacrine cells. It is very thick in the parafoveal region because of the accumulation of cells displaced away from the fovea.

The **nerve fiber layer** contains the axons of the ganglion cells and astrocytes. It is absent in the fovea and increases greatly in thickness as the optic disc is approached. Retinal nerve fibers from the periphery that arch above and below the fovea are called arcuate fibers. A lesion in the nerve fiber layer causes a blind spot or scotoma in the visual field corresponding to the denervated retina. Lesions on the nasal side of the disc produce wedge shaped scotomas. Lesions at the superior or inferior temporal borders of the disc produce curved or arcuate scotomas that arch above or below fixation. Small lesions at the temporal edge of the disc may cause a central scotoma involving the temporal half-field.

The **internal limiting membrane** is a noncellular basement membrane formed by the Müller cell endfeet. This membrane is the attachment site for the vitreous; it is involved in many retinal diseases associated with posterior vitreous detachment.

According to the layer primarily affected, the diseases are divided into seven anatomic categories: choroid, Bruch's membrane, retinal pigment epithelium (RPE), RPE-photoreceptor complex, photoreceptors, and inner retina. The seventh category includes retinal diseases that are associated with vitreous abnormalities, the so-called vitreoretinal diseases.

ORGANIZATION OF THE MANUAL

The manual is arranged in three parts. Following this introduction, Part II presents over 70 disease entities, each in a brief summary format: one page presents the essential characteristics of the disease; the following pages illustrate the basic fundus and angiographic findings. The page format has been designed to facilitate rapid scanning of the information essential to the diagnosis of each condition. The diseases are arranged in 14 groups based on which of the seven retinal layers is primarily involved: choroid, Bruch's membrane, retinal pigment epithelium (RPE), RPE-photoreceptor complex, photoreceptors, inner retina, and vitreoretinal diseases. Part III, the appendices, presents brief reviews of clinical visual electrophysiology (ERG, EOG, and VER) and the psychophysical tests used to evaluate color vision and dark adaptation.

We have approached the problem of diagnosis much as the practitioner must, by first considering possibilities suggested by the presenting symptoms and fundus appearance. This information should be enough to suggest the retinal layer or area primarily involved with the disease process (e.g., choroid or photoreceptors) and the disease category (e.g., choroidal atrophies). Table 1 should then be used as a guide to the section of the manual concerned with the implicated retinal layer and the primary disease groups within that layer.

The diseases listed in Table 1 are divided into 14 groups on the basis of clinical similarity or whether a particular retinal layer or the choroid is primarily involved. The assignment of some diseases to a particular group is somewhat arbitrary, and some appear in more than one group (fundus albipunctata appears in both the flecked retina and rod system groups). In addition to the diseases listed in the following table, we will also present summaries and illustrations for diseases related to congenital infections, toxic retinopathies, and nutritional deficiency.

After locating the appropriate layer and disease group, the flowcharts and tables listed below will lead the reader through a series of possible diagnoses within that group to the most probable diagnosis. Entrance to the flowcharts is by symptom (e.g., nyctalopia or color defect), by finding (e.g., bull's-eye retinopathy or pigmentary retinopathy), or by disease group (e.g., choroidal atrophies).

Flowcharts of symptoms
　　Stationary color vision defects, p. 188
　　Progressive nyctalopia, p. 123
　　Stationary nyctalopia, p. 177
　　Nystagmus, p. 190
　　Photophobia, p. 191

Table 1 DISORDERS OF THE CHOROID, RETINA, AND VITREOUS

LAYER	GROUP	DISEASE
I. Choroidal vessels	Choroidal atrophies (chorioretinal atrophies)	Choroideremia Gyrate atrophy Progressive bifocal chorioretinal dystrophy Diffuse choriocapillaris atrophy Central areolar choroidal dystrophy Peripapillary choroidal dystrophy Serpiginous, helicoidal, or geographic choroidal atrophy Circinate choroidal sclerosis Crystalline retinopathy of Bietti
II. Bruch's membrane	Bruch's membrane disorders	Angioid streaks Familial pseudoinflammatory macular dystrophy of Sorsby Dominant drusen (familial) Degenerative myopia
III. Retinal pigment epithelium	Macular pattern RPE dystrophies	Butterfly-shaped dystrophy Reticular dystrophy of Sjögren Macroreticular dystrophy (spider dystrophy) Adult-onset foveomacular vitelliform dystrophy of Gass Pattern dystrophy of the RPE of Marmor and Byers Reticular dystrophy of Benedikt and Werner Autosomal dominant dystrophy of the RPE of O'Donnell, Schatz, Reid, and Green Fundus pulverulentus (Slezak and Hommer) Dominant slowly progressive macular dystrophy of Singerman, Berkow, and Patz
	Generalized RPE dystrophy	Best's disease
	Focal RPE dystrophies	Central areolar pigment epithelial (CAPE) dystrophy Fenestrated sheen macular dystrophy Benign concentric annular macular dystrophy Lefler-Wadsworth-Sidbury dystrophy Stargardt's disease Dominant progressive foveal dystrophy (dominant Stargardt's disease) Pigment epithelial dystrophy of Noble-Carr-Siegel
	Congenital pigmentary anomalies	Albinism Congenital grouped albinotic spots Bear track–grouped pigmentation
IV. RPE-photoreceptor complex	Flecked retina diseases	Fundus flavimaculatus Retinitis punctata albescens* Fundus albipunctatus* Flecked retina of Kandori*
	Rod-cone dystrophies (retinitis pigmentosa)	Retinitis pigmentosa Retinitis pigmentosa sine pigmento Sector retinitis pigmentosa Unilateral retinitis pigmentosa Central retinitis pigmentosa (inverse RP) Pericentral retinitis pigmentosa Retinitis pigmentosa with PPRPE Retinitis punctata albescens* Senile retinitis pigmentosa Leber's congenital amaurosis Pigmented paravenous chorioretinal atrophy
	Rod-cone dystrophies (RP-associated syndromes)	Usher's syndrome Bardet-Biedl syndrome Kearns-Sayre syndrome Myotonic dystrophy of Steinert Refsum's disease Bassen-Kornzweig syndrome Olivopontocerebellar retinal degeneration
	Cone and cone-rod degenerations	Cone dystrophy Late-onset cone dystrophy with Mizuo phenomenon Cone-rod degeneration

*Included in more than one group.

Table 1 DISORDERS OF THE CHOROID, RETINA, AND VITREOUS—cont'd

LAYER	GROUP	DISEASE
V. Photoreceptors	Rod system disorders (congenital stationary night blindness [CSNB])	CSNB with normal fundus Oguchi's disease Fundus albipunctatus* Flecked retina of Kandori*
	Cone system disorders (stationary cone disorders)	Rod monochromatism Cone monochromatism Central cone monochromatism Blue cone monochromatism Dichromatism (protanopia, deuteranopia, tritanopia) Trichromatism (protanomaly, deuteranomaly, tritanomaly)
VI. Inner retina	Inner retinal diseases	Dominant cystoid macular dystrophy Familial foveal retinoschisis Gangliosidosis (Tay-Sachs disease)
VII. Vitreoretinal	Vitreoretinal dystrophies	X-linked juvenile retinoschisis Goldmann-Favre vitreoretinal dystrophy Wagner's vitreoretinal dystrophy Stickler's arthroophthalmopathy Snowflake virtreoretinal degeneration Familial exudative vitreoretinopathy Autosomal dominant vitreoretinochoroidopathy

Tables of symptoms
  Progressive nyctalopia, p. 120
  Stationary nyctalopia, p. 176

Flowcharts of defects or diseases
  Choroidal atrophies, p. 20
  Flecked retina diseases, p. 113

Tables of defects or diseases
  Albinism, pp. 102-103
  Bull's-eye maculopathy, pp. 166-167
  Choroidal atrophies, p. 19
  Flecked retina diseases, pp. 114-115
  Macular pattern dystrophies, p. 13
  Pigmentary retinopathy, secondary, pp. 118-119
  Retinal degeneration with deafness, pp. 150-151
  Stationary cone defects, p. 189
  Vitreoretinal dystrophies, p. 209

Disease summaries

Once an appropriate diagnosis is identified from a flowchart or table, details of the disease are found in the disease summary. Each of these summaries is complete, although many refer the reader to a table for complete differential diagnosis. Comparison of data concerning two diseases is facilitated by locating similar data in the same place on the summaries. Only data essential for differential diagnosis are presented. We have attempted to provide the essence of the disorder in a format that can be read and assimilated in about 2 minutes. Fundus photographs, angiograms, and drawings are also presented as standards for evaluating your own cases. Every attempt has been made to select typical data. Unfortunately, these diseases occur in a wide variety of expressions with all degrees of development. The symptoms and signs described are most relevant to a typical presentation of the disease.

Summary Page Format

The disease summaries consist of 13 summary categories (see sample below):

The group, referring to the 14 group categories of Table 1, is shown in small print at the top of the left-hand page.

Key symptoms include decreased visual acuity, color vision defects, nyctalopia, hemeralopia, photophobia, metamorphopsia, and visual field constriction. Only the three most important symptoms are listed. Some, such as nyctalopia and color vision defect, lead to a flowchart.

Key findings describe the most important physical signs associated with the disease. In most cases these findings refer to observations by funduscopy. Where appropriate, systemic findings are also included. This section is probably the single most

---

CHOROIDAL ATROPHIES

Choroideremia   FIGURE 1

KEY SYMPTOMS
Nyctalopia
Visual field constriction
Visual acuity reduced

KEY FINDINGS
Male propositus
Early
Salt and pepper pigmentation in the midperiphery
Focal RPE and choriocapillaris atrophy, peripapillary and equatorial choroidal vascular atrophy sparing the macula
Late
Macular choroidal atrophy and visual loss (after age 40)
Attenuation of vessels and pale disc, late
Choroidal atrophy is variable across the fundus
Female carriers usually show RPE granularity and pigment clumps and often have abnormal retinal function tests
Stage of choroidal atrophy varies greatly across the retina, unlike the case of gyrate atrophy

INHERITANCE	ONSET	PROGRESSION	PROGNOSIS
X-L	First decade	Slow	Light perception by age 50

LABORATORY STUDIES:

Visual Acuity	Normal to light perception
Refraction	Usually low myopia
Visual Fields	Constricted, often with scotomas
Color Vision	Normal to abnormal
Dark Adaptation	Abnormal
ERG	Abnormal scotopic to nonrecordable
EOG	Abnormal
Fluorescein Angiogram	*Early*
	Window defects, diffuse hyperfluorescence
	Late
	Hypofluorescence in areas of choroidal atrophy, retinal vessels are normal

TREATMENT	PATHOLOGY	SYNONYMS
None	Atrophy of the choroid, choriocapillaris and Bruch's membrane with loss of receptors and degeneration of the RPE, involving periphery more than central areas	Progressive chorioretinal degeneration-tapetoretinal dystrophy, diffuse total choroidal vascular atrophy of X-linked inheritance

DIFFERENTIAL DIAGNOSIS   **REFERENCES**
Gyrate atrophy   55, 166, 213, 225, 265,
Retinitis pigmentosa   308, 311, 352
Other choroidal atrophies (see Table 2, p. 19)

important in the book because many diagnoses must ultimately be based on the appearance of the fundus.

Inheritance is described with three abbreviations: "AD" means autosomal dominant, "AR" means autosomal recessive, and "XL" means sex chromosome–linked recessive inheritance. "Sporadic" refers to diseases that appear sporadically and cannot be classified as to inheritance, but which may be inherited. "Noninherited" is used in a few diseases that are known not to be inherited (e.g., vitamin A deficiency); these are included to support differential diagnosis. Inheritance patterns are of great importance in this group of diseases from the standpoint of both diagnosis and genetic counseling. A more complete review of ophthalmic genetics is presented below.

Onset is described as the decade in which the first symptoms or abnormality of the disease are most likely to appear. The term "congenital" is used here for diseases that are present at birth. Age at onset is crucial to the differentiation of certain diseases (e.g., rod monochromatism versus cone dystrophy).

Progression indicates an increase in abnormality with time and is a feature of all degenerations and dystrophies. Stationary defects are usually present from birth. Progression is described as "slow" (involving years) and "rapid" (involving weeks or months).

Prognosis is usually described as "good" for slowly progressive or stationary defects that do not threaten acuity and "poor" for sight threatening diseases. In some cases a probable final Snellen acuity is mentioned.

Laboratory studies include:

Visual acuity, as determined by Snellen chart, is usually presented as a range from the initial acuity decrement to that found in the fully developed disease. In some cases it is simply described as "decreased" if wide variability among patients is encountered.

Refraction: Hyperopia or myopia is noted for those diseases where it is an important diagnostic sign (e.g., Leber's amaurosis presents with hyperopia). Where it is not important, refraction is omitted.

Visual fields findings are usually "normal" or note scotomas or constriction, important findings in diseases such as the pigmentary retinopathies. Visual field changes may provide the only method for documenting progression in some diseases, such as retinitis pigmentosa, in an advanced stage.

Color vision, although usually abnormal in most diseases of the macula, is of great diagnostic importance in the cone disorders. The abnormalities listed are those detected with the pseudoisochromatic plates commonly used in most ophthalmologists' offices. Reference is also made to the less common Farnsworth-Munsell D-15 and 100-hue tests and tests with the anomaloscope. Color vision testing is described briefly in Appendix B.

Dark adaptometry is an essential test for patients complaining of nyctalopia. The instrument usually used for this test is the Goldmann-Weekers dark adaptometer, probably found only in large laboratories. Details of dark adaptometry testing are presented in Appendix B.

The electroretinogram, or *ERG*, is now a widely available test and provides essential information for the diagnosis of many of these diseases. Cone abnormality affects the photopic responses, rod abnormality affects the scotopic responses, and inner retinal abnormality selectively depresses the b-wave (as in X-L juvenile retinoschisis).

The electrooculogram, or *EOG*, is a second useful electrophysiology test. It is abnormal in diseases affecting the receptor-RPE complex and is diagnostic in Best's disease, in which the EOG is abnormal but the ERG is normal.

The visual evoked response, or *VER*, (also called the VEP), an evoked potential recorded from the scalp, provides an objective evaluation of the entire visual apparatus and can be used to assess visual acuity.

These electrophysiology tests are briefly described and their proper application is presented in Appendix A.

Fluorescein angiography is available to most ophthalmologists. The findings of particular importance are the retinal location of hyperfluorescence and hypofluorescence caused by choroidal atrophy, pigment clumping, or RPE atrophy.

Treatment is not available for most of these diseases, with a few exceptions that are appropriately noted.

Pathology descriptions are provided where known and where the pathology correlates well with clinical findings. Many diseases progress to virtually total retinal degeneration, but this advanced stage of pathology is not described because it has little diagnostic importance.

Synonyms exist in abundance for many of these diseases; the most common are listed.

Differential diagnosis in most cases refers to other diseases in the primary disease group, usually described in a table or flowchart to which the reader is referred. Only the most important alternatives are listed on the summary page.

References: More complete information concerning a particular disease is available through the references listed on the disease summary page. These references are to the original descriptions of the disease or to recent review articles. No attempt has been made to provide complete bibliographic documentation.

SUMMARY

If the diagnosis is known or strongly suspected, turn directly to the Index for the location of the disease summary.

If the presenting symptom or the defect revealed by examination of the fundus is included in the list on pp. 9-11, it may be possible to identify the disease group or the disease from the indicated flowchart or diagnostic table.

Finally, since the illustrations depict typical disease appearance, browsing through the disease summary photographs may lead to recognition of important characteristics of the diseased fundus and indicate the group in which the disease should be sought.

Good luck!

Part II **REVIEW OF DISEASES**

Abnormalities of Choroidal Vessels
Abnormalities of Bruch's Membrane
Abnormalities of Retinal Pigment Epithelium (RPE)
Abnormalities of the RPE-Photoreceptor Complex
Abnormalities of Photoreceptors
Abnormalities of the Inner Retina
Vitreoretinal Abnormalities
Other Causes of Retinal Diseases

Abnormalities of Choroidal Vessels

CHOROIDAL ATROPHIES

The choroidal and retinal vasculatures differ substantially. Either can be occluded without the other. Autoregulation is prominent in the retinal vessels but is probably absent in the choroid. Autoregulation refers to the ability of vessels to alter their dimensions as a result of local conditions such as oxygen tension or pH. The volume of choroidal flow is extremely high, and only a small percentage of the carried oxygen is removed during passage through it. Thus, autoregulation is probably unnecessary because the reserve of the system is so great.

The outer retina is dependent on the integrity of the choroidal vessels for its nourishment. Choroidal vascular disease is therefore devastating to retinal function; it causes gross changes in retinal function tests and visual loss.

CHOROIDAL ATROPHIES

Choroideremia
Gyrate atrophy
Progressive bifocal chorioretinal dystrophy
Diffuse choriocapillaris atrophy
Central areolar choroidal dystrophy
Peripapillary choroidal dystrophy
Serpiginous, helicoidal, or geographic choroidal atrophy
Circinate choroidal sclerosis (shown in Table 2, Flowchart 1)
Crystalline retinopathy of Bietti

This group includes the hereditary chorioretinal disorders in which atrophy of one or more of the choroidal layers is a prominent finding. The choroidal atrophy is always in association with secondary retinal atrophy and pigment clumping in the atrophic areas. This group was divided by Krill and Archer[213] according to the most affected layer and the extension of the disease in the fundus (see Flowchart 1 and Table 2).

Crystalline retinopathy of Bietti was not included in the original classification, but all reported cases of this disease have some degree of choriocapillaris atrophy, and until more information regarding its pathogenesis is obtained, it seems appropriate to classify Bietti's as a choroidal atrophy.

The most characteristic and common disorders of this group are choroideremia and gyrate atrophy, both of which show a well-defined fundus picture and inheritance pattern. In choroideremia, most of the female carriers can be detected by their fundus and electrophysiologic abnormalities (see Appendix A). Accurate diagnosis is most important as a basis for genetic counseling. Patients with gyrate atrophy show a specific elevation in serum ornithine levels and, in some patients, dietary restriction and the addition of vitamin B_6 can help reduce the progression of the disease.

Progressive bifocal choroidal dystrophy is a rare disease described by Douglas et al[92] in only one large family in Scotland.

Diffuse choriocapillaris atrophy is a rare disease with an autosomal dominant inheritance pattern, characterized by marked pigmentary changes and generalized atrophy of the choriocapillaris beginning in the posterior pole and extending to the periphery.

Central areolar choroidal dystrophy, peripapillary choroidal dystrophy, and circinate choroidal sclerosis probably represent variants of regional choriocapillaris atrophy. Circinate choroidal sclerosis is considered only in the table of choroidal atrophies. It is characterized by choriocapillaris atrophy surrounding the temporal vessels and the optic disc. Serpiginous, or geographic choroidal atrophy, is not a true dystrophy because the disease is not inherited. The etiology is unknown, but because it is a relatively common choroidal atrophy, serpiginous choroidal atrophy must be considered in the differential diagnosis of these conditions.

Table 2 CHOROIDAL ATROPHIES

The primary choroidal atrophies were classified by Krill and Archer in 1971 into four categories. They are first divided according to their extensiveness into two groups: regional (localized) and diffuse (generalized). Each group is further subdivided, depending on the choroidal vascular layers affected: choriocapillaris atrophy and total choroidal vascular atrophy (Table 8). The best way to classify these groups of disorders is by use of the fluorescein angiogram, which can delineate extension and layers affected. Choriocapillaris atrophy is always accompanied by RPE atrophy, so there is an easy visualization of medium and larger choroidal vessels during the fundus examination and in all phases of the angiogram. In total choroidal vascular atrophy, there is atrophy of larger and medium choroidal vessels, resulting in choriocapillaris and RPE atrophy, with visualization of some areas of sclera. Some larger vessels may not be affected.

NAME	INHERITANCE	PRINCIPAL FINDINGS
Diffuse Choroidal Vascular Atrophy		
Total		
Choroideremia	XL	Only males affected; areas of total choroidal vascular atrophy with macular sparing (early); after fourth decade, atrophy of the remaining macular choroidal vessels; various stages of atrophy are seen at the same time; female carriers may show pigmentary changes
Gyrate atrophy	AR	Nyctalopia, reduced visual field, and well-demarcated areas of total choroidal vascular atrophy with hyperpigmentation of residual areas; the macula is usually spared; hyperornithinemia
Choriocapillaris		
Diffuse choriocapillaris atrophy	AD	Nyctalopia, RPE, and choriocapillaris atrophy begin in macula or peripapillary area and spread to the periphery; pigmentary retinopathy
Regional Choroidal Vascular Atrophy		
Total		
Serpiginous, helicoidal, or geographic choroidal atrophy	Sporadic	Acute stage: yellow-gray lesions in the posterior pole or peripapillary area; with healing: atrophic hyperpigmented scar and areas of total choroidal vascular atrophy with serpiginous or geographic pattern; may remain inactive for long periods; mild vitreous reaction in acute stage
Progressive bifocal chorioretinal dystrophy	AD	Onset from birth with nystagmus, strabismus, temporal, and nasal areas of total choroidal vascular atrophy
Choriocapillaris		
Central areolar choroidal dystrophy	AD	Circular or oval area of macular, RPE, and choriocapillaris atrophy; the lesion is localized in the posterior pole
Peripapillary choroidal dystrophy	?	Choriocapillaris and RPE atrophy around the optic disc; very slow progression; may include the macula; occasionally, fingerlike extensions and angioid streaks may be present
Circinate choroidal sclerosis	?	Choriocapillaris and RPE atrophy in the posterior pole, surrounding abnormal macula, with pigmentary changes in the affected area
Other diseases with secondary choroidal atrophy		
Crystalline retinopathy of Bietti		
RP and associated syndromes		
Pigmented paravenous chorioretinal atrophy		
Snowflake vitreoretinal degeneration		
Olivopontocerebellar retinal degeneration		
Stargardt's disease		
Degenerative myopia		

REVIEW OF DISEASES

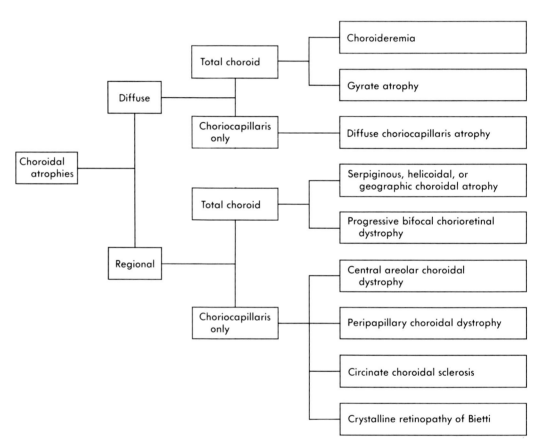

Flowchart 1

Flowchart 1
Choroidal atrophies
In diagnosing choroidal atrophies, the first consideration is whether the affliction is diffuse (involving most of the posterior pole) or regional (involving only a sector of the posterior pole). Next, it should be determined if only the choriocapillaris is abnormal or if all choroidal vessels are involved (total choroid). This distinction is generally made from the fluorescein angiogram.
Four subgroups are thus considered:
First subgroup: diffuse total vascular choroidal atrophies. The two diseases in this subgroup are choroideremia and gyrate atrophy. Choroideremia presents different degrees of choroidal atrophy at the same time. Gyrate atrophy shows the same degree of atrophy in all the lesions, which have sharply scalloped borders.
Second subgroup: diffuse choriocapillaris only. Diffuse choriocapillaris atrophy is the only disease in this subgroup and is characterized by a generalized RPE and choriocapillaris atrophy, but it spares the large choroidal vessels.
Third subgroup: regional total choroidal atrophy. The two diseases in this subgroup are serpiginous, helicoidal, or geographic choroidal atrophy and progressive bifocal chorioretinal dystrophy. In both diseases there are areas of total choroidal atrophy, localized primarily to the posterior pole. In the serpiginous form, the atrophy is present from the disc to the midperiphery; in progressive bifocal atrophy, two foci of atrophy are present—one in the nasal and one in the temporal choroid, often with a normal region intervening.
Fourth subgroup: regional choriocapillaris only. This subgroup includes central areolar choroidal dystrophy (macula), peripapillary choroidal dystrophy (surrounding the disc), circinate choroidal atrophy (surrounding temporal vessels), and crystalline retinopathy of Bietti (small intraretinal white dots and some areas of choriocapillaris and RPE atrophy in the posterior pole).

Choroideremia FIGURE 1

KEY SYMPTOMS
Nyctalopia
Visual field constriction
Visual acuity reduction

KEY FINDINGS
Male propositus
Early
Salt-and-pepper pigmentation in the midperiphery
Focal RPE and choriocapillaris atrophy, peripapillary and equatorial choroidal vascular atrophy sparing the macula
Late
Macular choroidal atrophy and visual loss (after age 40)
Attenuation of vessels and pale disc, late
Choroidal atrophy is variable across the fundus
Female carriers usually show RPE granularity and pigment clumps and often have abnormal retinal function tests
Stage of choroidal atrophy varies greatly across the retina, unlike the case of gyrate atrophy

INHERITANCE	ONSET	PROGRESSION	PROGNOSIS
X-L	First decade	Slow	Light perception by age 50

LABORATORY STUDIES
Visual Acuity	Normal to light perception
Refraction	Usually low myopia
Visual Fields	Constricted, often with scotomas
Color Vision	Normal to abnormal
Dark Adaptation	Abnormal
ERG	Abnormal scotopic to nonrecordable (see Figure 78, Appendix A)
EOG	Abnormal (see Figure 91, Appendix A)
Fluorescein Angiogram	*Early*
	Window defects
	Diffuse hyperfluorescence
	Late
	Hypofluorescence in areas of choroidal atrophy, retinal vessels are normal

TREATMENT	PATHOLOGY	SYNONYMS
None	Atrophy of the choroid, choriocapillaris, and Bruch's membrane, with loss of receptors and degeneration of the RPE, involving periphery more than central areas	Progressive chorioretinal degeneration Tapetoretinal dystrophy Diffuse total choroidal vascular atrophy of X-linked inheritance

DIFFERENTIAL DIAGNOSIS
Gyrate atrophy (p. 26)
Retinitis pigmentosa (p. 124)
Other choroidal atrophies (see Table 2, p. 19)

REFERENCES
55, 166, 213, 225, 265, 308, 311, 352

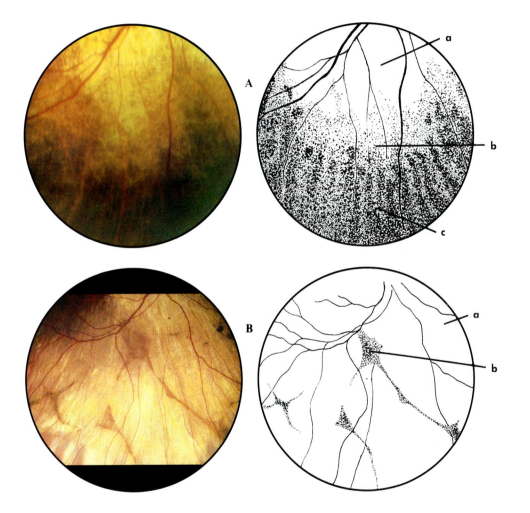

Figure 1
Chorioderemia

A, Fundus photograph showing different degrees of atrophy. Shown is an area of almost total loss of RPE and choroidal vessels, leaving areas of bare sclera *(a)*. There is no clear demarcation between the affected and less affected areas *(b)*. The retinal vessels show mild attenuation. There is increased pigmentation of the less affected retina *(c)*.

B, Generalized choroidal atrophy is seen near the equator; some areas of relatively unaffected RPE are present *(a)* and some pigment clumping is seen *(b)*. Retinal vessels are attenuated. (**B,** courtesy of Stephen Ryan, M.D.)

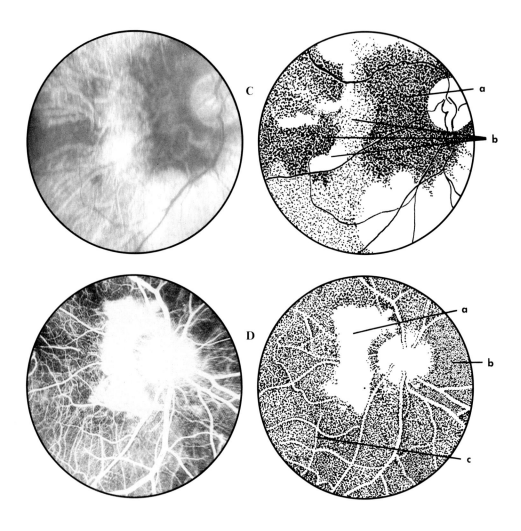

C-D, Fundus photograph and angiogram (OD) of a 42-year-old man with advanced choroideremia. Visual acuity: light perception OU. Family history: two brothers affected with the same condition; ERG nonrecordable.

C, There is an area of relative RPE preservation temporal to the optic disc *(a)*. Different degrees of atrophy are seen in the macular area *(b)*.

D, Angiogram showing a hyperfluorescent area of intact choriocapillaris temporal to the optic disc *(a)* and a relative hypofluorescent area caused by RPE and choriocapillaris atrophy *(b)*. Some large choroidal vessels remain unaffected *(c)*. Retinal vessels show mild attenuation.

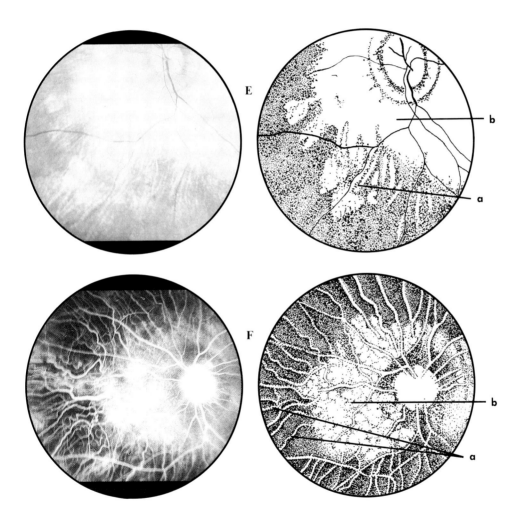

E, Fundus photograph and fluorescein angiogram of a 38-year-old man with visual acuity of hand motions, showing generalized chorioretinal atrophy *(a)*, with visualization of some areas of sclera *(b)*. Optic disc is pale and retinal vessels are narrow.

F, Angiogram shows almost total disappearance of RPE and choriocapillaris; some large choroidal vessels *(a)* and some choriocapillaris surrounding the optic disc remain *(b)*. (**E-F,** courtesy of Hugo Quiroz, M.D.)

Gyrate Atrophy FIGURE 2

KEY SYMPTOMS
Nyctalopia
Myopia
Visual field constriction
Late reduction in acuity

KEY FINDINGS
Midperipheral islands of chorioretinal atrophy, with sharply defined scalloped borders separated by normal retina
Extension and coalescence of islands form a "garland island"
Pigment clumps in atrophic areas; adjacent normal retinal areas have hyperpigmented edges
Late choroidal atrophy beneath the macula may expose the sclera
Stage of choroidal atrophy is relatively uniform in all affected areas, unlike choroideremia
Myopia in 90% of patients
Cataracts in 50% of patients after age 40
Pale discs and attenuated vessels are seen late
Hyperornithinemia caused by deficient ornithine aminotransferase
Carriers are asymptomatic but may have hyperornithinemia

INHERITANCE	ONSET	PROGRESSION	PROGNOSIS
AR	First decade	Slow	<20/200 by age 40

LABORATORY STUDIES
Visual Acuity	20/20 to light perception
Refraction	Myopia common (90% of patients)
Visual Fields	Constricted with scotomas
Color Vision	Normal to abnormal
Dark Adaptation	Abnormal, elevation of rod threshold early
ERG	Abnormal scotopic ERG early; nonrecordable later
EOG	Abnormal
Fluorescein Angiogram	Loss of choriocapillaris and RPE in affected areas, sparing large vessels; sharply demarcated intervening normal areas, with border leakage

TREATMENT
Pyridoxine; arginine-free diet to reduce ornithinemia; cataract extraction

PATHOLOGY
Not known

SYNONYMS
Diffuse total choroidal vascular atrophy of autosomal inheritance
Fuch's gyrate atrophy
Gyrate atrophy of the choroid and retina

DIFFERENTIAL DIAGNOSIS
Choroideremia (p. 22)
Retinitis pigmentosa (p. 124)
Choroidal atrophies (see Table 2, p. 19)

REFERENCES
27, 97, 165, 166, 193, 213, 225, 265, 352, 353, 354, 373, 374

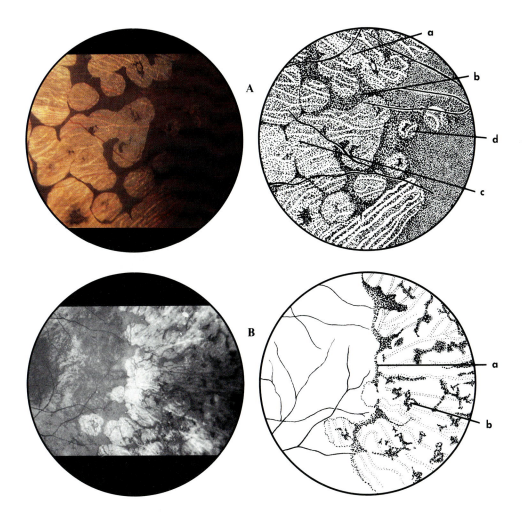

Figure 2
Gyrate Atrophy

A, Fundus photograph showing the characteristic areas of choroidal atrophy *(a)*, with hyperpigmentation of residual areas *(b)*. The underlying choroidal vessels appear "sclerotic" *(c)*. Affected areas are separated from normal-appearing retina by scalloped borders. Newly affected areas appear as isolated islands *(d)*. The retinal vessels look attenuated and cross over the affected areas.

B, Fundus photograph showing the scalloped border *(a)* between the normal and affected areas. Pigment clumping is seen in the area of chorioretinal atrophy *(b)*.

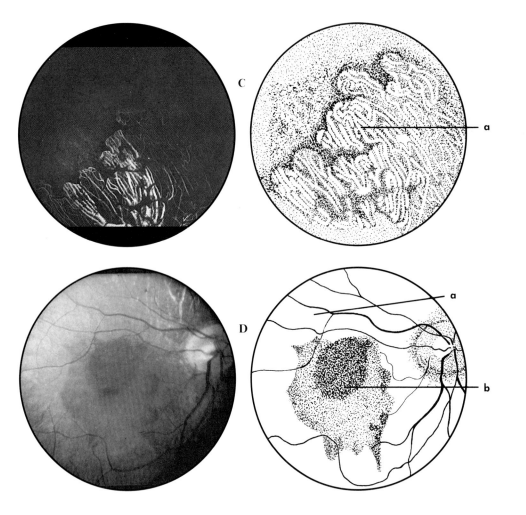

C, Angiogram in arterial phase shows a loss of choriocapillaris and RPE in the affected areas, with some large choroidal vessels remaining in atrophic areas *(a)*.

D, Fundus photograph showing late stages of chorioretinal atrophy from the periphery to the posterior pole *(a)*. The central macula is spared *(b)*. There is mild attenuation of the retinal vessels and mild optic disc pallor.

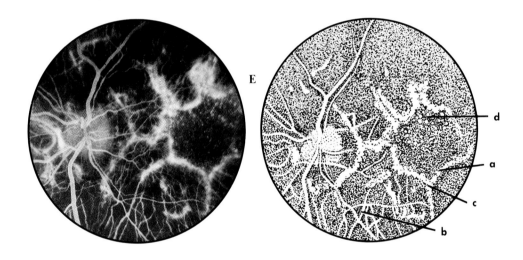

E, Fluorescein angiogram in late venous phase in one late stage case with the macula spared and a sharp demarcation between normal and affected retina *(a)*. In the affected area there is hypofluorescence caused by choriocapillaris and RPE atrophy. Some choroidal vessels are visible in these areas *(b)*. There is hyperfluorescence in the border of the central nonaffected macula *(c)*, probably caused by nonaffected choriocapillaris in the central macula. There is also a central nonfluorescent "normal appearing" macula caused by hyperpigmentation, with some "dots" of hyperfluorescence reflecting focal RPE atrophy *(d)*. (**A-D,** courtesy of Edgar Thomas, M.D.)

Progressive Bifocal Chorioretinal Dystrophy FIGURE 3

KEY SYMPTOMS
Very low visual acuity from birth

KEY FINDINGS
Pendular nystagmus, alternating esotropia

Large temporal area of choroidal atrophy surrounded occasionally by clumped pigment; probably begins at birth

Progression to equator in second decade

Nasal lesion develops later and spreads to equator

Fourth decade: total choroidal atrophy sparing only a narrow vertical strip of retina above and below the disc

Optic disc pallor and attenuated vessels

INHERITANCE	ONSET	PROGRESSION	PROGNOSIS
AD	Probably congenital	Slow	Poor

LABORATORY STUDIES
Visual Acuity	Decreased
Refraction	Myopia
Visual Fields	Scotomas
Color Vision	Abnormal
Dark Adaptation	Abnormal
ERG	Abnormal to nonrecordable
EOG	Probably abnormal
Fluorescein Angiogram	Large areas of hypofluorescence corresponding to choroidal atrophy

TREATMENT	PATHOLOGY	SYNONYMS
None	Not described	Progressive bifocal chorioretinal atrophy

DIFFERENTIAL DIAGNOSIS
Degenerative myopia (p. 56)

Choroidal atrophies (see Table 2, p. 19)

REFERENCES
92

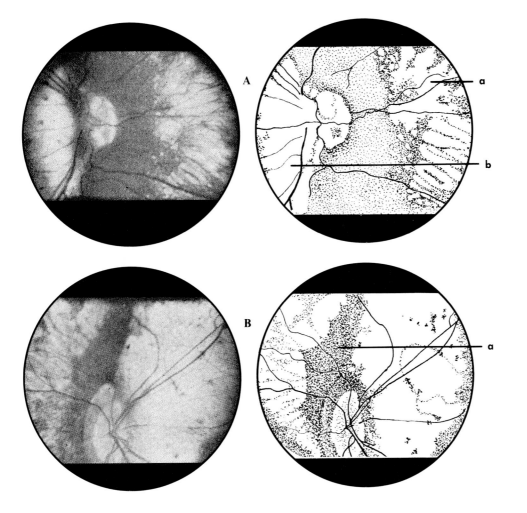

Figure 3
Progressive Bifocal Chorioretinal Dystrophy

A, Fundus photograph showing chorioretinal atrophy in the nasal *(a)* and temporal *(b)* retina.

B, Fundus photograph showing a more advanced stage; a vertical strip of retina about the optic disc is unaffected *(a)*. (**A-B,** reproduced and redrawn from Douglas AA, Waheed I, and Wyse CT: Progressive bifocal chorio-retinal atrophy: a rare familial disease of the eyes. Br J Ophthalmol 52:743, 1968.)

Diffuse Choriocapillaris Atrophy FIGURE 4

KEY SYMPTOMS
Visual acuity reduction
Nyctalopia
Visual field constriction

KEY FINDINGS
RPE atrophy; pigment stippling and mottling
Choroidal vessels are visible in involved areas
Starts centrally in the papillomacular area and spreads peripherally
Occasional peripheral lesions, spread centrally
Eventually the entire fundus shows choriocapillaris atrophy
Late
Retinal vessel attenuation and optic disc pallor

INHERITANCE	ONSET	PROGRESSION	PROGNOSIS
AD	First to fourth decade	Slow	Poor

LABORATORY STUDIES
Visual Acuity	Decreased
Visual Fields	Constricted with ring scotomas
Color Vision	May be abnormal
Dark Adaptation	Abnormal
ERG	Abnormal to nonrecordable
EOG	Abnormal very early in the disease
Fluorescein Angiogram	*Early*
	Diffuse hyperfluorescence caused by window defects (RPE atrophy)
	Late
	Hypofluorescence (combined choriocapillaris and RPE atrophy)

TREATMENT	PATHOLOGY	SYNONYMS
None	Not reported	Diffuse choroidal sclerosis
		Generalized choroidal sclerosis

DIFFERENTIAL DIAGNOSIS
Choroideremia (p. 22)
Choroidal atrophies (see Table 2, p. 19)
Retinitis pigmentosa (p. 124)

REFERENCES
166, 213, 265

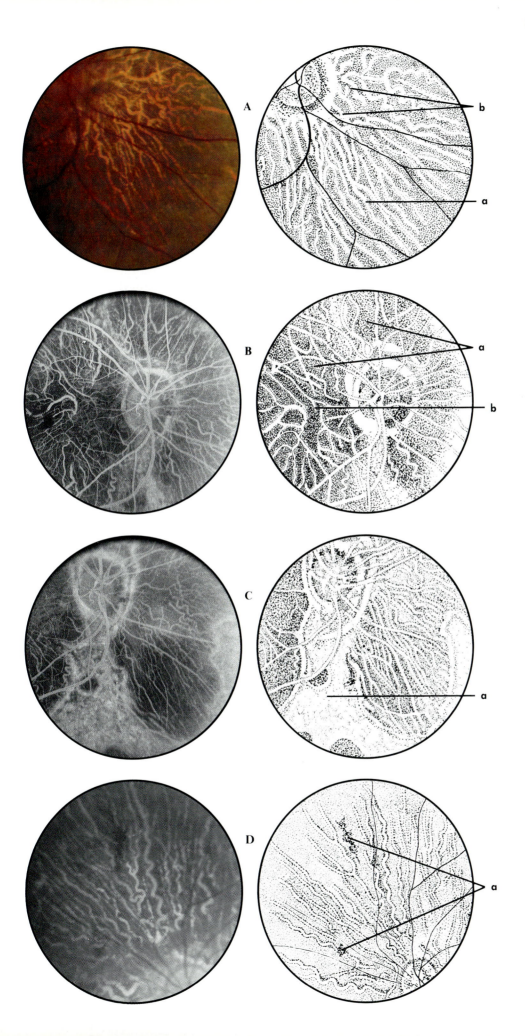

Figure 4
Diffuse Choriocapillaris Atrophy

A, A 35-year-old female with nyctalopia, photophobia, and low vision. One sister is similarly affected. Fundus photograph shows a diffuse loss of RPE revealing large choroidal vessels (a), some of which look "sclerotic" with a yellow-white appearance (b). The optic disc looks normal, but there is mild retinal vessel attenuation.

B, Angiogram shows loss of choriocapillaris and RPE (a), with irregular filling of the large choroidal vessels (b).

C, Angiogram showing an area of relatively nonaffected capillaris inferior to the optic disc (a).

D, Fundus photograph showing some irregular pigment clumping in the retina superior to the optic disc (a).

Central Areolar Choroidal Dystrophy FIGURE 5

KEY SYMPTOMS
Mild central vision loss

KEY FINDINGS
Early
Mild, nonspecific foveal pigment granularity
Late
A circular or oval area of RPE and choriocapillaris atrophy within the posterior pole
Underlying choroidal vessels appear yellowish-white through the defect, which usually has a sharp border
The peripheral retina is not involved

INHERITANCE	ONSET	PROGRESSION	PROGNOSIS
AD	Third decade	Very slow	Poor (20/200)

LABORATORY STUDIES
Visual Acuity	20/20 to 20/200
Visual Fields	Central scotoma
Color Vision	Abnormal
Dark Adaptation	Normal
ERG	Usually normal or mildly reduced; photopic
EOG	Normal to slightly abnormal
Fluorescein Angiogram	*Early*
	Faint transmission defects; may have bull's-eye
	Late
	Defective choriocapillaris filling and window defects caused by RPE atrophy

TREATMENT
None

PATHOLOGY
Sharply circumscribed area of loss of RPE and choriocapillaris; reduction in photoreceptor nuclei

SYNONYMS
Central choroidal vascular atrophy
Central areolar choroidal sclerosis
Central areolar pigment epithelial dystrophy and central areolar choroidal dystrophy are probably identical diseases

DIFFERENTIAL DIAGNOSIS
Choroidal atrophies (see Table 2, p. 19)

REFERENCES
7, 36, 51, 105, 213, 260, 265, 316, 317, 346, 371

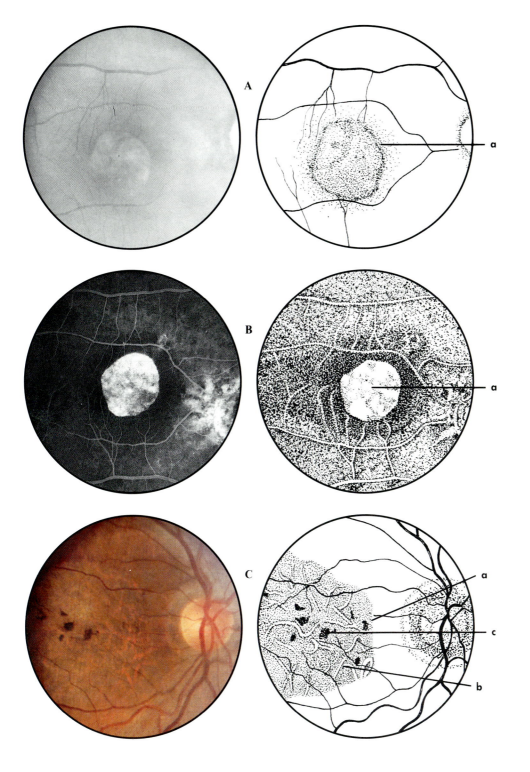

Figure 5
Central Areolar Choroidal Dystrophy

A 35-year-old female with a visual acuity of 20/100 OU. The ERG and EOG are normal. One brother is affected with the same condition.

A, Fundus photograph (OD) showing a central, well-demarcated area of RPE atrophy *(a)* with visualization of some large choroidal vessels. Retinal vessels look normal.

B, Angiogram (OD) in late phase showing a well-demarcated hyperfluorescent lesion *(a)*, probably caused by RPE atrophy, with preservation of some choriocapillaris.

C, Fundus photograph of a 48-year-old male, brother of the patient shown in **A**, with a visual acuity of 20/400 and normal electrophysiology tests. A large area of RPE atrophy is seen *(a)*, with visualization of large choroidal vessels *(b)* and some pigment clumping *(c)*.

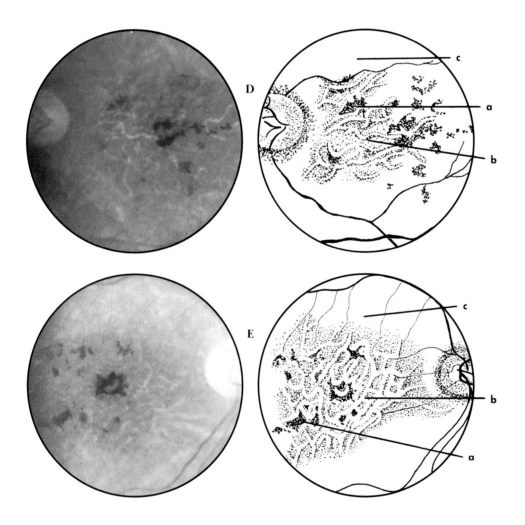

D-E, Fundus photographs (OD and OS) of a 52-year-old male with loss of central vision at the age of 30 years. No family members are affected. The ERG and EOG are normal. Fundus photographs show a large, symmetric, atrophic macular lesion *(a),* with visualization of choroidal vessels *(b)* and pigment clumps (OU). There are some RPE disturbances away from this area *(c).* Atrophic Stargardt's macular lesions must be considered in the differential diagnosis of this patient.

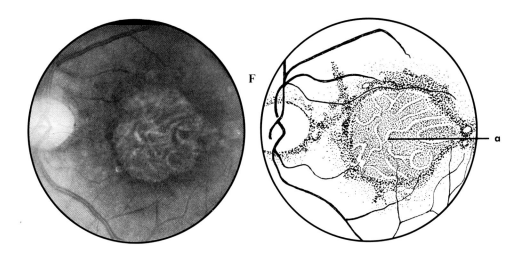

F, A 72-year-old male with a decrease in vision at age 66. Visual acuity is 20/200. Fundus photograph shows an atrophic macular lesion in the central macula *(a)* with visualization of choroidal vessels. This lesion corresponds to the areolar form of age-related macular degeneration.

Peripapillary Choroidal Dystrophy FIGURE 6

KEY SYMPTOMS
Asymptomatic or visual loss
Nyctalopia

KEY FINDINGS
RPE and choriocapillaris atrophy around optic disc, producing a peripapillary halo
Large choroidal vessels visible through defects
Slow progression toward macula and periphery
Lesion margins are poorly defined, in contrast to the lesions of central areolar choroidal dystrophy
Fingerlike lesions may extend from the optic disc
Angioid streaks may be present

INHERITANCE	ONSET	PROGRESSION	PROGNOSIS
Sporadic, AD	From age 20 to age 40	Very slow	Poor

LABORATORY STUDIES
Visual Acuity	20/20 to 20/400
Visual Fields	Central and paracentral scotomas
Color Vision	Normal to abnormal
Dark Adaptation	Normal to abnormal
ERG	Normal to abnormal
EOG	Normal to abnormal
Fluorescein Angiogram	Peripapillary hypofluorescence with visualization of large vessels caused by RPE and choriocapillaris atrophy

TREATMENT
None

PATHOLOGY
Loss of RPE, choriocapillaris, and photoreceptors, with breaks in Bruch's membrane; larger choroidal vessels are intact

SYNONYMS
None in general use

DIFFERENTIAL DIAGNOSIS
Choroidal dystrophies (see Table 2, p. 19)
Myopic conus (p. 56)
Senile peripapillary atrophy

REFERENCES
213, 262, 317

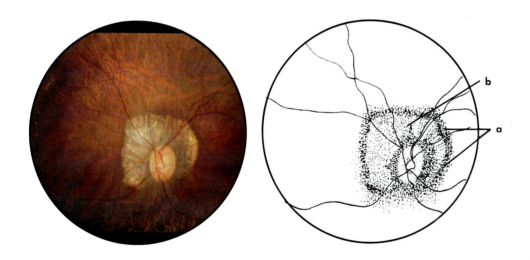

Figure 6
Peripapillary Choroidal Dystrophy

A 34-year-old female, asymptomatic with a corrected visual acuity of 20/20 OU, a refractive error −4.00 D, and normal ERG and EOG. Visual fields show a large blind spot. No family members are affected. Fundus photograph shows a well-demarcated area of RPE and choriocapillaris atrophy (a) surrounding the optic nerve. Large choroidal vessels are easily seen through this atrophic area (b).

Serpiginous, Helicoidal, or Geographic Choroidal Atrophy FIGURE 7

KEY SYMPTOMS
None or blurred vision
Visual acuity reduction
Scotomas

KEY FINDINGS
Yellow-gray lesions in the posterior pole (active lesions)
Episodic progression, with intervals of healing
Progresses from disc to periphery, leaving a tracklike scar with areas of total choroidal atrophy; the entire lesion may be active (geographic) or only the lesion tip (snakehead); remissions last months or years
Bilateral, but macula involvement usually asymmetric
Vitreous varies from clear to 2+ cells
Anterior segment not involved
Retinal vessels and optic nerve are normal
This disease is not a true dystrophy

INHERITANCE	ONSET	PROGRESSION	PROGNOSIS
None	Third to fourth decade	Slow	Poor

LABORATORY STUDIES
Visual Acuity	20/20 to 20/400
Visual Fields	Central and paracentral scotomas
Color Vision	Normal
Dark Adaptation	Normal
ERG	Normal to subnormal
EOG	Normal
Fluorescein Angiogram	Healed areas are hypofluorescent; active areas are nonfluorescent

TREATMENT	PATHOLOGY	SYNONYMS
None; steroids are not useful	RPE degeneration; choroidal and subretinal atrophy and scarring	Geographic choroidal atrophy Helicoid peripapillary choroidopathy

DIFFERENTIAL DIAGNOSIS
Choroidal atrophies (see Table 2, p. 19)
Acute posterior multifocal placoid pigment epitheliopathy
Presumed ocular histoplasmosis syndrome

REFERENCES
40, 158, 226, 319, 370, 379

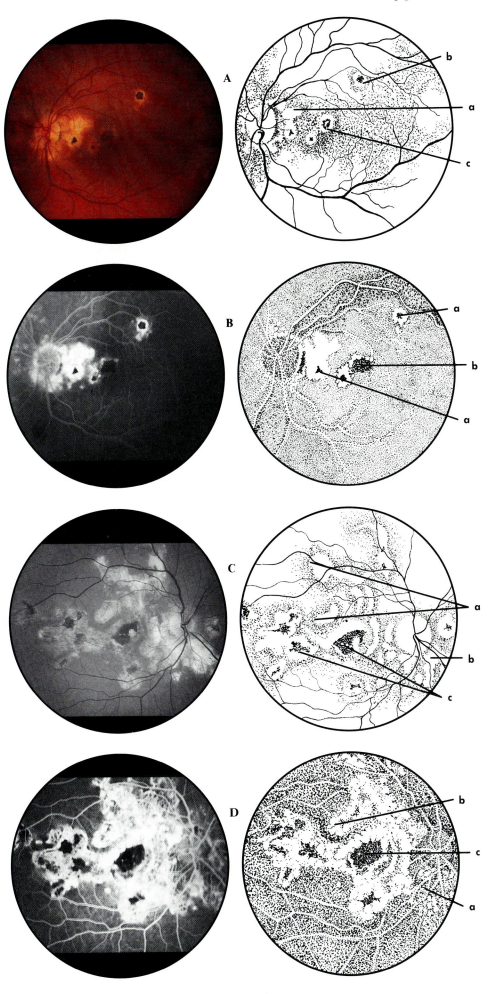

Figure 7
Serpiginous, Helicoidal, or Geographic Choroidal Atrophy

A 60-year-old female with a history of decrease in visual acuity OD of 10 years' duration and a recent onset of decreased visual acuity OS. Corrected acuity: counting fingers OD and 20/30 OS. ERG and EOG are normal.

A, Fundus photograph (OS) showing an inactive chorioretinal scar with pigment clumping surrounding the optic disc *(a)*; a second old scar near the superior temporal vessels showing hyperpigmentation surrounded by hypopigmentation is seen *(b)*. A third grayish, active lesion at the level of the RPE is seen in the central macular area *(c)*.

B, Angiogram (OS) showing hyperfluorescence in the old scars with two hypofluorescent spots caused by blockage by pigment *(a)* and a central hypofluorescent area corresponding to the active macular lesion *(b)*.

C, Fundus photograph (OD) showing a more advanced stage of atrophy. No active lesions but several "snakehead" areas are seen *(a)*, the bare sclera is visible in old scars near the optic disc *(b)*, and pigment clumps occur in some lesions *(c)*.

D, Angiogram showing hypofluorescence near the optic disc caused by choroidal atrophy *(a)*, hyperfluorescence caused by RPE atrophy *(b)*, and some areas of hypofluorescence caused by blockage by pigment *(c)*. (**A-D,** courtesy of Peter Liggett, M.D.)

Crystalline Retinopathy of Bietti FIGURE 8

KEY SYMPTOMS
Usually asymptomatic
Decreased vision (late)
Nyctalopia (late)

KEY FINDINGS
Posterior pole shows yellow glistening intraretinal crystals; many fine yellow refractile deposits in the RPE and inner retina
Sclerosis of choroidal vessels; RPE atrophy and choriocapillaris atrophy in many areas of the posterior pole
Tapetoretinal degeneration very similar in appearance to retinitis pigmentosa
Crystalline dystrophy of the cornea (not always present), which consists of yellowish-white dots in the superficial layers of the limbus
Optic disc and retinal vessels are normal

INHERITANCE	ONSET	PROGRESSION	PROGNOSIS
Uncertain: X-L or AD	First to third decade	Slow	Poor

LABORATORY STUDIES

Visual Acuity	20/20 to light perception
Visual Fields	Constriction and/or central scotoma
Color Vision	Normal to abnormal
Dark Adaptation	Normal to abnormal
ERG	Normal to subnormal
EOG	Normal to abnormal
Fluorescein Angiogram	Hyperfluorescence in areas of RPE atrophy; hypofluorescence in areas of choriocapillaris atrophy, with intervening areas of normal retina

TREATMENT	PATHOLOGY	SYNONYMS
None	Not known	Bietti's tapetoretinal degeneration with marginal corneal dystrophy

DIFFERENTIAL DIAGNOSIS	REFERENCES
Choroidal atrophies (see Table 2, p. 19) Pigmentary retinopathy (see Table 6, p. 118)	14, 29, 154, 164, 265, 372, 384

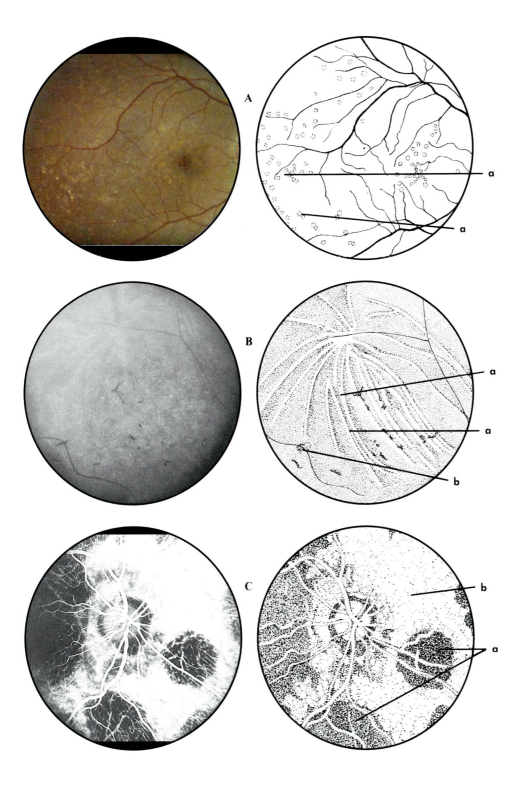

Figure 8
Crystalline Retinopathy of Bietti

A, Widespread intraretinal and subretinal crystalline deposits *(a)* in a 47-year-old male with no complaints. ERG and EOG were normal, and minimal atypical pigmentary changes were found in periphery.

B-C, A 52-year-old male with decrease in visual acuity, nyctalopia, central and paracentral scotomas, and reduced photopic and scotopic ERG.

B, Fundus photograph shows intraretinal crystalline bodies *(a)* and areas of RPE atrophy with pigment clumping *(b)*.

C, Angiogram shows areas of hypofluorescence caused by RPE and choriocapillaris atrophy *(a)* and areas of hyperfluorescence with normal choriocapillaris *(b)*.

Abnormalities of Bruch's Membrane

BRUCH'S MEMBRANE DISORDERS

The diseases included here have in common an important abnormality at the level of Bruch's membrane. In late stages the retina is affected, usually with subretinal neovascularization that develops in areas where the integrity of the membrane is interrupted; this results in secondary visual loss.

BRUCH'S MEMBRANE DISORDERS

Angioid streaks
Familial pseudoinflammatory macular dystrophy of Sorsby
Dominant drusen (familial)
Degenerative myopia

Angioid streaks are the classical abnormality of this layer. They are usually present in association with a systemic disease. The ocular diagnosis is made by fundus examination. The principal complications are hemorrhage and development of subretinal neovascularization.

Familial pseudoinflammatory macular dystrophy of Sorsby is a rare disease with a dominant inheritance pattern and the development of an acute serous and hemorrhagic detachment of the retina. This disease is somewhat similar to dominant drusen.

Dominant or familial drusen is a relatively common disease characterized by an autosomal dominant inheritance, early onset of drusen, and the development of an early subretinal neovascularization. Dominant drusen and senile drusen are identical, but family history and age at onset differentiate the two.

Degenerative myopia presents with lacquer cracks of Bruch's membrane, as well as changes in retinal and choroidal layers. It is usually characterized by high myopia, vitreous abnormalities, posterior staphyloma, subretinal neovascularization, and retinal detachment. All types of inheritance patterns are found.

Angioid Streaks FIGURE 9

KEY SYMPTOMS
Usually asymptomatic
Metamorphopsia
Micropsia
Visual acuity reduction

KEY FINDINGS
Irregular red-brown lines radiate from the optic disc, most prominent in the posterior pole
Subretinal neovascularization (SRN) is common
50% of patients develop macular hemorrhage
Angioid streaks are associated with several retinal abnormalities, including drusen, serous detachment of the RPE, choroidal atrophy, hyperpigmentation, retinal fibrosis, optic disc drusen, "peau d'orange" mottling of the RPE, and crystalline bodies
Usually associated with systemic diseases such as pseudoxanthoma elasticum, Paget's disease, Ehlers-Danlos syndrome, Marfan's syndrome, sickle cell disease, and senile elastosis

INHERITANCE	ONSET	PROGRESSION	PROGNOSIS
Primary disease AR or AD	Third to sixth decade	Slow	Poor

LABORATORY STUDIES
Visual Acuity	20/20 to 20/400
Visual Fields	Central or paracentral scotoma; large blind spot
Color Vision	Normal to abnormal
Dark Adaptation	Normal to abnormal
ERG	Usually normal
EOG	Usually normal
Fluorescein Angiogram	Streak hyperfluorescence; SRN may show leakage and pooling; hypofluorescence if hemorrhage is present

TREATMENT
Treat SRN with photocoagulation in some cases

PATHOLOGY
Fragmentation of Bruch's membrane caused by degeneration of elastic layers; subretinal proliferation of fibrovascular tissue

SYNONYMS
Choroidal elastosis
Melanosis vasculorum retinae

DIFFERENTIAL DIAGNOSIS
Trauma
Choroidal tears
Myopia
Lacquer cracks
Macular pattern dystrophies (p. 60)
Associated systemic conditions

REFERENCES
69, 72, 86, 104, 143, 145, 152, 153, 205, 221, 330, 339

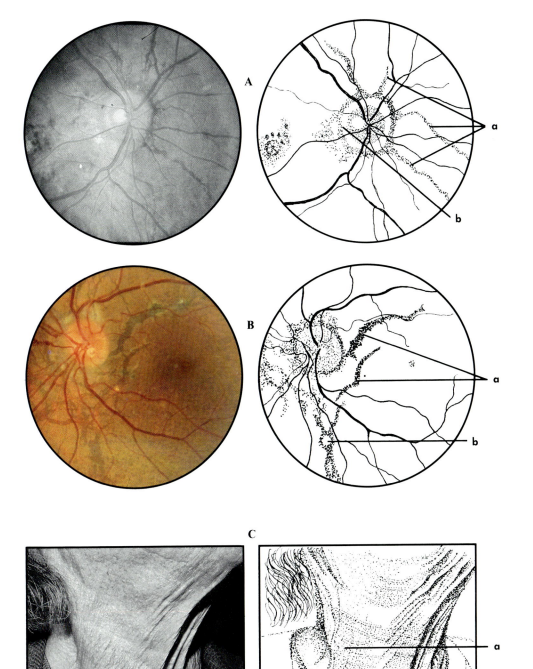

Figure 9
Angioid Streaks

A, Fundus photograph showing narrow, reddish, angioid streaks extending from the optic disc to the equator (a). In this case the streaks resemble the retinal vessels. There is also an area of peripapillary atrophy (b).

B, A 45-year-old female with pseudoxanthoma elasticum and angioid streaks (see also **C**). Fundus photograph shows wider angioid streaks (a), with a grayish-green to brownish-red color, enclosing some islands of "normal" retina (b). Note mottled appearance of the fundus ("peau d'orange"). An area of peripapillary atrophy is also present nasally.

C, Photograph of the neck region of a 45-year-old female with pseudoxanthoma elasticum (see also **B**). The skin is lax and shows multiple folds (a) with the characteristic "plucked-chicken" appearance.

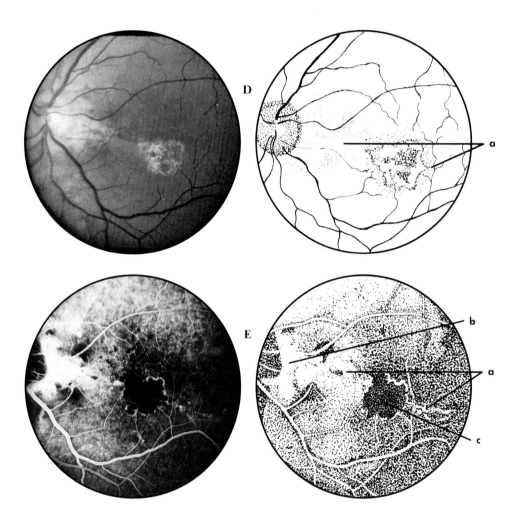

D-E, A 41-year-old male with pseudoxanthoma elasticum, angioid streaks, and secondary SRN. He has a 1-year history of metamorphopsia and decreased vision. Visual acuity is 20/70.

D, OS shows an angioid streak *(a)* running through the central macula after photocoagulation of SRN.

E, Angiogram of the same eye in late venous phase showing hyperfluorescence of the macular angioid streak *(a)* and from the peripapillary atrophy *(b)*; a central, nonfluorescent spot corresponds to the area of photocoagulation of the SRN *(c)*. (**D-E,** courtesy of Peter Liggett, M.D.)

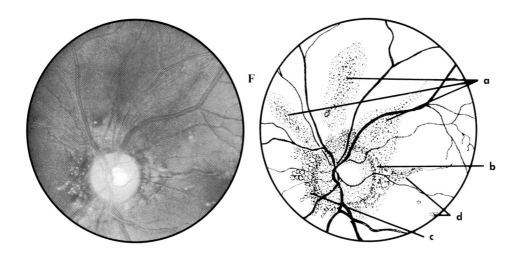

F, Fundus photograph showing subretinal hemorrhages extending from the disc, following some angioid streaks *(a)*. An area of peripapillary atrophy is also present *(b)*, with multiple white subretinal crystalline bodies *(c)* and some lesions with cometlike white tails *(d)*. This type of subretinal hemorrhage may occur after a minimal ocular contusion.

Familial Pseudoinflammatory Macular Dystrophy of Sorsby FIGURE 10

KEY SYMPTOMS
Acute visual loss

KEY FINDINGS
Central scotoma with mottling of the fundus
An inflammatory-like macular lesion with edema, exudate, and hemorrhage
Widely scattered drusen are common
Serous and hemorrhagic detachment of the RPE (SRN)
Rapid development of a hypertrophic macular scar
Slow extension over many years to periphery, with total choroidal vascular atrophy and pigment deposition
Optic disc, vessels, and vitreous are normal
This disease closely resembles dominantly inherited drusen with SRN

INHERITANCE	ONSET	PROGRESSION	PROGNOSIS
AD	From age 30 to age 40	Rapid	Poor

LABORATORY STUDIES
Visual Acuity	20/100 to light perception
Visual Fields	Central scotoma
Color Vision	Normal to abnormal
Dark Adaptation	Normal
ERG	Normal to abnormal
EOG	Normal to abnormal
Fluorescein Angiogram	Central hypofluorescence because of RPE and choroidal atrophy; extensive window defects; leakage from SRN

TREATMENT	PATHOLOGY	SYNONYMS
None	Typical choroidal neovascularization and drusen with pigment epithelial changes	None in general use

DIFFERENTIAL DIAGNOSIS
Dominant drusen (p. 54)
Disciform macular degeneration
Nonspecific chorioretinitis

REFERENCES
125, 135, 187, 309, 347

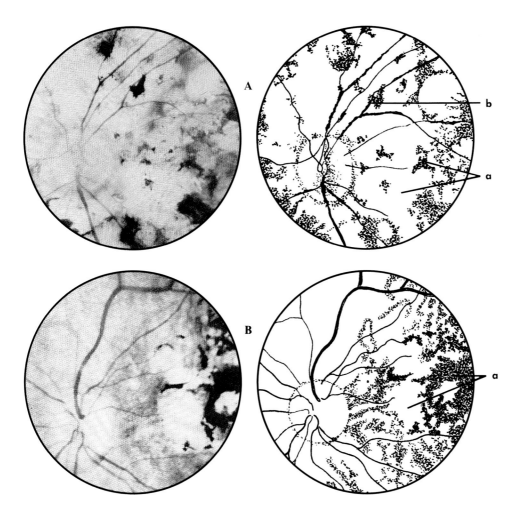

Figure 10
Familial Pseudoinflammatory Macular Dystrophy of Sorsby

A, A 65-year-old father of 8 affected children experienced a sudden decrease in vision at age 50. His visual acuity at age 65 was 20/40 OD and 20/50 OS. At age 77, acuity was counting fingers at 1m OD and at 30cm OS. Fundus photograph shows scattered atrophy of the retina and choroid *(a)*, with attenuation of retinal vessels and pigment clumps in the posterior pole *(b)*.

B, This female noted the first abnormality at 33 years of age. At 36 years of age, large pigmented areas were found in both maculas and her visual acuity was 20/60 OU. At 38 years of age her corrected visual acuity was 20/150 OD and 20/60 OS. Large areas of chorioretinal atrophy were noted at 46 years of age. At 60 years of age her visual acuity was counting fingers at 20cm OU. Fundus photograph (OD) at 47 years of age shows a large scar in the macula *(a)*. (**A-B,** reproduced and redrawn from Forsius HR, Erikson AW, Suvanto EA, and Alanko HI: Pseudoinflammatory fundus dystrophy with autosomal recessive inheritance, Am J Ophthalmol 94:634, 1982. Published with permission from The American Journal of Ophthalmology. Copyright by the Ophthalmic Publishing Company.)

Dominant Drusen (Familial) FIGURE 11

KEY SYMPTOMS
None, early
Metamorphopsia and/or central scotoma, late

KEY FINDINGS
Multiple Drusen
Small white or yellow oval or round lesions seen at level of the RPE
Familial macular drusen appear in the third decade; best seen by angiogram
Drusen are most common at the posterior pole
Drusen may become confluent after the fourth decade
Eventual central vision loss correlates with macular involvement
Late
SRN may lead to serous detachment and hemorrhage; drusen may calcify, with associated pigmentary changes
Drusen nasal to the disc were considered pathognomonic of dominant or familial drusen but also are present in senile drusen
Senile drusen are common in the elderly and can be distinguished from dominant drusen only on the basis of family history

INHERITANCE	ONSET	PROGRESSION	PROGNOSIS
AD	Second to third decade	Slow	20/200 by age 60

LABORATORY STUDIES
Visual Acuity	20/20 to 20/200
Amsler Grid	Normal, or central or paracentral distortion
Visual Fields	Normal or paracentral and central scotomas
Color Vision	Normal
Dark Adaptation	Normal
ERG	Normal
EOG	Normal to abnormal (dissociated ERG/EOG)
Fluorescein Angiogram	Fluorescence block, early
	Window defects, late
	SRN
	Early hyperfluorescence and late staining

TREATMENT
None or photocoagulation of SRN

PATHOLOGY
Amorphous sub-RPE material, remnants of the RPE; atrophy of the RPE overlying the drusen; fibrovascular membranes (SRN)

SYNONYMS
Familial drusen
Doyne's honeycomb degeneration
Guttate choroiditis
Holthouse-Batten superficial choroiditis or macular degeneration
Hutchinson-Tays choroiditis
Malattia-leventinese

DIFFERENTIAL DIAGNOSIS
Flecked retina diseases (see Table 5, p. 114)
Fundus flavimaculatus and albipunctatus (pp. 116, 184)
Early angioid streaks—orange peel spots (p. 48)

REFERENCES
85, 99, 100, 114, 136, 137, 138, 220, 257, 281

Figure 11
Dominant Drusen (Familial)

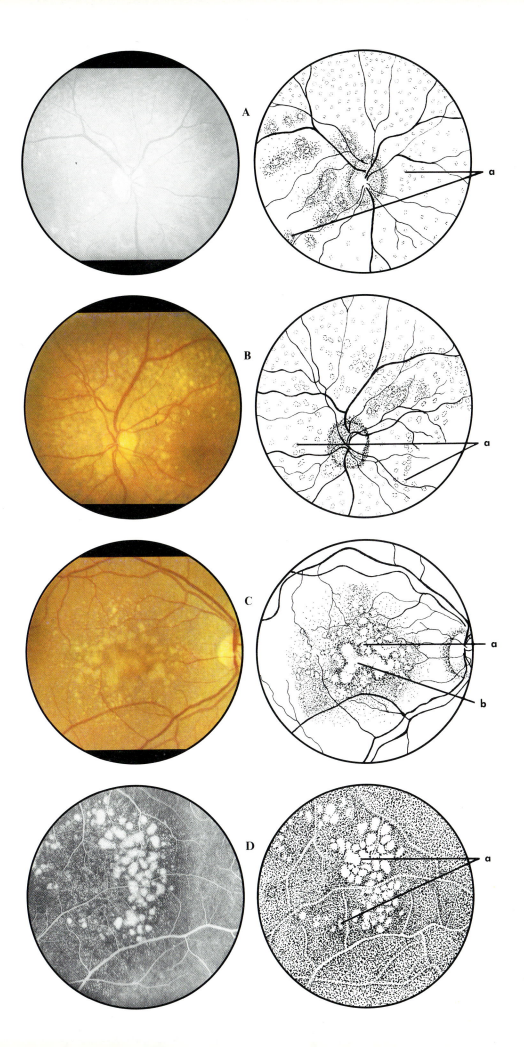

A-B, A 33-year-old male, asymptomatic with a visual acuity of 20/20 OU. He has a family history of drusen and early macular degeneration. Widespread drusen are seen in the nasal and temporal retina *(a);* some drusen in the macular area are calcified.

C, Confluent drusen *(a)* and yellow subretinal exudate *(b)* are seen in the macular area OD of this 37-year-old female with metamorphopsia and a visual acuity of 20/70.

D, Angiogram showing multiple drusen of different sizes *(a)* with variation in the fluorescent pattern. The angiogram may delimit the affected area.

Degenerative Myopia FIGURE 12

KEY SYMPTOMS
Visual acuity reduction
Nyctalopia

KEY FINDINGS
Myopic Conus
A white semilunar area on the temporal side or surrounding the optic disc
Peripapillary atrophy of RPE and choriocapillaris exposing large choroidal vessels or even bare sclera
Posterior staphyloma and breaks in Bruch's membrane (lacquer cracks), through which subretinal neovascularization may occur
Macular Pigmented Scar
Fuchs-Foster spots
Periphery
Lattice, snail track, paving stone degeneration
White without pressure and pigmentary degeneration
Retinal holes and detachment are common
Posterior vitreous detachment and fibrillar degeneration

INHERITANCE	ONSET	PROGRESSION	PROGNOSIS
AR (X-L or AD; rare)	First decade	Slow	Poor

LABORATORY STUDIES
Visual Acuity	20/20 (corrected) to hand motions
Refraction	High myopia
Visual Fields	Enlarged blind spot, occasional scotomas
Color Vision	Normal to abnormal
Dark Adaptation	Normal to subnormal
ERG	Normal to severely abnormal
EOG	Usually normal
Fluorescein Angiogram	Areas of hyperfluorescence and hypofluorescence, SRN may leak; blocked fluorescence in areas of hemorrhage

TREATMENT	PATHOLOGY	SYNONYMS
None (prophylactic cryopexy and retinal surgery for detachment)	RPE and choriocapillaris atrophy with receptor degeneration in involved areas	Pathologic progressive myopia

DIFFERENTIAL DIAGNOSIS
Choroidal atrophies (see Table 2, p. 19)

REFERENCES
11, 34, 90, 159, 188, 203, 230, 289

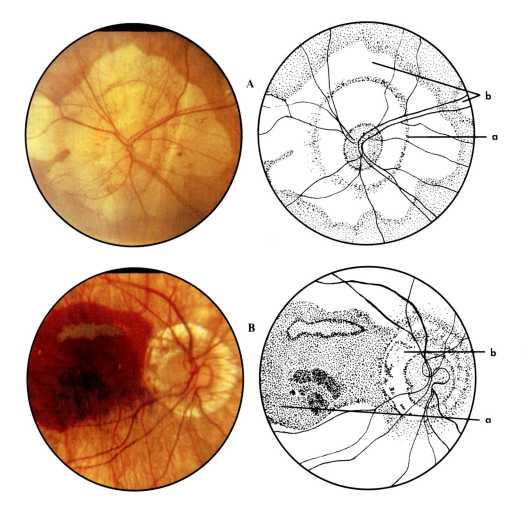

Figure 12
Degenerative Myopia

A, Left eye of a 24-year-old female with a large posterior staphyloma (a) and multifocal choroidal atrophy (b). Refractive error: −18.00 D.

B, Right eye of a 27-year-old male with subretinal macular hemorrhage (a) and myopic conus (b). Refractive error: −12.00 D.

Abnormalities of Retinal Pigment Epithelium (RPE)

MACULAR PATTERN RPE DYSTROPHIES
GENERALIZED RPE DYSTROPHY
FOCAL RPE DYSTROPHIES
CONGENITAL PIGMENTARY ANOMALIES

Diseases of the RPE are subdivided into four subgroups distinguished by differences in the extent of RPE involvement, which is generally indicated by EOG test results (see Appendix A). Only the generalized RPE dystrophies show consistently abnormal EOGs. The congenital anomalies are nonprogressive, with the exception of some types of albinism, and thus are easily distinguished. The macular pattern dystrophies are generally mild afflictions with a striking pattern of RPE involvement that is particularly apparent in the angiogram and minimal changes in the ERG and EOG. The focal RPE dystrophies include several conditions not easily placed in the other subgroups, but each is characterized by RPE changes.

MACULAR PATTERN RPE DYSTROPHIES	Butterfly-shaped dystrophy Reticular dystrophy of Sjögren Macroreticular dystrophy (spider dystrophy) Adult-onset foveomacular vitelliform dystrophy of Gass Pattern dystrophy of the RPE of Marmor and Byers Reticular dystrophy of Benedikt and Werner Autosomal dominant dystrophy of the RPE of O'Donnell, Schatz, Reid, and Green Fundus pulverulentus (Slezak and Hommer) Dominant slowly progressive macular dystrophy of Singerman, Berkow, and Patz

These macular dystrophies are relatively benign disorders presenting an abnormality at the level of the RPE, usually with hyperpigmentation. The lesions are clearly seen in the angiogram. The patients are asymptomatic and usually have normal vision. The ERG is always normal and the EOG may be normal or slightly subnormal (Table 3). These diseases probably represent only variants of the same process, and it is common to find several of the diseases in the same family and occasionally in the fellow eye of the same patient.

The most common patterns observed are butterfly-shaped dystrophy, reticular dystrophy of Sjögren, macroreticular dystrophy (spider dystrophy) and adult-onset foveomacular vitelliform dystrophy of Gass. The remaining five disorders are rare, each having been observed in only one family. Two of them are presented below as examples of the pattern dystrophies: pattern dystrophy of the RPE of Marmor and Byers and dominant slowly progressive macular dystrophy of Singerman, Berkow, and Patz.

The remaining three disorders, reticular dystrophy of Benedikt and Werner, autosomal dominant dystrophy of O'Donnell, Schatz, Reid, and Green,[271] and fundus pulverulentus[334] are considered only in Table 3.

Table 3 MACULAR PATTERN DYSTROPHIES OF THE PIGMENT EPITHELIUM

This group of macular disorders is characterized by the following: lack of symptoms, usually normal vision or slight decrease in vision, dominant inheritance, posterior pole hyperpigmentation believed to be at the level of RPE and more clearly visible with fluorescein angiography, usually normal ERG and abnormal EOG. The disc, retinal vessels, and peripheral retina are normal. The presence of several family members affected with different pattern dystrophies suggests that these diseases are variants of a single pathogenetic mechanism.

NAME	INHERITANCE	PRINCIPAL FINDINGS	ERG	EOG
Butterfly-shaped dystrophy	AD	Onset second decade; asymptomatic, normal vision, hyperpigmented lesion of the fovea with a butterfly shape; more clearly visible with fluorescein angiogram	Normal	Abnormal
Reticular dystrophy of Sjögren	AD, AR	Onset first decade; usually asymptomatic, normal visual acuity (two reported older cases with low vision); hyperpigmented bands arranged in a reticular pattern, giving the fundus the appearance of a "fishnet" with "knots;" the abnormality is more clearly visible with fluorescein angiography	Normal	Normal to abnormal
Macroreticular dystrophy (spider dystrophy)	AD	Onset fifth decade; asymptomatic to mild visual loss; pigmented bands arranged in a reticular pattern in the posterior pole	Normal	Normal to abnormal
Adult-onset foveomacular vitelliform dystrophy of Gass	AD	Onset after fourth decade; asymptomatic or metamorphopsia; visual acuity: 20/20 to 20/40; yellowish oval subretinal macular lesion about one third disc diameter in size with a central dark spot within the fovea	Normal	Normal to abnormal
Pattern dystrophy of the RPE of Marmor and Byers	AD	Onset second to fourth decade; asymptomatic; normal vision; granular pigmentation within the central macula in a reticular pattern; peripheral pigmentary retinopathy	Normal	Abnormal
Reticular dystrophy of Benedikt and Werner	AD	Asymptomatic with normal vision; hyperpigmented bands arranged in reticular pattern (similar to Sjögren's reticular dystrophy), with the appearance of a "fishnet" with "knots;" the pigmentary changes are more obvious than in Sjögren's dystrophy	Normal	—
Autosomal dominant dystrophy of the RPE of O'Donnell, Schatz, Reid, and Green	AD	Salt-and-pepper fundus appearance, subretinal patterned pigment figures; the lesion is more obvious with fluorescein angiography	Normal or photopic reduced	Abnormal
Fundus pulverulentus (Slezak and Hommer)	AD?	Asymptomatic; spotty and mottled pigmentation in the posterior pole and midperiphery; optic disc and vessels are normal	Normal	Abnormal
Dominant slowly progressive macular dystrophy of Singerman, Berkow, and Patz	AD	Onset fifth decade; asymptomatic, slight decrease in vision; RPE defects measuring less than one disc diameter with a central round spot; associated or no flecks	Normal to abnormal	Usually normal

Butterfly-Shaped Dystrophy FIGURE 13

KEY SYMPTOMS
Asymptomatic
Metamorphopsia
Photophobia (rare)

KEY FINDINGS
Bilaterally symmetrical reticular pattern of pigmentation in the central macula
This hyperpigmented lesion usually has a butterfly shape
The lesion can be seen more clearly during fluorescein angiography
This lesion may also be seen in patients with Best's disease or with other pattern macular dystrophies of the RPE

INHERITANCE	ONSET	PROGRESSION	PROGNOSIS
AD	Second to fifth decade	None or very slow	Good

LABORATORY STUDIES
Visual Acuity	20/20 to 20/30
Visual Fields	Normal
Color Vision	Normal
Dark Adaptation	Normal
ERG	Normal
EOG	Slightly abnormal
Fluorescein Angiogram	Reticular pattern of hyperfluorescence surrounding a central hypofluorescent lesion with a butterfly shape

TREATMENT	PATHOLOGY	SYNONYMS
None	None reported	Butterfly-shaped pigment dystrophy of the fovea

DIFFERENTIAL DIAGNOSIS
Macular pattern RPE dystrophies (see Table 3, p. 61)

REFERENCES
12, 76, 83, 89, 146, 156, 189, 246, 301, 365

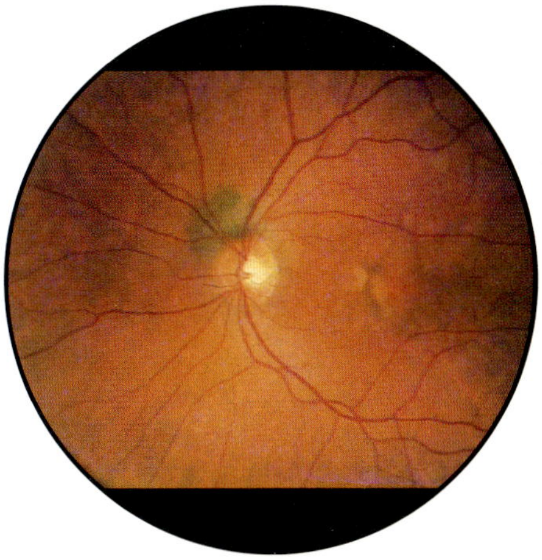

Butterfly-Shaped Dystrophy 63

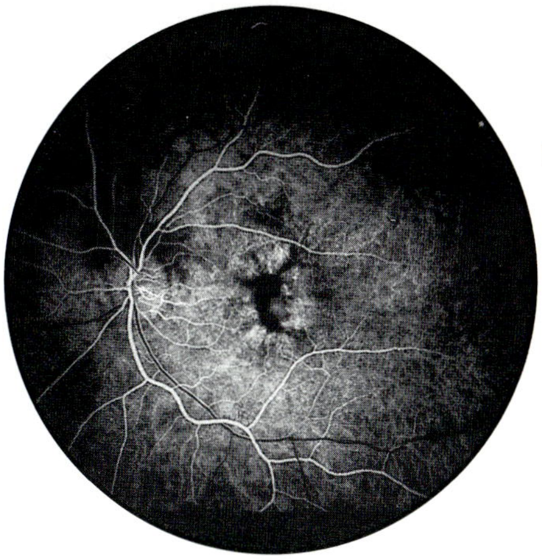

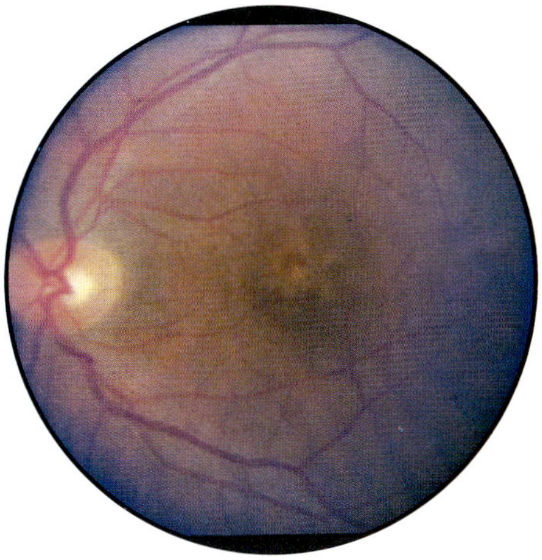

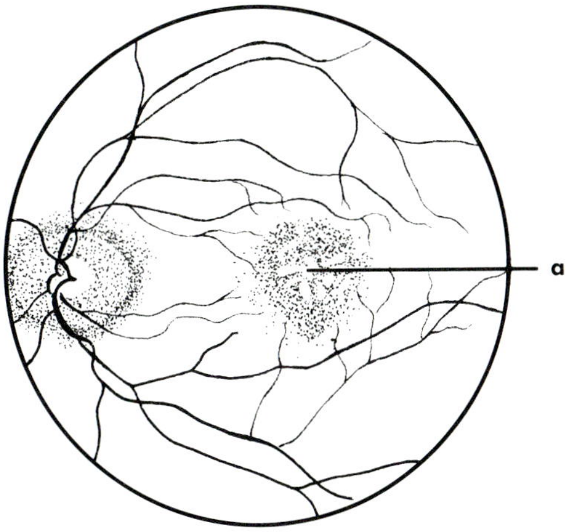

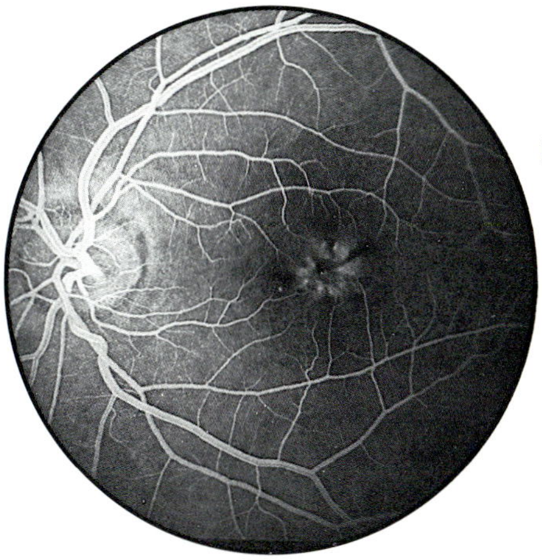

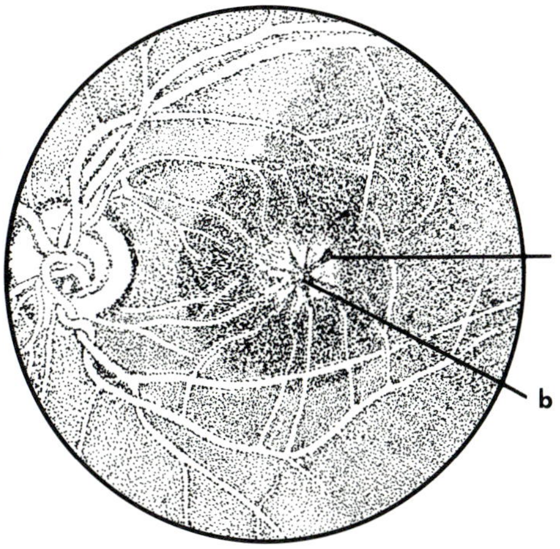

Figure 13
Butterfly-shaped Dystrophy

A, Fundus photograph (OS) showing an irregular pigmented macular lesion partially surrounded by a yellow lesion.

B, Angiogram (OS) in early venous phase showing hyperfluorescence caused by window defects surrounding a central irregular area of hypofluorescence. See Figure 16, **C-D,** for fellow eye with foveomacular vitelliform dystrophy. (**A-B,** courtesy of John Lean, M.D.)

C-D, A typical lesion of an adult-onset foveomacular vitelliform dystrophy. This is an example of the interrelationship between the macular pattern dystrophies, with two expressed in the same patient.

C, Fundus photograph (OS) showing an irregular yellowish lesion (a) with some pigmentary changes in the macular area.

D, Angiogram (OS) showing an irregular hyperfluorescent lesion (a) with some "branches" surrounding a central nonfluorescent lesion (b).

Reticular Dystrophy of Sjögren FIGURE 14

KEY SYMPTOMS
Usually asymptomatic
Decreased vision (late)
Nyctalopia (rare)

KEY FINDINGS
The initial lesion is a darkly pigmented spot within the central macula, 1-disc diameter in size; a reticular network of pigment granules eventually extends from the spot into the periphery
Pigmented knobs at intersecting lines of granules give an appearance of a fishnet with knots
The network is oval, 5-disc diameters in vertical and 7-disc diameters in horizontal dimension
The network never extends beyond the equator
Optic disc, retinal vessels, and choroidal vessels are normal
Drusen appear in the late stages of the disease
Only two cases with substantial visual acuity loss have been reported
The lesion is most clearly seen in fluorescein angiography

INHERITANCE	ONSET	PROGRESSION	PROGNOSIS
AR	First decade	Very slow	Good

LABORATORY STUDIES
Visual Acuity	Usually normal
Visual Fields	Normal
Color Vision	Normal
Dark Adaptation	Normal
ERG	Normal
EOG	Normal to abnormal
Fluorescein Angiogram	Netlike hypofluorescence pattern; intervening areas may hyperfluoresce; no dye staining or pooling

TREATMENT	PATHOLOGY	SYNONYMS
None	Not known	Sjögren's reticular dystrophy Dystrophia reticularis laminae pigmentosae

DIFFERENTIAL DIAGNOSIS
Macular pattern RPE dystrophies (see Table 3, p. 61)

REFERENCES
66, 76, 83, 122, 189, 201

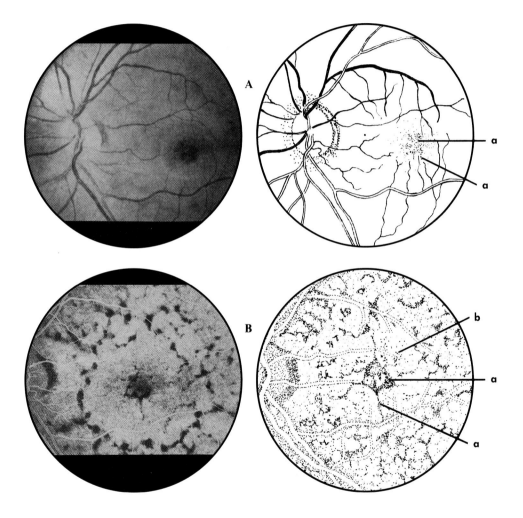

Figure 14
Reticular Dystrophy of Sjögren

A 24-year-old female with a visual acuity of 20/15 OU. Her family history showed affected members in three generations.

A, Fundus photograph showing a dark clump of pigment in the fovea and a reticular pattern of pigment clumping at the level of the RPE. The reticular spaces are about 0.25- to 1.25-disc diameters in size, and there is a knotlike accumulation of pigment where pigmented lines cross. The reticular pattern (fishnet) is most pronounced around the macula *(a)*.

B, Angiogram showing an accentuated reticular pattern of pigmentary clumping in retrofluorescence *(a)*. Integrity of the underlying choriocapillaris within the reticular spaces is demonstrated *(b)*. (**A-B,** reproduced and redrawn from Kingham JD, Fenzl RE, Willerson D, and Aaberg TM: Reticular dystrophy of the retinal pigment epithelium: a clinical and electrophysiologic study of three generations, Arch Ophthalmol 96:1177, 1978. Copyright 1978, American Medical Association.)

Macroreticular Dystrophy (Spider Dystrophy) FIGURE 15

KEY SYMPTOMS
Asymptomatic (early)
Mild visual loss (late)

KEY FINDINGS
Posterior pole pigment bands with a reticular pattern; described as spiderlike, propeller-like, or hot-cross-bun–like
Pigmentary changes involve the RPE
Peripheral pigmentary stippling is seen in some patients
Reticular pattern more easily seen with angiography
Different macular pattern RPE dystrophies may be seen in the same family (see Table 3, p. 61)

INHERITANCE	ONSET	PROGRESSION	PROGNOSIS
AD	Probably second decade	Slow	Good

LABORATORY STUDIES
Visual Acuity	20/30 to 20/70
Visual Fields	Relative central scotoma
Color Vision	Mild protan or tritan defect
Dark Adaptation	Normal
ERG	Normal
EOG	Normal
Fluorescein Angiogram	Reticular pattern of blocked fluorescence; intervening areas are hyperfluorescent and larger than those areas found in Sjögren's dystrophy

TREATMENT	PATHOLOGY	SYNONYMS
None	Unknown	Spider dystrophy

DIFFERENTIAL DIAGNOSIS
Macular pattern dystrophies of the RPE (see Table 3, p. 61)

REFERENCES
76, 112, 146, 189

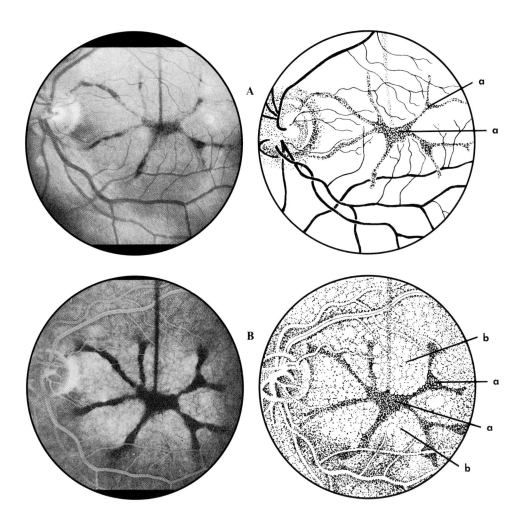

Figure 15
Macroreticular Dystrophy (Spider Dystrophy)

A-B, A 21-year-old female with a visual acuity of 20/20 OD and 20/40 OS with relative amblyopia OS because of anisometropia. Three different macular pattern dystrophies were found in the family of this patient: macroreticular dystrophy (butterfly shaped), Sjögren's reticular dystrophy, and macroreticular dystrophy (spider dystrophy).

A, Fundus photograph (OS) showing a black spiderlike lesion *(a)* radiating from the macular (foveal) area, composed of clumps of pigment seen beneath the sensory retina and superficial to the choroidal pattern.

B, Angiogram (OS) showing that the lesion densely obstructed the choroidal flush. Immediately adjacent to the nonfluorescent bands *(a)*, areas of hyperfluorescence are found *(b)*. (**A-B,** reproduced and redrawn from Hsieh RC, Fine BS, and Lyons JS: Patterned dystrophies of the retinal pigment epithelium, Arch Ophthalmol 95:429, 1977. Copyright 1977, American Medical Association.)

Adult-onset Foveomacular Vitelliform Dystrophy of Gass FIGURE 16

KEY SYMPTOMS
Usually asymptomatic
Mild visual blurring
Metamorphopsia

KEY FINDINGS
Symmetric yellowish, oval or round subretinal macular lesion, often with central gray or orange spot
Macular lesion is one third disc diameter in size; slightly elevated
Larger lesions may resemble those of Best's disease
Drusenlike paracentral spots are occasionally seen
Lesion area eventually becomes depigmented
Subretinal neovascularization in the area of the lesion is a rare complication
This disease may be related to the macular pattern dystrophies of the RPE (see Table 3, p. 61)

INHERITANCE	ONSET	PROGRESSION	PROGNOSIS
AD; sporadic	From age 30 to age 50	Slow	Good

LABORATORY STUDIES
Visual Acuity	20/20 to 20/200 (rare)
Visual Fields	Small central scotoma
Color Vision	Normal to moderate tritan defect
Dark Adaptation	Normal
ERG	Normal
EOG	Normal to slightly subnormal
Fluorescein Angiogram	Hyperfluorescent annulus around a hypofluorescent spot; some cases may not show fluorescence

TREATMENT	PATHOLOGY	SYNONYMS
None	RPE atrophy and loss of some foveal cones	Gass' adult-onset foveomacular vitelliform dystrophy

DIFFERENTIAL DIAGNOSIS
Best's disease (p. 76)
Macular pattern dystrophies of the RPE (see Table 3, p. 61)

REFERENCES
96, 139, 186, 240, 279, 360, 362

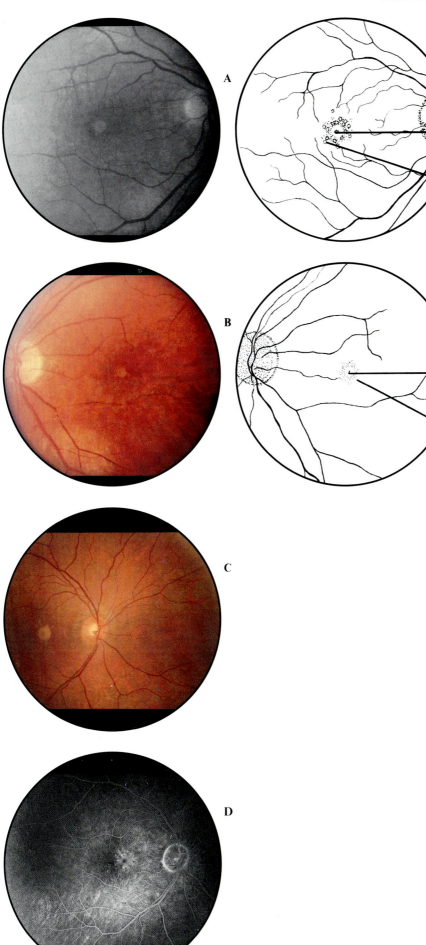

Figure 16
Adult-onset Foveomacular Vitelliform Dystrophy of Gass

A-B, A 43-year-old female with a visual acuity of 20/300 OU. ERG and EOG are normal. Fundus photographs (OD and OS) showing symmetric bilateral involvement. There are small, central vitelliform lesions with a central grayish spot *(a)*. Small paracentral drusen surround the central lesion *(b)*.

C, Fundus photograph (OD) showing a typical .33-disc diameter vitelliform lesion with a central pigmented dark spot. Small paracentral drusen surround the lesion.

D, Angiogram (OD) showing a ring of hyperfluorescence surrounding a central nonfluorescent spot (see also Figure 13, *A-B)*. (**C-D,** courtesy of John Lean, M.D.)

Pattern Dystrophy of the RPE of Marmor and Byers FIGURE 17

KEY SYMPTOMS
Usually asymptomatic
Mild visual acuity reduction
Metamorphopsia and photophobia

KEY FINDINGS
Young Patients
Granular macular pigmentation
Later
Patterned pigment deposition in the posterior pole with branching and a partial network
Granular pigmentation or areas of depigmentation in the periphery
The macular pattern lesion is more easily seen in the angiogram

INHERITANCE	ONSET	PROGRESSION	PROGNOSIS
AD	Second to fourth decade	Very slow	Good

LABORATORY STUDIES
Visual Acuity	20/20 to 20/30
Visual Fields	Normal
Color Vision	Normal
Dark Adaptation	Normal
ERG	Normal
EOG	Abnormal
Fluorescein Angiogram	Hypofluorescence corresponding to the macular areas of hyperpigmentation, with hyperfluorescence surrounding the hyperpigmentation

TREATMENT	PATHOLOGY	SYNONYMS
None	Not described; abnormal EOG suggests a generalized RPE dysfunction	None in general use

DIFFERENTIAL DIAGNOSIS
Macular pattern RPE dystrophies (see Table 3, p. 61)

REFERENCES
241

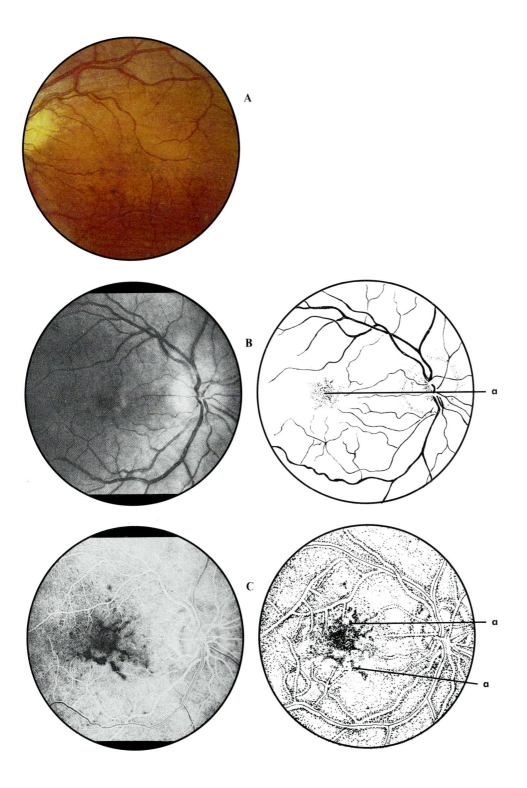

Figure 17
Pattern Dystrophy of the RPE of Marmor and Byers

A, Fundus photograph (OS) of a 20-year-old male, asymptomatic with a corrected visual acuity of 20/25 OU. His fundi showed a demarcated pigment pattern in the macular area in both eyes. The macular lesions showed little progression over 3 years. EOGs were subnormal, and several family members in different generations were affected.

B, Fundus photograph (OD) showing pigmentary changes in the macula *(a)*.

C, Angiogram (OD) reveals a more apparent pattern, showing diffuse damage to the pigment epithelium without leakage or accumulation of dye *(a)*. (**A-C,** reproduced and redrawn from Marmor MF, and Byers B: Pattern dystrophy of the pigment epithelium, Am J Ophthalmol 84:32, 1977. Published with permission from The American Journal of Ophthalmology. Copyright by the Ophthalmic Publishing Company.)

Dominant Slowly Progressive Macular Dystrophy of Singerman, Berkow, and Patz FIGURE 18

KEY SYMPTOMS
Asymptomatic or mild visual acuity reduction
Metamorphopsia

KEY FINDINGS
Early
Subtle RPE mottling in the fovea
Late
Type 1: Ovoid area of macular RPE atrophy, less than 1-disc diameter in size with a central yellow or grayish spot; no flecks in the posterior pole
Type 2: Macular lesion similar to Type 1; flecks seen throughout posterior pole
Lesions may predispose to development of macular degeneration and subretinal neovascularization (SRN)

INHERITANCE
AD

ONSET
Second to sixth decade

PROGRESSION
Slow

PROGNOSIS
Good

LABORATORY STUDIES
Visual Acuity	20/25 to 20/60
Visual Fields	Constricted with paracentral scotomas
Color Vision	Normal
Dark Adaptation	Not described
ERG	Normal photopic; subnormal scotopic
EOG	Usually normal
Fluorescein Angiogram	Ovoid central hyperfluorescence and late staining; central spot hypofluorescence; flecks may stain (Type 2)

TREATMENT
None or photocoagulation of SRN

PATHOLOGY
Not described

SYNONYMS
Singerman-Berkow-Patz-dominant slowly progressive macular dystrophy

DIFFERENTIAL DIAGNOSIS
Pattern dystrophies of the RPE (see Table 3, p. 61)

REFERENCES
329, 365

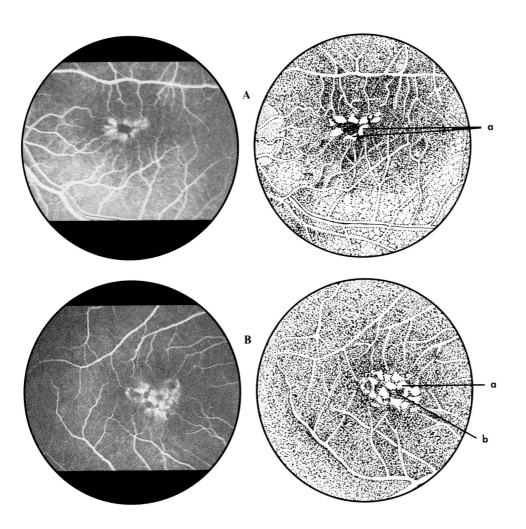

Figure 18
Dominant Slowly Progressive Macular Dystrophy of Singerman, Berkow, and Patz

This 47-year-old female with a corrected visual acuity of 20/20 OU complained of metamorphopsia. The fundus showed an ovoid area of pigment epithelial disturbance surrounding the fovea (OU). In the center of this oval area was a round deposit of darker gray material.

A, Angiogram (OS) shows clearly defined areas of hyperfluorescence *(a)* in an ovoid configuration surrounding the fovea with fluorescence early in the arterial phase.

B, Angiogram (OD) shows a more irregular and larger hyperfluorescent area in the macula *(a)* with a central hypofluorescent spot *(b)*. (**A-B,** reproduced and redrawn from Singerman LJ, Berkow JW, and Patz A: Dominant slowly progressive macular dystrophy, Am J Ophthalmol 83:680, 1977. Published with permission from The American Journal of Ophthalmology. Copyright by the Ophthalmic Publishing Company.)

GENERALIZED RPE DYSTROPHY

Best's Disease

Although the lesions of vitelliform macular dystrophy, or Best's disease, appear to be focal, the generalized nature of the abnormality and its involvement of the retinal pigment epithelium is clearly demonstrated by the abnormal EOG that is the hallmark of the disease (see Appendix A). The abnormal EOG also indicates that classification of Best's disease as a generalized RPE abnormality is appropriate. The ERG and the EOG are summed retinal responses and reflect total retinal function; these tests are insensitive to focal abnormalities. Thus, the obvious macular lesions of Best's disease have no effect on the electrophysiological tests. The basis of dissociation of the ERG, which is normal in these patients, and the EOG, which is abnormal, is not known. It must represent abnormality at the level of the RPE cell membrane that does not affect its ability to service the photoreceptors. This dystrophy is relatively common, but most patients are asymptomatic.

Best's Disease FIGURE 19

KEY SYMPTOMS
Asymptomatic (early)
Metamorphopsia
Central vision decreased (late)

KEY FINDINGS

Subclinical Stage

Fundus appears normal and only the EOG is abnormal; most patients remain in this stage as carriers

Clinical Stage

Vitelliform lesion

"Sunnyside-up egg yolk"—Yellow-orange macular cyst measuring 1- to 5-disc diameters, usually bilateral and symmetric; mild visual loss (20/40); cyst may remain stable for many years; multifocal lesions may be seen

"Scrambled egg"—Granular lumpy appearance of the cyst (later)

Pseudohypopyon—Cyst partially liquefied and reabsorbed

Atrophic Stage

Eventual rupture or reabsorption of the cyst, leaving an oval area of RPE atrophy and loss of central vision (20/200)

Subretinal neovascularization (SRN) may occur

Adult-onset Best's disease may occur after third decade

INHERITANCE	ONSET	PROGRESSION	PROGNOSIS
AD	First or second decade	Slow	Poor

LABORATORY STUDIES

Visual Acuity	20/30 to 20/200
Refraction	Mild hyperopia
Visual Fields	Normal to central scotoma
Color Vision	Normal to abnormal
Dark Adaptation	Normal
ERG	Normal; dissociation between ERG and EOG
EOG	Abnormal (see Figure 92, Appendix A)
Fluorescein Angiogram	*Cyst Stage*
	Central fluorescence blocked early
	Cyst Rupture Stage
	Window defect; SRN may leak

TREATMENT
None

PATHOLOGY
RPE and photoreceptor atrophy in the central macula (the abnormal EOG shows the presence of RPE abnormality involving the entire retina)

SYNONYMS
Vitelliform macular dystrophy
Vitelleruptive macular dystrophy

DIFFERENTIAL DIAGNOSIS
Other vitelliform lesions
Serous RPE detachment
Stargardt's disease (p. 92)

REFERENCES
39, 96, 120, 133, 146, 156, 185, 224, 235, 240, 250, 251, 255, 332, 345, 368, 378

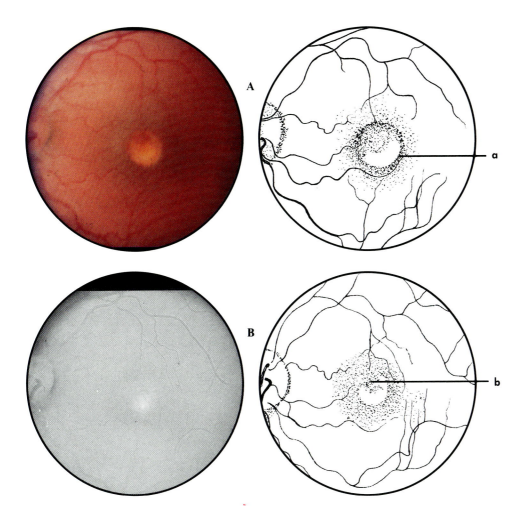

Figure 19
Best's Disease

A–E, The evolution of Best's disease in a 12-year-old female is illustrated in these fundus photographs taken at successive intervals. The patient had a sudden decrease in vision in 1984. She has a family history positive for Best's disease. The ERG is normal, and the EOG is severely abnormal.

A, Fundus photograph (OS) showing the typical "sunnyside-up" vitelliform lesion in the central macula, measuring 1-disc diameter in size. The cyst is uniform with a yellow-orange color and with regular borders *(a)*. Visual acuity is 20/300 OD and 20/25 OS. (January 1985.)

B, Vision is unchanged. There is a partial reabsorption of the superior portion of the cyst *(a)* and a mild reduction in size, and the color is yellow. (March 1986.)

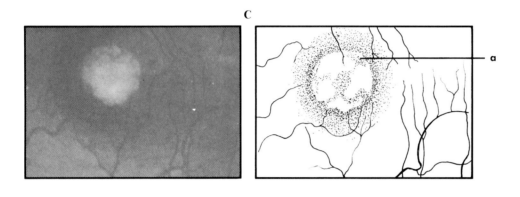

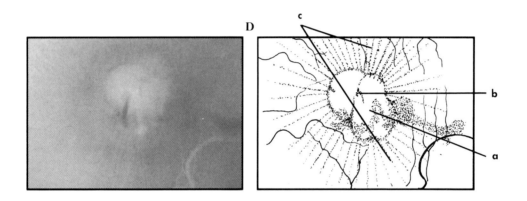

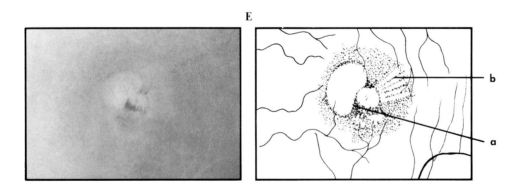

C, Enlarged view of the macular area showing an increase in size, irregularity in the superior border *(a)*, and a return to the yellow-orange color. Vision remains stable. (April 1986.)

D, A sudden decrease in central vision has occurred. The cyst has been spontaneously ruptured *(a)*, some hemorrhages are present *(b)*, and a radial wrinkling of the internal limiting membrane is seen *(c)*. (May 1986.)

E, An atrophic, hyperpigmented macular scar has developed *(a)*, and the wrinkling of the internal limiting membrane is present only on the temporal side *(b)*. (June 1986.) (**A-E,** courtesy of Edgar Thomas, M.D.)

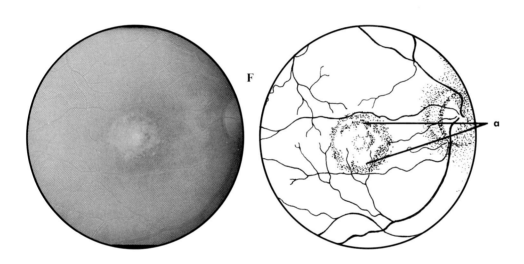

F, Fundus photograph (OD) of a 14-year-old male showing the end-stage of a vitelliform lesion with spontaneous reabsorption, leaving an atrophic macular area *(a).* Visual acuity is 20/200.

80 GENERALIZED RPE DYSTROPHY

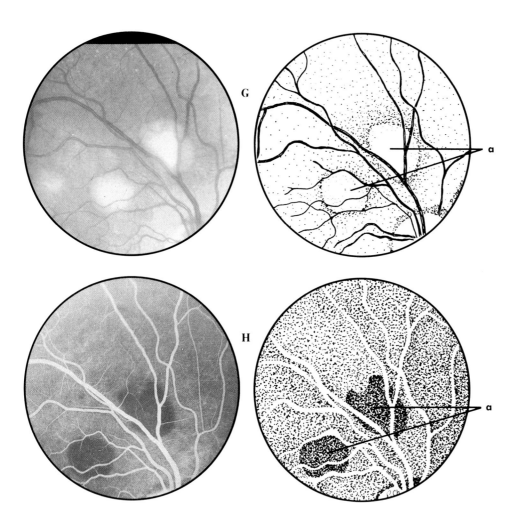

G, Fundus photograph (OD) showing multifocal extramacular vitelliform lesions *(a)* beneath the superior temporal arcades.

H, Angiogram (OD) showing two areas of blockage of fluorescence at the level of the RPE *(a)*. Note the normal fluorescence of the retinal vessels crossing over the lesions.

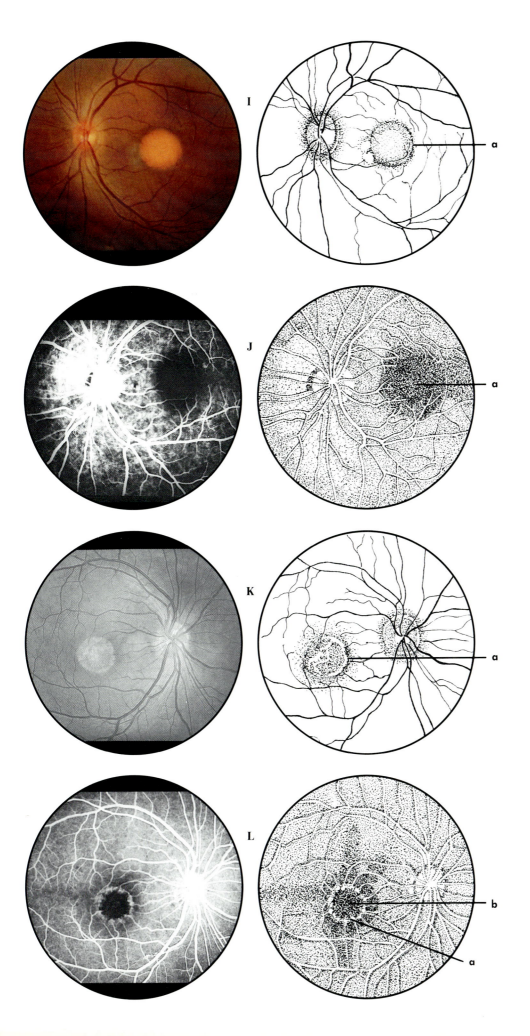

I-L, A 34-year-old female with a visual acuity of 20/40 OD and 20/20 OS. She has no family history of Best's disease. The EOG is severely abnormal, and the ERG is normal. This case represents typical Best's disease with late onset.

I, Fundus photograph (OS) showing a 2-disc diameter "sunnyside-up" vitelliform lesion *(a)*.

J, Angiogram (OS) showing hypofluorescence *(a)* of the central macula.

K, Fundus photograph (OD) showing an apparent partially reabsorbed lesion with a small yellow spot in the center.

L, Angiogram (OD) showing an atypical pattern of fluorescence, with hyperfluorescence *(a)* surrounding a central area of complete blockage of fluorescence *(b)*.

FOCAL RPE DYSTROPHIES   This group of retinal pigment epithelial diseases is defined by limited involvement of the posterior pole and macula.

> Central areolar pigment epithelial (CAPE) dystrophy
> Fenestrated sheen macular dystrophy
> Benign concentric annular macular dystrophy
> Lefler-Wadsworth-Sidbury dystrophy
> Stargardt's disease
> Dominant progressive foveal dystrophy (dominant Stargardt's disease)
> Pigment epithelial dystrophy of Noble-Carr-Siegel

This is a group of autosomal dominant, mild, slowly progressive macular dystrophies. The patients are often asymptomatic or show only a mild visual loss. The exception is Stargardt's disease, which is inherited as an autosomal recessive dystrophy, progresses rapidly, and causes severe loss of central vision. Several of the diseases resemble a bull's-eye maculopathy; yellow flecks or drusenoid lesions occur in some; and all show pigmentary changes in the macula. Angiograms show macular abnormality early in all the diseases. Electrophysiology (see Appendix A) is normal or mildly abnormal except in pigment epithelial dystrophy of Noble-Carr-Siegel, where the ERG may be nonrecordable late, when the disease becomes generalized.

Central areolar pigment epithelial dystrophy shows a central loss of the RPE and can probably be considered a variant of central areolar choroidal dystrophy. Fenestrated sheen macular dystrophy presents with areas of RPE defects in the macula, sparing the central fovea in a characteristic pattern. Benign concentric annular macular dystrophy is distinguished by an area of RPE atrophy with a typical bull's-eye pattern and mild visual loss. Lefler-Wadsworth-Sidbury dystrophy presents a picture varying from drusen in the posterior pole to the presence of colobomas in the macular area.

Stargardt's disease, or juvenile macular degeneration, is an autosomal recessive disease and probably the most common macular dystrophy. It is characterized by the presence of a macular lesion that is usually associated with flecks in the posterior pole. If the flecks become extensive, the disease is called fundus flavimaculatus. Only Stargardt's disease is described in this section. Fundus flavimaculatus is described under flecked retina diseases. Dominant progressive foveal dystrophy (dominant Stargardt's), also mentioned under flecked retina diseases, is clinically identical to fundus flavimaculatus and typical Stargardt's disease but is distinguished by a late onset and autosomal dominant inheritance.

Pigment epithelial dystrophy of Noble-Carr-Siegel is very rare and presents a focal or generalized RPE and retinal abnormality at an early age.

Central Areolar Pigment Epithelial (CAPE) Dystrophy FIGURE 20

KEY SYMPTOMS
Asymptomatic

KEY FINDINGS
Early
Fine mottled areolar depigmentation of the fovea
Late
Depigmented area is sharply demarcated and involves the RPE
The central lesion is surrounded by fine drusenlike lesions
Subretinal neovascular membrane can occur

INHERITANCE	ONSET	PROGRESSION	PROGNOSIS
AD	First decade	None	Good

LABORATORY STUDIES

Visual Acuity	Normal
Visual Fields	Normal
Color Vision	Normal
Dark Adaptation	Normal
ERG	Normal
EOG	Normal
Fluorescein Angiogram	Central window defects correspond to depigmented areas; SRN may show leaking and pooling of dye

TREATMENT	PATHOLOGY	SYNONYMS
None	Not known; this disease may represent a form of Lefler-Wadsworth-Sidbury dystrophy	CAPE dystrophy (central areolar pigment epithelial dystrophy) and central areolar choroidal dystrophy are probably identical diseases

DIFFERENTIAL DIAGNOSIS
Lefler-Wadsworth-Sidbury dystrophy (p. 90)
Central areolar choroidal dystrophy (p. 34)

REFERENCES
91, 107

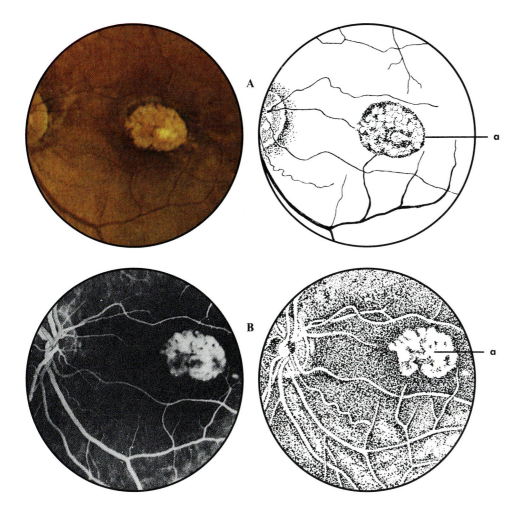

Figure 20

Central Areolar Pigmented Epithelial (CAPE) Dystrophy

A, Fundus photograph (OS) of the macula of a 13-year-old male with a visual acuity of 20/25. Four family members in three generations were affected. The macula shows a central 1-disc diameter zone of RPE atrophy with excavation into the choroid *(a)*. Optic disc and retinal vessels are normal.

B, Fluorescein angiogram (OS) showing a central area of hyperfluorescence with a well-circumscribed border corresponding to the area of RPE atrophy *(a)*. (A-B, reproduced and redrawn from Fetkenhour CL, Gurney N, Dobbie JG, and Choromokos E: Central areolar pigment epithelial dystrophy, Am J Ophthalmol 81:745, 1976. Published with permission from The American Journal of Ophthalmology. Copyright by the Ophthalmic Publishing Company.)

86 FOCAL RPE DYSTROPHIES

Fenestrated Sheen Macular Dystrophy FIGURE 21

KEY SYMPTOMS
Asymptomatic
Paracentral scotomas (late)

KEY FINDINGS
Early
Yellowish refractile sheen with red fenestrations in the macula
Paracentral RPE atrophy, annulus of hypopigmentation; this progressively enlarges in the third decade
Late
Bull's-eye maculopathy appearance caused by hyperpigmentation surrounding hypopigmented annulus
Good visual acuity despite appearance of macula

INHERITANCE	ONSET	PROGRESSION	PROGNOSIS
AD	First decade	Very slow	Good

LABORATORY STUDIES

Visual Acuity	20/20 to 20/50
Visual Fields	Normal or paracentral scotoma
Color Vision	Normal
Dark Adaptation	Normal
ERG	Normal to subnormal
EOG	Normal to subnormal
Fluorescein Angiogram	*Early*
	Normal
	Late
	Shows multiple window defects in annular area surrounded by hypofluorescence caused by hyperpigmentation

TREATMENT	PATHOLOGY	SYNONYMS
None	Not described	Fenestrated sheen macular dystrophy of O'Donnell and Welch

DIFFERENTIAL DIAGNOSIS
Stargardt's disease (p. 92)
Central areolar RPE dystrophy (p. 34)
Cone dystrophy (p. 168)
Benign concentric annular macular dystrophy (p. 88)

REFERENCES
80, 272, 276, 333

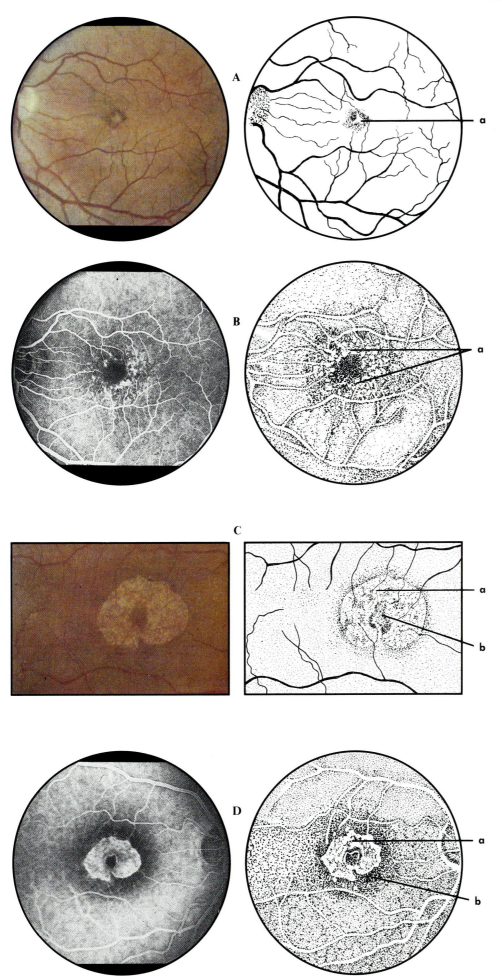

Figure 21
Fenestrated Sheen Macular Dystrophy

A, Fundus photograph: yellowish lesion is visible in the foveal area *(a)*. Fundus photography does not show the full extent of sensory retina lesion, nor does it demonstrate refractile appearance of the sheen.

B, Angiogram of the same eye in arteriovenous phase showing annular zone of punctate choroidal hyperfluorescence *(a)*.

C, Fundus photograph (OD) of patient's father. Complete ring of hypopigmentation *(a)* surrounds the central area of preserved RPE *(b)*. The sensory retinal sheen is yellowish.

D, Angiogram of eye shown in **C.** Arteriovenous phase shows choriocapillaris perfusion at macula seen through hypopigmented RPE *(a)*. Notice annulus of increased pigmentation of RPE, causing subnormal choroidal fluorescence around zone of increased transmission *(b)*. (**A-D,** reproduced and redrawn from O'Donnell FE, Jr, and Welch RB: Fenestrated sheen macular dystrophy: a new autosomal dominant maculopathy, Arch Ophthalmol 97:1292, 1979. Copyright 1979, American Medical Association.)

Benign Concentric Annular Macular Dystrophy FIGURE 22

KEY SYMPTOMS
Early
Asymptomatic or mildly decreased vision
Nyctalopia
Late
Dyschromatopsia

KEY FINDINGS
Bull's-eye maculopathy (circular or ovoid zone of retinal pigment epithelium atrophy surrounding an intact central area) (see Figure 22, C)
Slight narrowing of arterioles
Mild midperipheral stippling
Occasionally small paramacular drusen
The macular lesion most closely resembles that of chloroquine toxicity and cone dystrophy
Optic disc is normal
Late
Macular pigmentary changes and peripheral pigmentary retinopathy

INHERITANCE	ONSET	PROGRESSION	PROGNOSIS
AD	Second decade	Slow	Good

LABORATORY STUDIES
Visual Acuity	20/20 to 20/25
Refraction	Emmetropia or hyperopia
Visual Fields	Annular paracentral scotoma
Color Vision	Mild protan or deutan defects
Dark Adaptation	Normal to abnormal
ERG	Normal to subnormal
EOG	Normal to abnormal
Fluorescein Angiogram	Hypofluorescence of the central intact zone surrounded by hyperfluorescent annulus of RPE atrophy

TREATMENT	PATHOLOGY	SYNONYMS
None	Not described	Bull's-eye maculopathy of Deutman

DIFFERENTIAL DIAGNOSIS	REFERENCES
See Table 9, p. 166, for list of conditions causing bull's-eye maculopathy	62, 75, 84, 359, 369

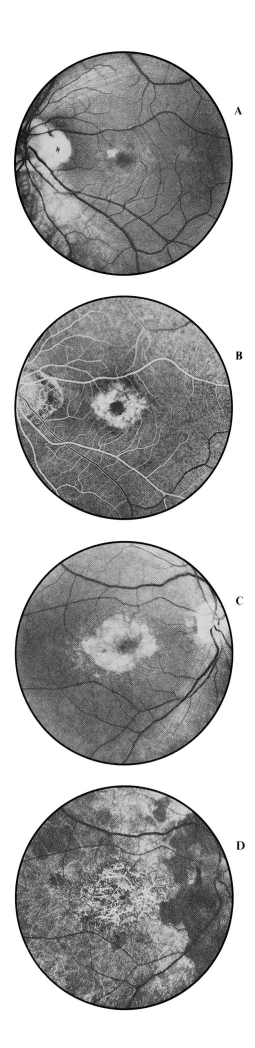

Figure 22
Benign Concentric Annular Macular Dystrophy

A 26-year-old male with a visual acuity of 20/150 OU and a subnormal ERG and EOG.

A, Red-free fundus photograph (OS) showing a pericentral area of depigmentation and attenuated vessels; there is also peripapillary atrophy.

B, Angiogram (OS) in the venous phase showing a pericentral area of hyperfluorescence surrounding a central, nonfluorescent spot (bull's-eye).

C, Red-free photograph of 54-year-old mother of patient shown in **A** and **B,** with a visual acuity of 20/40 showing a bull's-eye pattern of RPE atrophy.

D, Angiogram (OD) in the early phase showing atrophy of the RPE and choriocapillaris. (**A-D,** reproduced and redrawn from Van den Biesen PR, Deutman AF, and Pinckers AJLG: Evolution of benign concentric annular macular dystrophy, Am J Ophthalmol 100:73, 1985. Published with permission from The American Journal of Ophthalmology. Copyright by the Ophthalmic Publishing Company.)

Stargardt's Disease FIGURE 24

KEY SYMPTOMS
Visual acuity reduction
Mild color vision defect
Photophobia (not always present)

KEY FINDINGS
Early
Reduced visual acuity before age 20
Loss of foveal reflex, fundus otherwise normal
Late
Fovea: granular appearance
Macula: varnished appearance common; some patients have bull's-eye maculopathy
Later: beaten-bronze appearance caused by RPE atrophy
Yellow-to-brown flecks may surround macular lesion and may extend to the periphery
Central retina: may resemble choroidal atrophy with sclerosis of the choroidal vessels
Pigmentary changes of midperiphery occur in advanced disease; typical fundus flavimaculatus may eventually develop

INHERITANCE	ONSET	PROGRESSION	PROGNOSIS
AR	First or second decade	Rapid	20/200 by second decade

LABORATORY STUDIES
Visual Acuity	20/25 to 20/200
Refraction	Emmetropia to low myopia
Visual Fields	Central scotoma (relative to absolute)
Color Vision	Abnormal early
Dark Adaptation	Normal until extensive peripheral involvement
ERG	Normal; abnormal in patients with extensive peripheral involvement (about 20%)
EOG	Normal; abnormal in patients with extensive peripheral involvement (about 20%)
Fluorescein Angiogram	*Early*
	Normal macula, pericentral window defects and hyperfluorescence if bull's-eye type
	Late
	Central hyperfluorescence from RPE defect

TREATMENT	PATHOLOGY	SYNONYMS
None	Total loss of RPE and receptors in the macula; inner retina may show cystoid degeneration and calcium deposits	Juvenile macular degeneration

DIFFERENTIAL DIAGNOSIS
Best's disease (p. 76)
Cone degenerations (pp. 168-172)
X-L juvenile retinoschisis (p. 210)
Fundus flavimaculatus (p. 116)

REFERENCES
62, 157, 218, 263, 282

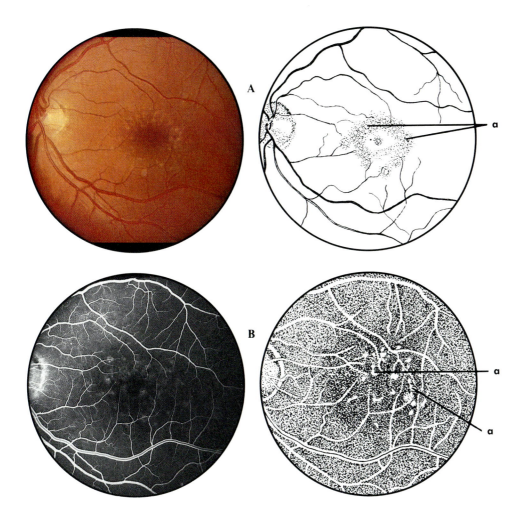

Figure 24
Stargardt's Disease

A-B, A 12-year-old male with a visual acuity of 20/100 OU, mild photophobia, and no pertinent family history. The ERG and EOG are normal.

A, Fundus photograph (OS) shows perifoveal mottled depigmentation of the RPE *(a)* principally in the superior half of the central macula that corresponds to **B,** the areas of transmission defects in the angiogram *(a)*. Optic disc and vessels are normal.

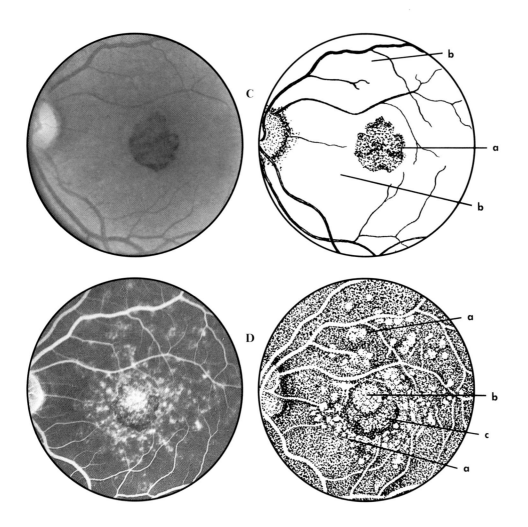

C-D, A 25-year-old female with a history of low vision for the last 12 years, with a visual acuity of 20/200 OU. One brother is affected with a similar condition. The ERG and EOG are normal.

C, Fundus photograph shows a central area of hyperpigmentation *(a)* surrounded by yellow-white flecks *(b)* in the posterior pole; optic disc and vessels are normal.

D, Angiogram in late venous phase shows multiple areas of hyperfluorescence *(a)* corresponding to the flecks, a central area with hyperfluorescence caused by RPE atrophy *(b)*, and hypofluorescence caused by blockage of fluorescence by pigment *(c)*. This patient's condition represents an intermediate stage between Stargardt's disease and fundus flavimaculatus.

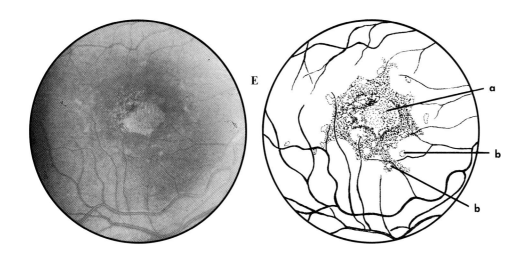

E, Fundus photograph showing the typical "beaten-bronze" area of atrophy *(a)* surrounded by one line of paracentral yellow flecks in a characteristic arrangement *(b)*. No other flecks are seen in the posterior pole or periphery. This patient has typical Stargardt's disease without fundus flavimaculatus.

Dominant Progressive Foveal Dystrophy FIGURE 25

KEY SYMPTOMS
Visual acuity reduction
Abnormal color vision
Central scotoma

KEY FINDINGS
Atrophic macular degeneration with prominent yellow flecks in the macula and/or posterior pole
Appearance is identical to Stargardt's disease but onset is later and progression is slower
This disease is much more rarely seen than Stargardt's disease, which has autosomal recessive inheritance (see Stargardt's disease)

INHERITANCE	ONSET	PROGRESSION	PROGNOSIS
AD	Second to fourth decade	Slow	Poor

LABORATORY STUDIES

Visual Acuity	20/20 to 20/200
Refraction	Usually low myopia
Visual Fields	Central scotoma
Color Vision	Abnormal
Dark Adaptation	Normal
ERG	Usually normal
EOG	Usually normal
Fluorescein Angiogram	*Early*
	Numerous paramacular window defects
	Late
	Central hyperfluorescence and hypofluorescence caused by RPE and choriocapillaris atrophy

TREATMENT	PATHOLOGY	SYNONYMS
None	RPE atrophy involving the macula with degeneration of overlying receptors	Dominant Stargardt's disease

DIFFERENTIAL DIAGNOSIS
Stargardt's disease (recessive juvenile macular degeneration) (p. 92)

REFERENCES
67

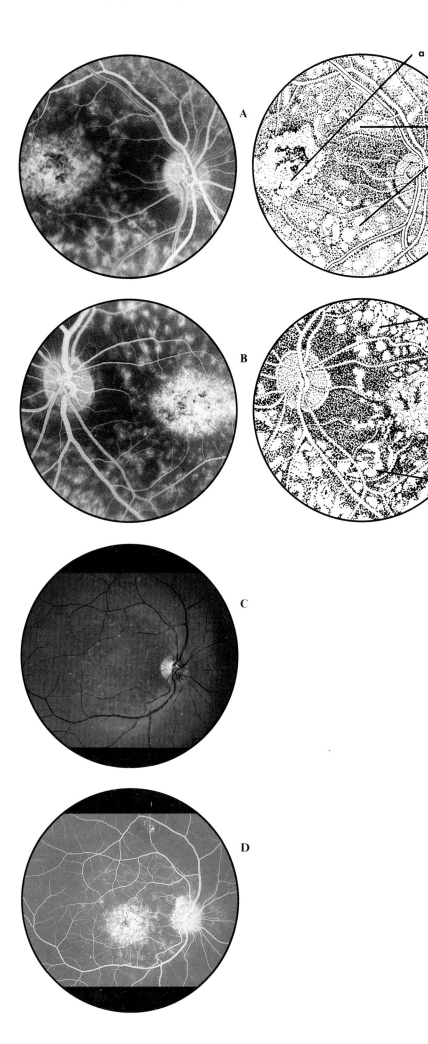

Figure 25
Dominant Progressive Foveal Dystrophy

A-B, A 27-year-old male with loss of central vision since age 20. Visual acuity is 20/200 OU. His mother is affected with a similar condition, and there is no history of consanguinity. (This case probably represents a dominant inheritance.) Angiograms (OD and OS) show a central area of RPE atrophy *(a)* and multiple window defects in the posterior pole *(b)* identical to those seen in fundus flavimaculatus. Note the relative peripapillary sparing.

C, Fundus photograph (OD) of a 44-year-old male with possible dominant Stargardt's disease and onset of symptoms at age 40. His visual acuity is 20/60. Note the linear yellow flecks surrounding a central macular lesion.

D, The angiogram shows a hyperfluorescent pattern characteristic of combined Stargardt's disease and fundus flavimaculatus. (**C-D,** courtesy of Peter Liggett, M.D., and Oscar Vergara, M.D.)

98 FOCAL RPE DYSTROPHIES

Pigment Epithelial Dystrophy of Noble-Carr-Siegel   FIGURE 26

KEY SYMPTOMS
Visual acuity reduction
Nystagmus

KEY FINDINGS
Foveal reflex abnormal or absent
Abnormal peripapillary sheen
RPE degeneration in advanced cases
Choroidal vessels visible because of RPE atrophy
Pigment clumping at the posterior pole
Myopia
NOTE: Presentation of this disease is variable because of differences in expression

INHERITANCE	ONSET	PROGRESSION	PROGNOSIS
AD	Birth to 1 year	No progression or slow	Good to poor

LABORATORY STUDIES
Visual Acuity	20/20 to hand motion
Refraction	Myopia; more than 8.00 D in half of all patients
Visual Fields	Central scotoma
Color Vision	Normal to abnormal
Dark Adaptation	Normal
ERG	Subnormal to nonrecordable
EOG	Normal to abnormal
Fluorescein Angiogram	Window defects in areas of RPE atrophy; pigmented areas block fluorescence

TREATMENT	PATHOLOGY	SYNONYMS
None	Not described	None in general use

DIFFERENTIAL DIAGNOSIS
Leber's congenital amaurosis (p. 146)
Pigmentary retinopathy (see Table 6, p. 118)
Progressive nyctalopia (p. 120)

REFERENCES
266

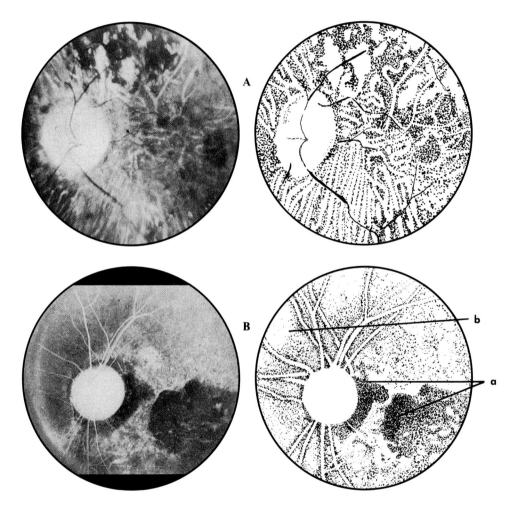

Figure 26
Pigment Epithelial Dystrophy of Noble-Carr-Siegel

A, Fundus photograph showing marked pigmentary changes, diffuse chorioretinal atrophy associated with pigment clumping, and arteriolar narrowing.

B, Late venous-phase angiogram showing mottled hyperfluorescence caused by RPE atrophy. There is peripapillary and macular hypofluorescence caused by pigment accumulation *(a)*. The superior nasal quadrant shows a normal fluorescent pattern *(b)*. (**A-B,** reproduced and redrawn from Noble KG, Carr RE, and Siegel IM: Pigment epithelial dystrophy, Am J Ophthalmol 83: 751, 1977. Published with permission from The American Journal of Ophthalmology. Copyright by the Ophthalmic Publishing Company.)

CONGENITAL PIGMENTARY ANOMALIES	Albinism Congenital grouped albinotic spots Bear track–grouped pigmentation

Albinism, or congenital hypopigmentation, is divided into cases of true albinism and cases of albinoidism. True albinism includes oculocutaneous albinism and ocular albinism (see Table 4 and Flowchart 2). Albinoidism resembles albinism without macular hypoplasia and includes four autosomal dominant syndromes. Congenital grouped albinotic spots and bear track–grouped pigmentation are congenital localized pigmentary disorders that are included here for convenience. They are nonprogressive and are probably related anomalies.

Albinism is a metabolic defect characterized by a deficiency or absence of melanin in melanocytes and other pigmented cells such as the RPE. The melanin defect results from an inability to convert the amino acid *tyrosine* into dopa (3,4-dihydroxyphenylalanine), a precursor of melanin. Albinism occurs in various forms, affecting either only the eyes or the eyes, skin, and hair. It is inherited as an autosomal dominant, autosomal recessive, or X-L recessive trait. The most important ocular findings of albinism are nystagmus (associated with macular hypoplasia) and photophobia.

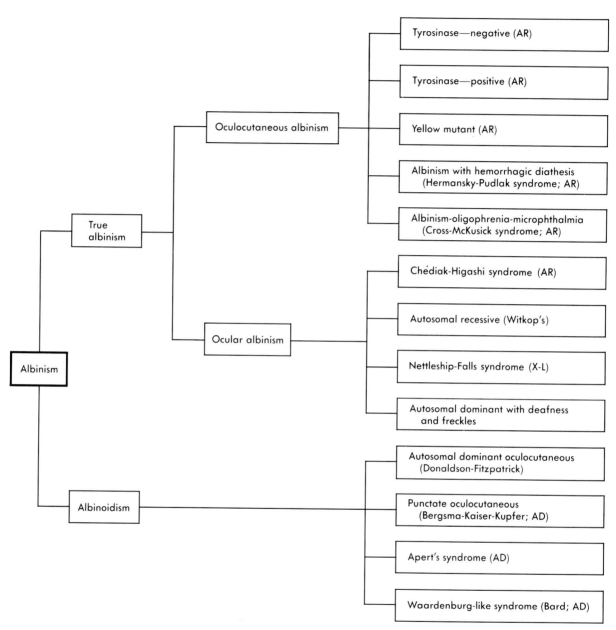

Flowchart 2

True albinism is divided into oculocutaneous albinism, in which there are both ocular and cutaneous manifestations of the abnormality, and ocular albinism, in which all abnormalities are confined to the eyes. Albinoidism is very rare and resembles albinism in some respects, but it is without macular hypoplasia.

Table 4 TYPES OF ALBINISM

Any congenital hypopigmentation is a form of albinism. Two types of albinism affect the eye: true albinism and albinoidism.
1. True albinism has been subdivided into (1) oculocutaneous albinism (skin and eyes affected), and (2) ocular albinism (only the eyes are clinically affected). True albinism manifests with congenitally abnormal visual acuity, photophobia, nystagmus, and foveal hypoplasia (absence of the foveal reflex and yellow macular pigment).
2. Albinoidism manifests with photophobia. The fovea and visual acuity are close to normal, so no nystagmus occurs.

NAME	INHERITANCE	CLINICAL FINDINGS	LABORATORY FINDINGS
Oculocutaneous Albinism			
Tyrosinase-negative (incomplete universal albinism)	AR	Pink skin, white hair, light blue irides with marked transillumination, macular hypoplasia, poor vision, nystagmus, usually myopia; carriers may show partial transillumination of iris	Tyrosinase activity: negative (hair) Melanosomes in skin: no melanin
Tyrosinase-positive (incomplete universal albinism)	AR	The ocular findings are similar to those found in tyrosinase-negative patients, but with some degree of pigmentation in the skin and hair	Tyrosinase activity: positive Melanosomes in skin: trace melanin
Yellow-mutant	AR	Complete albinism at birth, some degree of pigmentation with age; yellow hair, skin a creamy color, easily sunburned and does not tan; blue translucent irides, nystagmus, and photophobia	Tyrosinase activity: intermediate reaction (trace) Melanosomes in skin: incompletely melanized (hair bulb incubated in L-cysteine develops increased pigment)
Albinism with hemorrhagic diathesis (Hermansky-Pudlak syndrome)	AR	Variation in pigmentation, easily bruised, epistaxis, hemoptysis, eye color blue-gray to brown, mild to severe nystagmus and photophobia, moderate decrease in visual acuity	Tyrosinase activity: normal Melanosomes in skin: incompletely melanized Platelet defect, catechol-like material in urine
Albinism-oligophrenia-microphthalmia (Cross-McKusick syndrome)	AR	Severe nystagmus and blindness, microphthalmia, gray-blue eye color, cataracts, leukomas, hair white to light blonde, pink to white skin, freckles, oligophrenia	Tyrosinase activity: positive Scanty melanosomes

Table 4 TYPES OF ALBINISM—cont'd

NAME	INHERITANCE	CLINICAL FINDINGS	LABORATORY FINDINGS
Ocular Albinism			
Chédiak-Higashi syndrome	AR	Partial albinism, photophobia, nystagmus, light blue to brown irides, iris transillumination moderate; diminished uveal and retinal pigmentation, neurologic defects, hepatosplenomegaly, lymphadenopathy, early death (8 to 10 years) from infections, leukemia or lymphoma	Tyrosinase activity: positive Melanosomes in skin: macromelanosomes Neutropenia with lymphocytosis, anemia, thrombocytopenia
Autosomal recessive ocular albinism	AR	Normal hair, normal skin, easily sunburned, irides normal or transilluminated; females affected as severely as males; foveal hypoplasia; visual acuity: 20/100 to 20/400	Tyrosinase activity: normal Melanosomes in skin: normal
Nettleship-Falls X-linked ocular albinism	X-L	Males: decreased visual acuity, nystagmus, photophobia, iris transillumination, normal skin pigmentation Carriers may manifest iris transillumination, macular hypoplasia, nystagmus, photophobia, near vision better than distant, normal hair	Tyrosinase activity: normal Melanosomes in skin: macromelanosomes
Autosomal dominant ocular albinism with deafness and freckles	AD	Ocular albinism with congenital sensorineural deafness, cutaneous lentigines	Tyrosinase activity: positive Melanosomes in skin: macromelanosomes
Albinoidism			
Autosomal dominant oculocutaneous (Donaldson-Fitzpatrick)	AD	Diffuse iris transillumination, fundus hypopigmentation, no nystagmus, normal visual acuity	Tyrosinase activity: positive Melanosomes in skin: normal
Punctate oculocutaneous (Bergsma-Kaiser-Kupfer)	AD	Diffuse iris transillumination, punctate window defects in RPE without congenital nystagmus or foveal hypoplasia	Tyrosinase activity: positive
Apert's syndrome	AD	Abnormal iris transillumination, fundus hypopigmentation, low fertility	Tyrosinase activity: positive
Waardenburg-like syndrome (Bard)	AD	Congenital sensorineural deafness, broad nasal root, white forelock, segmented iris heterochromia, normal inner canthi, strabismus, iris transillumination, fundus hypopigmentation	Tyrosinase activity: positive

Albinism FIGURE 27

KEY SYMPTOMS
Severe photophobia
Low vision

KEY FINDINGS
Nystagmus, iris transillumination, hypopigmentation of the fundus (large choroidal vessels are easily seen except in the macular area), absence of foveal reflex (macular hypoplasia), strabismus
Types of Albinism with Ocular Involvement (See Table 4, p. 102)
Oculocutaneous albinism: clinical hypopigmentation of the skin, hair, and eyes
Ocular albinism: hypopigmentation is mostly confined to the eyes
Albinoidism: mild decrease in vision, absence of nystagmus, and no foveal hypoplasia

INHERITANCE	ONSET	PROGRESSION	PROGNOSIS
AR, AD, X-L	Congenital	None	Good to poor

LABORATORY STUDIES
Visual Acuity	20/40 to 20/200
Refraction	Myopia and astigmatism
Visual Fields	Normal or central scotoma
Color Vision	Normal to abnormal with low vision
Dark Adaptation	Normal
ERG	Normal, supernormal, or abnormal
EOG	Normal (large ratios)
Fluorescein Angiogram	Background fluorescence brighter than normal; choroidal vessels visible in the venous phase

TREATMENT	PATHOLOGY	SYNONYMS
Dark glasses	Foveomacular dysplasia; foveola absent	Oculocutaneous albinism Ocular albinism

DIFFERENTIAL DIAGNOSIS
See "Albinism" in Table 4, p. 102

REFERENCES
61, 98, 222, 232, 242, 270, 273, 274, 275

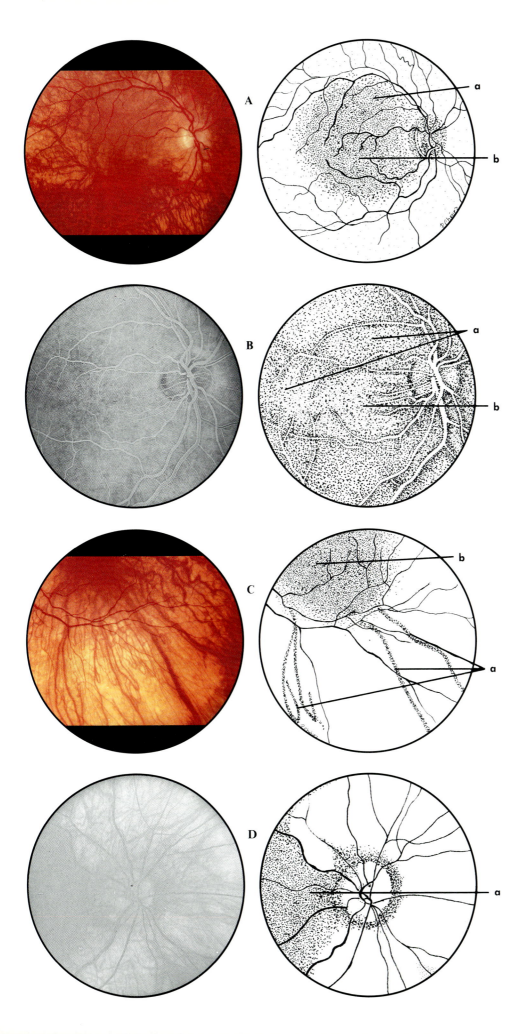

Figure 27
Albinism

A-23-year-old female with photophobia, nystagmus, and loss of vision since birth. Corrected visual acuity is 20/200 OU; partial iris transillumination is present.

A, Fundus photograph shows hypopigmentation with visualization of choroidal vessels throughout the fundus except in the macula *(a)*. There is no well-defined foveal depression *(b)*.

B, Angiogram in early venous phase shows diffuse hyperfluorescence throughout the fundus *(a)*. The capillary free zone is not visualized *(b)*.

C, Fundus photograph (OS) of the inferotemporal retina shows easy visualization of choroidal vessels *(a)* throughout the fundus except in the macula *(b)*. (A-C, courtesy of Peter Liggett, M.D.)

D, Fundus photograph (OD) of a patient with oculocutaneous albinism showing the albinotic appearance sparing the central area *(a)*.

Congenital Grouped Albinotic Spots FIGURE 28

KEY SYMPTOMS
Asymptomatic

KEY FINDINGS
Polar bear tracks

Multiple white, variable-sized spots involving the RPE in a pattern similar to that of bear track–grouped pigmentation

These lesions tend to be more numerous and larger in the periphery; the macular area is usually spared

Usually bilateral

In some cases the underlying choroidal vessels are visible through the lesions

INHERITANCE	ONSET	PROGRESSION	PROGNOSIS
None	Congenital	None	Good

LABORATORY STUDIES
Visual Acuity	Normal
Visual Fields	Normal
Color Vision	Normal
Dark Adaptation	Normal
ERG	Normal
EOG	Normal
Fluorescein Angiogram	Variable degrees of transmission of choroidal fluorescence through the lesions

TREATMENT
None

PATHOLOGY
Peripheral retinal albinotic spots; flattened RPE cells with loss of pigment granules; Bruch's membrane, choriocapillaris, and photoreceptors are normal

SYNONYMS
Congenital grouped albinotic retinal pigment epithelium spots

Polar bear tracks

DIFFERENTIAL DIAGNOSIS
Flecked retina diseases (see Table 5, p. 114)

REFERENCES
142, 321

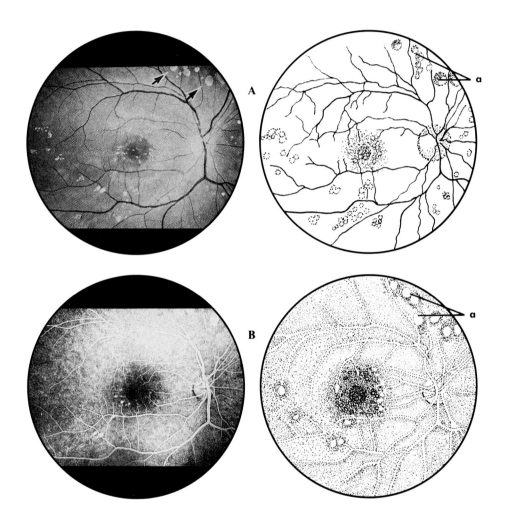

Figure 28
Congenital Grouped Albinotic Spots

A, Fundus photograph (OD) showing the distribution of multiple irregular white spots. Note the peripheral distribution of white material in some of the larger spots *(a)*.

B, Angiogram (OD) showing variable transmission of choroidal fluorescence through the spots *(a)*. (**A-B,** reproduced and redrawn from Gass JDM: Stereoscopic atlas of macular diseases, diagnosis and treatment, St. Louis, 1987, The C.V. Mosby Co.)

Bear Track–Grouped Pigmentation FIGURE 29

KEY SYMPTOMS
Asymptomatic

KEY FINDINGS
Distinctive pigment changes that resemble bear tracks within a triangular area of retina; the apex of the area points to the macula
Usually involves upper or lower temporal sectors
Unilateral in 85% of patients
Sharply defined affected areas; intervening areas of retina are normal
Pigment clump size varies from .1- to 1-disc diameter
Normal vessels and optic disc

INHERITANCE	ONSET	PROGRESSION	PROGNOSIS
None	Congenital	None	Good

LABORATORY STUDIES
Visual Acuity	Normal
Visual Fields	Normal
Color Vision	Normal
Dark Adaptation	Normal
ERG	Normal
EOG	Normal
Fluorescein Angiogram	Hypofluorescence corresponding to the pigment clumps

TREATMENT	PATHOLOGY	SYNONYMS
None	Hypertrophy of the RPE with large pigment granules; the overlying receptors may show degeneration	Bear tract pigmentary retinopathy

DIFFERENTIAL DIAGNOSIS
Pigmentary retinopathy (see Table 6, p. 118)

REFERENCES
288, 325, 328, 350

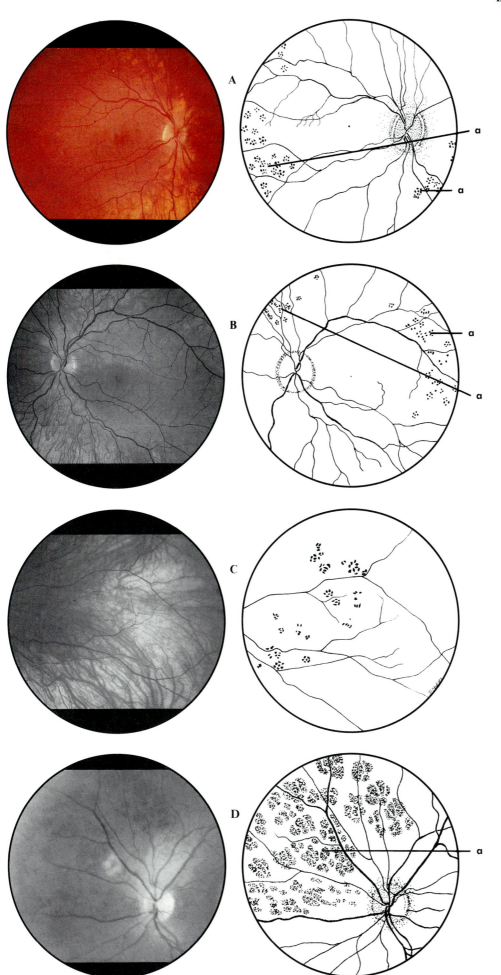

Figure 29
Bear Track–Grouped Pigmentation

A-C, Bilateral involvement without macular lesions in this asymptomatic patient. The bear tracks surround the posterior pole *(a)*.

D, Larger grouped pigmentations *(a)* in the inferonasal quadrant of this asymptomatic patient.

Abnormalities of the RPE-Photoreceptor Complex

FLECKED RETINA DISEASES
ROD-CONE DYSTROPHIES (RETINITIS PIGMENTOSA)
ROD-CONE DYSTROPHIES (RP-ASSOCIATED SYNDROMES)
CONE AND CONE-ROD DEGENERATIONS

The RPE-photoreceptor complex group includes those diseases in which photoreceptor abnormality is the principal finding and is always associated with RPE degeneration.

The flecked retina diseases group is included here in accordance with previous classifications. The diseases in this group represent various pathogenetic mechanisms. Their only commonality is the presence of white dots in the fundus.

The rod-cone dystrophies group includes classical retinitis pigmentosa and its variants.

The rod-cone dystrophies/RP-associated syndromes group includes systemic diseases with a retinal degeneration similar to that seen in retinitis pigmentosa.

The cone and cone-rod degenerations group includes those diseases in which cone degeneration occurs early and is the most important finding.

FLECKED RETINA DISEASES

Fundus flavimaculatus
Retinitis punctata albescens
Fundus albipunctatus
Flecked retina of Kandori

Flecked retina diseases also include dominant drusen, which is found in the section on Diseases of Bruch's Membrane. As we prefer to classify diseases on the basis of the structure primarily involved, fundus albipunctatus and flecked retina of Kandori are found in the section on Diseases of the Rod System. Retinitis punctata albescens is found in the section on Rod-Cone Dystrophies.

Flowchart 3 shows some of the symptoms, as well as clinical and laboratory findings, used to distinguish among these diseases.

We divide the flecked retinas into two groups based on the symptom of nyctalopia. When nyctalopia is absent and the flecks are round, yellow, and located in the posterior pole with or without SRN, drusen is suggested. When nyctalopia is absent and the flecks are linear or have fishtail configurations without a macular lesion, the picture suggests fundus flavimaculatus. If a macular lesion is present, Stargardt's disease with fundus flavimaculatus must be considered.

When progressive nyctalopia is present with severely abnormal adaptometry and ERG tests (see Appendices A and B), the picture suggests retinitis punctata albescens. If stationary nyctalopia is found with normal cone function and subnormal or delayed rod function, the probable diagnosis is fundus albipunctatus.

Table 5 includes some diseases that must be considered in the differential diagnosis of the flecked retina diseases.

Abnormalities of the RPE-Photoreceptor Complex

```
Flecked retina
├── No nyctalopia
│   ├── Round yellow flecks, SRN may be seen ──→ Drusen, dominant or senile
│   └── Irregular linear or fishtail flecks
│       ├── No macular lesion ──→ Fundus flavimaculatus
│       └── Atrophic macular lesion ──→ Stargardt's disease ──→ Fundus flavimaculatus
└── Nyctalopia
    ├── ERG/EOG, adaptometry severely abnormal, Fields constricted ──→ Retinitis punctata albescens
    └── Cone ERG often normal, Rod ERG very abnormal with delayed adaptation, Photopic fields normal, Scotopic fields abnormal ──→ Fundus albipunctatus
```

Flowchart 3

The flecked retina diseases are easily divided on the basis of symptoms of night blindness, the nature of the flecks, and the results of electrophysiologic recordings.

Table 5 FLECKED RETINA DISEASES

The term *flecked retina syndrome* was applied by Krill and Klien in 1965 to several conditions having a related fundus appearance. This term has been used with increasing frequency to describe the appearance of certain disorders in which the fundi are characterized by widespread posterior distribution of deep yellowish-white spots of various sizes and configurations. The classic syndrome includes fundus flavimaculatus, fundus albipunctatus, familial drusen, and retinitis punctata albescens. Other diseases with similar fundus abnormalities are included in the differential diagnosis.

NAME	INHERITANCE	PRINCIPAL FINDINGS
Fundus flavimaculatus (Stargardt's disease)	AR AD (uncommon)	Asymptomatic or decrease in vision; yellowish-white spots in the posterior pole with linear or fishtail configuration; in 50% of the patients, macular lesion is present (Stargardt's disease)
Fundus albipunctatus (stationary albipunctate degeneration)	AR AD (uncommon)	Asymptomatic or stationary nyctalopia; uniform white dots in the midperiphery; central macula is free of flecks; dark adaptation and ERG abnormal
Retinitis punctata albescens (progressive albipunctate degeneration)	AR	Progressive nyctalopia; visual field reduction; small white dots generally spare the posterior pole; optic disc pale with narrow vessels; dark adaptation and ERG abnormal
Dominant drusen (familial)	AD	Onset in second decade, symptomatic in fourth or fifth decades; metamorphopsia and decrease in vision; flecks are round and yellowish, with greatest concentration in the posterior pole; subretinal neovascular membrane formation common
Flecked retina of Kandori	AR	Stationary nyctalopia; normal vision; irregular large and small flecks; dark adaptation and ERG abnormal

Table 5 FLECKED RETINA DISEASES—cont'd

NAME	INHERITANCE	PRINCIPAL FINDINGS
Hallervorden-Spatz syndrome	AR	Onset in first decade; rigidity of extremities; dysarthria and dementia; retinal degeneration with flecks; bull's-eye macular lesion
Crystalline retinopathy (Bietti's tapetoretinal degeneration with marginal corneal dystrophy)	AD	Asymptomatic or decreased vision; yellow glistening intraretinal crystals in the posterior pole; tapetoretinal degeneration with choroidal atrophy; superficial whitish dots in the cornea
Vitamin A retinopathy	—	Night blindness; xerophthalmia; small white flecks in the midperiphery; dark adaptation, ERG, and visual field abnormal; abnormalities disappear after vitamin A therapy
Primary hyperoxaluria (oxalosis)	AR	Oxalate urolithiasis and nephrocalcinosis; type I: glycolic aciduria; type II: glyceric aciduria; crystals in the macular area, iris, ciliary body, and choroid
Kjellin syndrome	AR	Spastic paraplegia; dementia; few yellow perifoveal flecks; hyperfluorescence surrounding flecks
Secondary oxalosis caused by methoxyflurane toxicity	—	Postoperative renal failure from renal oxalosis, with deposit of crystals in the retina
Tamoxifen retinopathy	—	After prolonged use (more than 1 year), retinopathy is characterized by fine, white, refractile, superficial flecks in the posterior pole
Alport's syndrome	AD X-L	Hereditary chronic nephritis associated with neurosensory deafness; multiple, small, yellow-white lesions in the superficial retina in the macula; microspherophakia; cataracts

Fundus Flavimaculatus FIGURE 30

KEY SYMPTOMS
Early
Asymptomatic
Late
Mild visual acuity reduction

KEY FINDINGS
Posterior pole retina shows multiple irregular, linear, and round yellow-white flecks deep in the retina
The flecks vary in size; many have fishtail configuration
Involved retina is sharply demarcated from normal retina
Growth of flecks may lead to confluency; spread into the fovea may decrease acuity to 20/100
Macular lesion identical to that of Stargardt's disease occurs in 50% of patients with fundus flavimaculatus
RPE atrophy and pigmentary changes may occur late; SRN has been reported
In fundus flavimaculatus, flecks are prominent and macular involvement occurs late or not at all; macular disease and decreased vision at an early age indicate Stargardt's disease

INHERITANCE	ONSET	PROGRESSION	PROGNOSIS
AR	Occurs at 8 to 15 years	Slow	50%—good 50%<20/200

LABORATORY STUDIES
Visual Acuity	20/20 to 20/200 (if macula involved)
Refraction	Hyperopia or emmetropia
Visual Fields	Normal, or central or paracentral scotomas
Color Vision	Normal unless macula involved
Dark Adaptation	Abnormal with delayed rod threshold
ERG	Normal (mild b-wave loss in about 20% of cases)
EOG	Normal early, abnormal with extensive RPE loss
Fluorescein Angiogram	Window defects in affected areas, which are sharply delimited; no leakage; early flecks do not hyperfluoresce

TREATMENT	PATHOLOGY	SYNONYMS
None	RPE atrophy; deposits of lipofuscin in the RPE; RPE shows pleomorphic changes with variability of cell size and nuclear displacement	Stargardt's disease

DIFFERENTIAL DIAGNOSIS	REFERENCES
Stargardt's disease (p. 92) Flecked retina diseases (see Table 5, p. 114)	94, 109, 113, 123, 128, 157, 204, 206, 220, 257, 263, 358

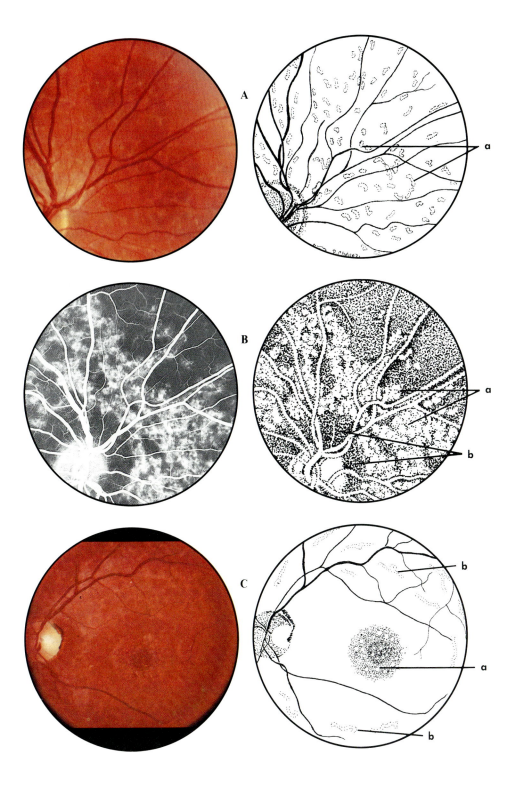

Figure 30

Fundus Flavimaculatus

A, Fundus photograph showing typical linear and fishtail yellow-white flecks *(a)* in the superonasal quadrant outside the macular area. The optic disc and vessels are normal.

B, The angiogram demonstrates transmission defects *(a)* corresponding to the observed flecks and sparing the peripapillary area *(b)*.

C, Fundus photograph of a 24-year-old female with a visual acuity of 20/100 OU, showing mottled pigmentary changes surrounding the central macula *(a)* and yellow linear flecks outside the arcades *(b)*.

**ROD-CONE DYSTROPHIES
(RETINITIS PIGMENTOSA)**

Retinitis pigmentosa
Retinitis pigmentosa sine pigmento
Sector retinitis pigmentosa
Unilateral retinitis pigmentosa
Central retinitis pigmentosa (inverse RP)
Pericentral retinitis pigmentosa
Retinitis pigmentosa with PPRPE
Retinitis punctata albescens
Senile retinitis pigmentosa
Leber's congenital amaurosis
Pigmented paravenous chorioretinal atrophy

Retinitis pigmentosa (RP) is the most common retinal dystrophy and is usually incapacitating. All forms of inheritance patterns are observed in this disease. The most common forms are sporadic and autosomal recessive; less common are autosomal dominant and X-linked cases. The clinical, electrophysiologic, and psychophysical findings usually confirm the diagnosis (see Appendices A and B). The classic findings are nyctalopia, "bone-spicule" pigmentation, attenuated vessels, waxy pallor of the optic disc, visual field constriction, and a nonrecordable ERG.

Several diseases must be considered in the differential diagnosis, including some choroidal atrophies, the stationary rod system abnormalities, RP-associated syndromes, and some vitreoretinal dystrophies. Diseases with pigmentary retinopathy are listed in Table 6. Some diseases with progressive nyctalopia are mentioned in Table 7 and Flowchart 4.

Table 6 CAUSES OF PIGMENTARY RETINOPATHY

This table includes multiple causes of pigmentary retinopathy that must be considered in the differential diagnosis of the primary and secondary pigmentary retinopathies.

NAME (CAUSE)	INHERITANCE	PRINCIPAL FINDINGS
Abetalipoproteinemia (Bassen-Kornzweig syndrome)	AR	Acanthocytosis, vitamin A deficiency, spinocerebellar degeneration, abetalipoproteinemia; dark adaptation restored with high levels of vitamin A
Alport's syndrome	AD, AR, X-L	Lenticonus, spherophakia, cataract, myopia, deafness, hemorrhagic nephritis, retinal detachment; mild in women and severe in men
Alström syndrome	AR	Deafness, obesity, diabetes mellitus, cataract, nephropathy, acanthosis nigricans
Arteriohepatic dysplasia (Alagile's syndrome)	AD	Intrahepatic cholestatic syndrome, embryotoxon, cataract, myopia, retinal degeneration
Autosomal dominant vitreoretinochoroidopathy	AD	Pigmentary degeneration from vortex veins to ora serrata, arteriolar occlusion, cystoid macular edema, vitreous condensations and hemorrhage, cataract, neovascularization
Batten disease (amaurotic idiocy, neuronal ceroid lipofuscinosis)	AR	Late infantile and juvenile forms of amaurotic idiocy or Batten-Spielmeyer-Vogt syndrome; red spot in macula and retinal degeneration
Bardet-Biedl syndrome	AR	Obesity, polydactyly, hypogenitalism, mild mental retardation
Carotinemia (familial)	—	Retinal degeneration from vitamin A deficiency, failure of cleavage of beta-carotene
Cerebrohepatorenal syndrome (Zellweger syndrome)	AR	Nystagmus, cataract, congenital glaucoma, microphthalmia, retinal degeneration, epicanthal folds, hypertelorism, hepatomegaly, nephropathy, mental retardation, muscular hypotony, early death
Charcot-Marie-Tooth disease (progressive neuritic muscular atrophy)	AR, AD, X-L	Reduced vision, nystagmus, optic atrophy, atrophy of small muscles of hands and feet
Cockayne's syndrome	AR	Deafness, dwarfism, progeria, oligophrenia, optic atrophy, cataract, photophobia

Table 6 CAUSES OF PIGMENTARY RETINOPATHY—cont'd

NAME (CAUSE)	INHERITANCE	PRINCIPAL FINDINGS
Crystalline retinopathy of Bietti	AR? X-L?	Intraretinal crystals with tapetoretinal degeneration, areas of choriocapillaris atrophy, crystalline deposits in cornea in some patients
Cystinosis	AR	Cystine crystals in cornea and conjunctiva, retinal pigmentary degeneration in periphery, polyuria, progressive renal failure
Dysplasia spondyloepiphysiana congenita	AD	Dwarfism, mild deafness, cleft palate, congenital high myopia with associated retinal degeneration, cataract, glaucoma
Flynn-Aird syndrome	AD	Cataract, myopia, ataxia, dementia, epilepsy, nerve deafness, skin atrophy, baldness, cystic bone changes, peripheral neuropathy
Friedreich's ataxia	AR	Optic atrophy, nystagmus, ataxia, spinocerebellar degeneration
Fundus flavimaculatus (Stargardt's disease)	AR	Linear or fishtail flecks in the posterior pole, macular lesion (Stargardt's disease); pigment patches of "bone spicules" can be seen in periphery
Goldmann–Favre disease	AR	Juvenile retinoschisis, vitreous degeneration, preretinal strands
Hallervorden-Spatz syndrome	AR	Extrapyramidal signs related to degenerative changes in the basal ganglia
Hallgren's syndrome (Usher's III, Merin classification)	AR	Congenital deafness, vestibulocerebellar ataxia, psychoses, dementia
Homocystinuria	AR	Myopia, subluxation or dislocated lenses, peripheral cystic degeneration of retina, glaucoma, marfanoid appearance, cardiovascular abnormalities, mental retardation, osteoporosis, fine fair hair
Hooft disease	AR	Atypical pigmentary retinopathy, panhypolipidemia, hypoglycemia, mental retardation, skin rash, death by age 3
Hyperostosis corticalis deformans (juvenile Paget's disease)	AR	Large head, expanded and bowed extremities, chronic idiopathic hyperphosphatemia, retinal degeneration, angioid streaks
Incontinentia pigmenti (Bloch-Sulzberger syndrome)	X-D	Corneal opacities, cataract, nystagmus, blue sclerae, myopia, pseudoglioma, dental abnormalities, abnormal skin pigmentation, mental deficiency; only females (lethal in males)
Imidazole aminoaciduria	AR	Seizures, mental deterioration, excess carnosine and anserine in urine
Infantile phytanic acid storage	AR?	Hypotony, hearing loss, pigmentary retinopathy, neuropathy; serum phytanic acid levels are elevated, ERG is abnormal
Kartagener's syndrome	AR	Dextrocardia, bronchiectasis, sinusitis
Kearns-Sayre syndrome	?	Progressive external ophthalmoplegia, ptosis, heart block, deafness, weakness of trunk and extremity musculature, small stature
Laurence-Moon syndrome	AR	Hypogenitalism, mental retardation, spastic paraplegia
Leber's congenital amaurosis	AR, AD	Low vision from birth with normal or abnormal fundi; may develop pigmentary retinopathy in second decade
Lignac-Fanconi syndrome	AR	Renal dwarfism, osteoporosis, chronic nephritis
Mannosidosis	X-L	Small lens opacities, optic disc pale with blurred margins, macroglossia, flat nose, psychomotor retardation, muscular hypotony
Marinesco-Sjögren syndrome	AR	Congenital cataracts, oligophrenia, cerebellar ataxia
Mucopolysaccharidoses I. Hurler syndrome (MPS I) (gargoylism)	AR	Ptosis, corneal clouding, strabismus, glaucoma, optic atrophy, deafness, mental retardation, hepatosplenomegaly, dwarfism, skeletal abnormalities
IS. Scheie's syndrome	AR	Corneal clouding, open-angle glaucoma, normal intelligence, aortic valve disease, bone cyst, stiff joints
II. Hunter's syndrome	X-L	Little corneal clouding, mild clinical course, mental retardation
III. Sanfilippo's syndrome	AR	Little corneal clouding, optic atrophy, mental retardation
Myopia, high	Sporadic, AR, AD	Pigmentary retinal degeneration may occur, usually associated with lattice degeneration
Myotonic dystrophy of Steinert	AD	Lens opacities, myotonia, frontal baldness, endocrinopathy, macular changes, testicular atrophy
Oculodentodigital dysplasia (Meyer-Schwickerath and Weyers syndrome)	AD	Microphthalmos, microcornea, congenital glaucoma and lens opacities, typical facies, thin nose, hypoplastic alae, syndactyly, hypoplastic dental enamel
Olivopontocerebellar retinal degeneration	AD	Macular degeneration, cerebellar ataxia, progression to quadriplegia, mental retardation
Osteopetrosis (Albers-Schönberg disease)	AR	Retinal degeneration, defective resorption of immature bone, macrocephaly, progressive deafness, hepatosplenomegaly, anemia
Osteoporosis (infantile and mild forms)	AR, AD	Optic atrophy, large head, frequent fractures, cranial nerve palsies
Pallidal degeneration and retinitis pigmentosa	AR	Extrapyramidal rigidity, dysarthria, destruction of globus pallidus and substantia nigra

Continued.

Table 6 CAUSES OF PIGMENTARY RETINOPATHY—cont'd

NAME (CAUSE)	INHERITANCE	PRINCIPAL FINDINGS
Paget's disease	AD	Occasionally angioid streaks
Pelizaeus-Merzbacher disease	X-L	Pigmentary retinopathy with absent foveal reflex, mental retardation, extrapyramidal signs
Pierre Marie syndrome	AD	Cone-rod degeneration, bitemporal hemianopsia, choked disc, disturbed hair growth, acromegaly
Paravenous chorioretinal atrophy	Sporadic AD, AR	Bone spicule pigmentation along the distribution of one or more veins
Pseudoxanthoma elasticum (Grönblad-Strandberg syndrome)	AD, AR	Angioid streaks, possible pigmentary changes in the streaks, characteristic plaquelike skin lesions on the neck
Refsum's disease (heredopathia atactica polyneuritiformis)	AR	Deafness, cerebellar ataxia, baldness, ichthyosis, muscular weakness, peripheral neuropathy
Renal dysplasia and retinal aplasia	AR	Congenital blindness, developmental renal abnormalities
Reticular degeneration	—	Reticular pigmentary degeneration in the midperiphery with drusen that increase with age
Saldino-Mainzer syndrome	AR	Skeletal dysplasia, familial juvenile nephrophthisis, cerebellar ataxia, short stature, congenital onset of retinal degeneration, nystagmus
Senior-Loken syndrome	AR	Childhood onset of nephrophthisis and congenital onset of retinal degeneration, nystagmus
Snowflake vitreoretinal degeneration	—	"White with pressure" with small peripheral yellow-white crystalline spots, vitreous degeneration, sheathing of retinal vessels, pigment clumping in stage III
Stickler syndrome (progressive arthroophthalmopathy)	AD	Progressive myopia, secondary glaucoma, retinal detachment, deafness, cleft palate, Pierre Robin anomaly
Turner's syndrome	—	Infertility, short stature, shield chest, low hairline
Usher's syndrome	AR	Familial congenital deafness (see Table 8, p. 150, Deafness and Pigmentary Retinopathy)
Waardenburg syndrome	AD	Hypertelorism, blepharophimosis, heterochromia iridis, hyperplasia of eyebrows medially, white forelock, broad nasal root, deafness (cochlear)
Wagner's hereditary vitreoretinal dystrophy	AD	Narrowed and sheathed retinal vessels, pigmented spots in the retinal periphery and along retinal vessels, choroidal and optic atrophy, vitreous degeneration
X-linked juvenile retinoschisis	X-L	Macular schisis, peripheral retinoschisis (50%), vitreous veils and strands; diffuse pigmentary changes may occur

Other causes of pigmentary retinopathy:
- Chloroquine
- Tamoxifen
- Rubella
- Vascular occlusion
- Metallosis
- Tilorane
- Syphilis
- Retinal detachment
- Phenothiazine
- Toxoplasmosis
- Trauma
- Choroidal detachment

Retinitis pigmentosa sine pigmento presents the same clinical picture as does RP but with pigment migration not occurring or only occurring in late stages; early cases of classic RP are also sine pigmento.

In *unilateral retinitis pigmentosa*, most of the cases considered as unilateral pigmentary degeneration are probably secondary to an inflammatory process. It is necessary to provide long-term follow-up care in suspected cases to rule out asymmetric onset of RP.

Sector retinitis pigmentosa is a pigmentary retinopathy that affects only a portion of the fundus. Typical bone spicules and arterial narrowing resemble the changes of RP and are associated with visual field changes. The ERG is only slightly abnormal, and this can distinguish sector RP from a generalized RP with asymmetric or slow onset, in which the ERG is severely abnormal.

Central retinitis pigmentosa, or *inverse RP*, is a rod-cone degeneration that begins in the posterior pole; however, its differentiation from cone-rod degeneration is not clear.

Table 7 PROGRESSIVE NYCTALOPIA (NIGHT BLINDNESS)

Progressive nyctalopia includes all the retinal and choroidal dystrophies with onset after birth and with a progressive course. In all cases, dark adaptation is abnormal and the ERG is usually abnormal (see Appendices A and B).

NAME (CAUSE)	INHERITANCE	PRINCIPAL FINDINGS
Retinitis pigmentosa (RP) (classic RP)	AR, AD, X-L	Progressive nyctalopia, visual field constriction, symmetric pigmentary retinopathy—"bone spicules," narrow vessels, pale optic disc, posterior vitreous detachment, pigment in vitreous, posterior subcapsular cataract; ERG severely abnormal to extinguished, EOG abnormal
RP Variants		
Retinitis punctata albescens	AR	Progressive nyctalopia, visual field constriction, numerous white dots in the posterior pole, optic disc pale and narrow vessels; may be associated with pigmentary retinopathy; ERG severely abnormal
Retinitis pigmentosa sine pigmento	AD, AR	Progressive nyctalopia, visual field constriction; normal fundus early; narrow vessels and pale optic disc in late stage; ERG severely abnormal
Unilateral retinitis pigmentosa	?	Typical pigmentary retinopathy of classic retinitis pigmentosa, but only one eye is affected; for the diagnosis, it is necessary to exclude an inflammatory process in the affected eye, and a long period of observation is needed to rule out delayed onset of RP in the unaffected eye; ERG in unaffected eye should be normal
Sector retinitis pigmentosa	AD, AR	Typical bone spicule pigmentary changes in only one sector of the retina (usually bilateral); the remainder of the retina is normal; ERG is usually subnormal
Pericentral retinitis pigmentosa	AR	Asymptomatic or nyctalopia; pigmentary retinopathy similar to RP, but occurs only in the pericentral retina; ERG usually normal
Central retinitis pigmentosa (inverse RP)	AR	Decrease in central vision, occasionally nyctalopia; the pigmentary changes occur only in the macular area; ERG usually normal
Leber's congenital amaurosis	AR, AD (uncommon)	Progressive nyctalopia; very low vision from birth and during the first years; nystagmus, photophobia, fundus normal or abnormal (salt-and-pepper), macular colobomas, pigmentary retinopathy in second decade, oculodigital sign of Franceschetti, cataract, mental retardation; ERG severely abnormal
Crystalline retinopathy (Bietti's tapetoretinal degeneration with marginal corneal dystrophy)	AD	Asymptomatic or progressive nyctalopia; intraretinal crystals with tapetoretinal degeneration, areas of choriocapillaris atrophy and crystalline dystrophy of the cornea; ERG normal to abnormal
Retinitis pigmentosa with preserved para-arteriolar retinal pigment epithelium (PPRPE)	AR	Similar to retinitis pigmentosa with low hypermetropia; the bone spicule pigment avoids the area surrounding arterioles; ERG severely abnormal
Goldmann–Favre vitreoretinal dystrophy	AR	Progressive nyctalopia, central and peripheral retinoschisis, vitreous degeneration, pigmentary retinopathy; ERG severely abnormal
Usher's syndrome	AD, AR, ?	Progressive nyctalopia, congenital deafness, pigmentary retinopathy similar to that of RP (see Table 8, p. 150, Deafness and Pigmentary Retinopathy); ERG severely abnormal
Bardet-Biedl syndrome (Laurence-Moon-Bardet-Biedl)	AR	Progressive nyctalopia, pigmentary retinopathy, obesity, mental retardation, polydactyly, hypogenitalism; ERG severely abnormal
Bassen-Kornzweig syndrome (abetalipoproteinemia)	AR	Progressive nyctalopia, pigmentary retinopathy, neuromuscular disturbances, gastrointestinal abnormalities, vitamin A deficiency, acanthocytosis; ERG severely abnormal
Refsum's disease (heredopathia atactica polyneuritiformis)	—	Progressive nyctalopia, pigmentary retinopathy, miosis, dental abnormalities, sensory loss and weakness, finally quadriplegia; excess of phytanic acid; ERG severely abnormal
Other diseases		
Pigmented paravenous chorioretinal atrophy	Sporadic, AD (rare), AR (rare)	Usually asymptomatic, nyctalopia and progression have been reported; bone spicule pigmentation along the distribution of one or more veins; ERG usually normal
Myotonic dystrophy (Steinert's disease)	AD	Myotonia and muscular weakness; nyctalopia has been reported; progressive ophthalmoplegia, lens abnormalities, pigmentary retinopathy, baldness; ERG normal to abnormal
Sjögren's reticular dystrophy	AD, AR	Usually asymptomatic, nyctalopia has been reported; RPE: hypopigmented network with the appearance of fishnet with knots; ERG normal; EOG normal to abnormal

Continued.

Table 7 PROGRESSIVE NYCTALOPIA (NIGHT BLINDNESS)—cont'd

NAME (CAUSE)	INHERITANCE	PRINCIPAL FINDINGS
Other diseases—cont'd		
Degenerative myopia	Sporadic AR	Nyctalopia, decrease in visual acuity, myopic conus, posterior staphyloma, breaks in Bruch's membrane with SRN and hemorrhage, hyperpigmented scar in macula (Foster-Fuchs spot), posterior vitreous detachment, lattice degeneration, and retinal holes
Choroideremia	X-L	Progressive nyctalopia, visual field constriction; affects only males; areas of choroidal atrophy with macular sparing (early); macula is affected in the fifth decade; various stages of atrophy are seen at the same time; ERG severely abnormal; female carriers may have an abnormal fundus
Gyrate atrophy	AR	Progressive nyctalopia, areas of total choroidal atrophy with scalloped borders; macula usually spared; cataracts; ERG abnormal
Diffuse choriocapillaris atrophy	AD	Decrease in vision and progressive nyctalopia, areas of choriocapillaris atrophy and RPE atrophy (increased visibility of large choroidal vessels); ERG abnormal to nonrecordable
Peripapillary choroidal sclerosis	—	Decrease in vision and occasionally nyctalopia, choriocapillaris, and RPE atrophy around the optic disc and macular area; ERG normal to abnormal

Pericentral retinitis pigmentosa is a variant of rod-cone degeneration that begins in the posterior pole, usually sparing the macula. It has a good prognosis and minimal symptoms and findings.

Retinitis pigmentosa with preserved para-arteriolar retinal pigment epithelium (PPRPE) is a variant of RP, was described by Heckenlively,[168] and consists of RP presenting with hyperopia with a preservation of the RPE beneath the arterioles. It appears that, in later stages, the RPE is more generally affected. The inheritance is autosomal recessive.

In *retinitis punctata albescens* the symptoms and test results are the same as those in classic RP but the presence of multiple small white dots in the fundus provides the key to diagnosis. Fundus albipunctatus or stationary albipunctate degeneration must be considered in the differential diagnosis.

Senile retinitis pigmentosa, a generalized form of retinal degeneration, has been described in four families, usually in the absence of nyctalopia; the pathogenesis is not clear and may correspond to advanced cases of cone-rod degeneration. This disease is not described in the summaries.

Leber's congenital amaurosis is a severe, early rod-cone degeneration with onset usually occurring in the first year of life. There is very low vision, nystagmus, photophobia, variable fundus appearance, and severely abnormal or extinguished ERG. Some diseases with low vision, photophobia, and nystagmus that must be considered in the differential diagnosis are mentioned in Flowcharts 2, p. 101 and 6, p. 188.

Pigmented paravenous chorioretinal atrophy is not a true rod-cone dystrophy because it is usually stationary, but progression has also been documented. It is included here because it forms part of the differential diagnosis of RP.

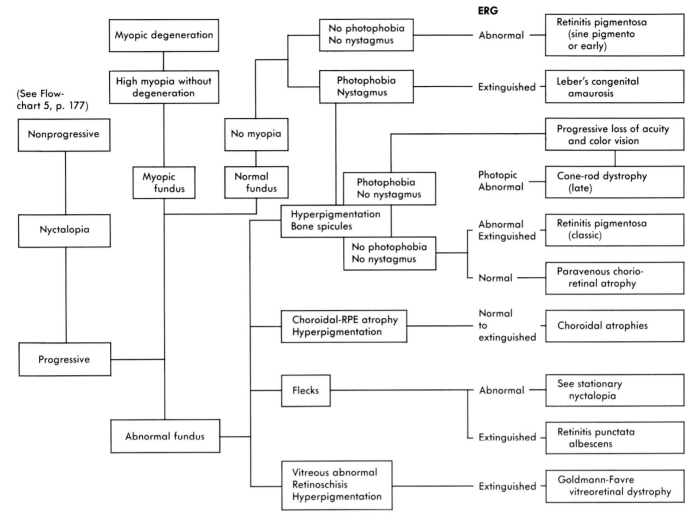

Flowchart 4

Progressive Nyctalopia

In a patient with progressive nyctalopia, the fundus examination gives the first key to the diagnosis. Three principal groups are identified:

1. High myopic fundus suggests a degenerative myopia.
2. Normal fundus with low myopia or hyperopia with the presence of photophobia, nystagmus, low vision, and extinguished ERG suggests Leber's congenital amaurosis; the absence of photophobia and nystagmus with severely abnormal ERG suggests retinitis pigmentosa sine pigmento or early classic RP.
3. When the fundus is abnormal, four categories of fundus appearance are considered: hyperpigmentation, choroidal atrophy, flecks and vitreoretinal degeneration.

Bone spicule hyperpigmentation suggests three alternatives:

1. Photophobia and nystagmus with extinguished ERG suggest Leber's congenital amaurosis; nyctalopia is not a complaint in most patients with this condition.
2. Photophobia and no nystagmus with progressive loss of central vision and with a photopic ERG more abnormal than the scotopic ERG suggest cone-rod dystrophy; nyctalopia is present only in late stages of this disease.
3. The absence of photophobia and nystagmus with severely abnormal ERG suggests classic RP; this is the most common cause of progressive nyctalopia.

Paravenous chorioretinal atrophy is suggested if the pigmentation is only surrounding veins and the ERG is normal; however, nyctalopia is not common in this disease.

If the principal fundus abnormalities are large areas of choroidal-RPE atrophy with hyperpigmentation and with a normal to extinguished ERG, three choroidal atrophies must be considered: choroideremia, gyrate atrophy, and diffuse choriocapillaris atrophy.

If the principal finding is flecks with an extinguished ERG, retinitis punctata albescens is suggested. An abnormal scotopic ERG suggests fundus albipunctatus (see Stationary Nyctalopia, Flowchart 5, p.177).

If the principal abnormalities are vitreous degeneration, macular retinoschisis, and bone spicule hyperpigmentation with an extinguished ERG, Goldmann-Favre vitreoretinal dystrophy is a likely diagnosis.

Retinitis Pigmentosa FIGURE 31

KEY SYMPTOMS
Nyctalopia
Visual field constriction
Visual acuity reduction

KEY FINDINGS
Pigmentary changes (bone spicules) in midperipheral retina, pigment clumps spread slowly toward the posterior pole and periphery; usually the pigment surrounds vessels

Early
Vessel attenuation

Late
Waxy pallor of the optic disc
Macular involvement
Posterior vitreous detachment, pigment in vitreous, and vitreous degeneration are common
Posterior subcapsular cataract is common
Cystoid macular edema, evident by angiography, is common and is the principal cause of early decrease in central vision
Areas of RPE and choriocapillaris atrophy
Optic disc drusen and epiretinal membranes

INHERITANCE	ONSET	PROGRESSION	PROGNOSIS
Sporadic, AD, AR, X-L	First to third decade	Slow	AR or X-L—poor AD—better

LABORATORY STUDIES
Visual Acuity	20/20 to no light perception
Refraction	Low myopia and astigmatism
Visual Fields	Constricted with scotomas
Color Vision	Usually abnormal
Dark Adaptation	Abnormal rod function (early) (see Figure 111, Appendix B)
ERG	Abnormal to extinguished (early) (see Figure 78, Appendix A)
EOG	Abnormal (see Figure 91, Appendix A)
Fluorescein Angiogram	Diffuse hyperfluorescence resulting from RPE defects; hypofluorescence resulting from pigment clumping and occasional choriocapillaris and RPE atrophy

TREATMENT	PATHOLOGY	SYNONYMS
None	Degeneration of photoreceptors, inner retinal layers, and RPE with pigment clumping and migration around vessels; glial proliferation and gliosis in optic disc; hyalinization of vessels	Primary retinal dystrophy Tapetoretinal dystrophy or degeneration

DIFFERENTIAL DIAGNOSIS
Pigmentary retinopathy (see Table 6, p. 118)
Progressive nyctalopia (see Table 7, p.120)

REFERENCES
16, 22, 23, 25, 32, 106, 110, 111, 115, 116, 121, 155, 215, 239, 243, 278, 283, 284, 303, 331

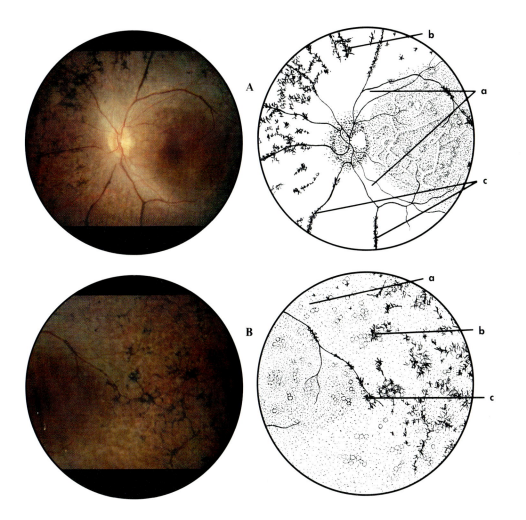

Figure 31
Retinitis Pigmentosa

A 27-year-old female with nyctalopia for the past 8 years. Visual acuity is 20/30, with visual field constriction and a nonrecordable ERG.

A-B, Fundus photograph (OS) showing a large area of mottled RPE disturbance *(a)* sparing the macular area. This RPE abnormality is often the first finding in the fundus of eyes with pigmentary retinopathy. The typical bone spicule pattern is seen *(b)*. This pattern is characteristic but not pathognomonic of RP. Some pigment clumps follow the vessels *(c)*, which are attenuated; the optic disc shows minimal pallor until late in the disease.

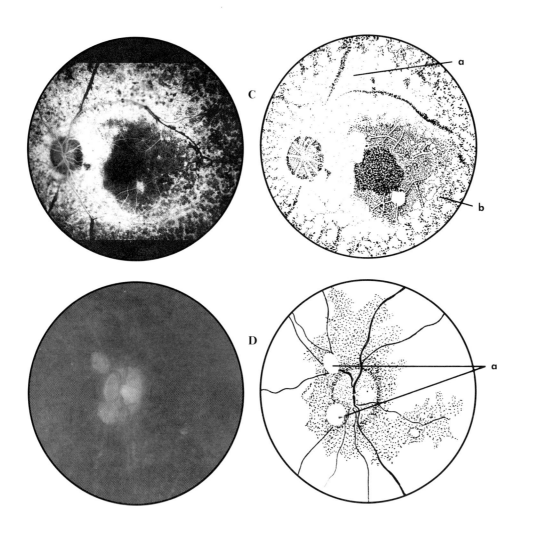

C, Angiogram (OS) in early venous phase of the same eye showing widespread transmission defects *(a)*, with relative sparing of the macular area and fluorescence blockage by pigment *(b)*.

D, Optic nerve drusen or hyaline bodies *(a)* are commonly seen in patients with RP.

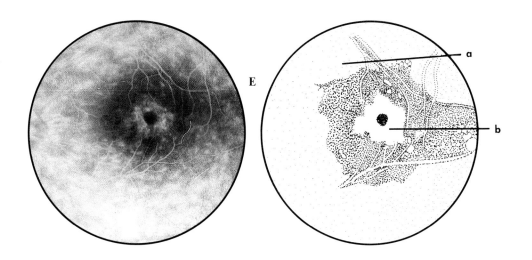

E, Angiogram showing a diffuse hyperfluorescence from the retinal vessels *(a)* and a macular hypofluorescent lesion with a bull's-eye pattern *(b)*. These lesions and cystoidlike macular edema are causes of loss of central vision in patients with RP.

Retinitis Pigmentosa Sine Pigmento FIGURE 32

KEY SYMPTOMS
Nyctalopia
Tunnel vision
Vision reduction (late)

KEY FINDINGS
Early
Fundus normal with greenish-gray reflex
Late
Optic disc pallor; vessel attenuation
Occasionally white spots resulting from hypopigmentation
Fundus changes are mild and develop late after nyctalopia and visual field constriction
NOTE: Early classic retinitis pigmentosa may also show a normal fundus (sine pigmento)

INHERITANCE	ONSET	PROGRESSION	PROGNOSIS
AD, AR	First to second decade	Slow	Poor

LABORATORY STUDIES

Visual Acuity	20/20 to light perception
Refraction	Emmetropia or low myopia
Visual Fields	Constricted
Color Vision	Normal to abnormal
Dark Adaptation	Abnormal rod function
ERG	Abnormal to nonrecordable
EOG	Abnormal
Fluorescein Angiogram	Widespread window defects resulting from RPE atrophy

TREATMENT	PATHOLOGY	SYNONYMS
None	Widespread RPE atrophy with loss of photoreceptors, with microscopic evidence of pigment migration into the retina	None in general use

DIFFERENTIAL DIAGNOSIS
Pigmentary retinopathy (see Table 6, p. 118)
Progressive nyctalopia (see Table 7, p. 120)

REFERENCES
108, 287

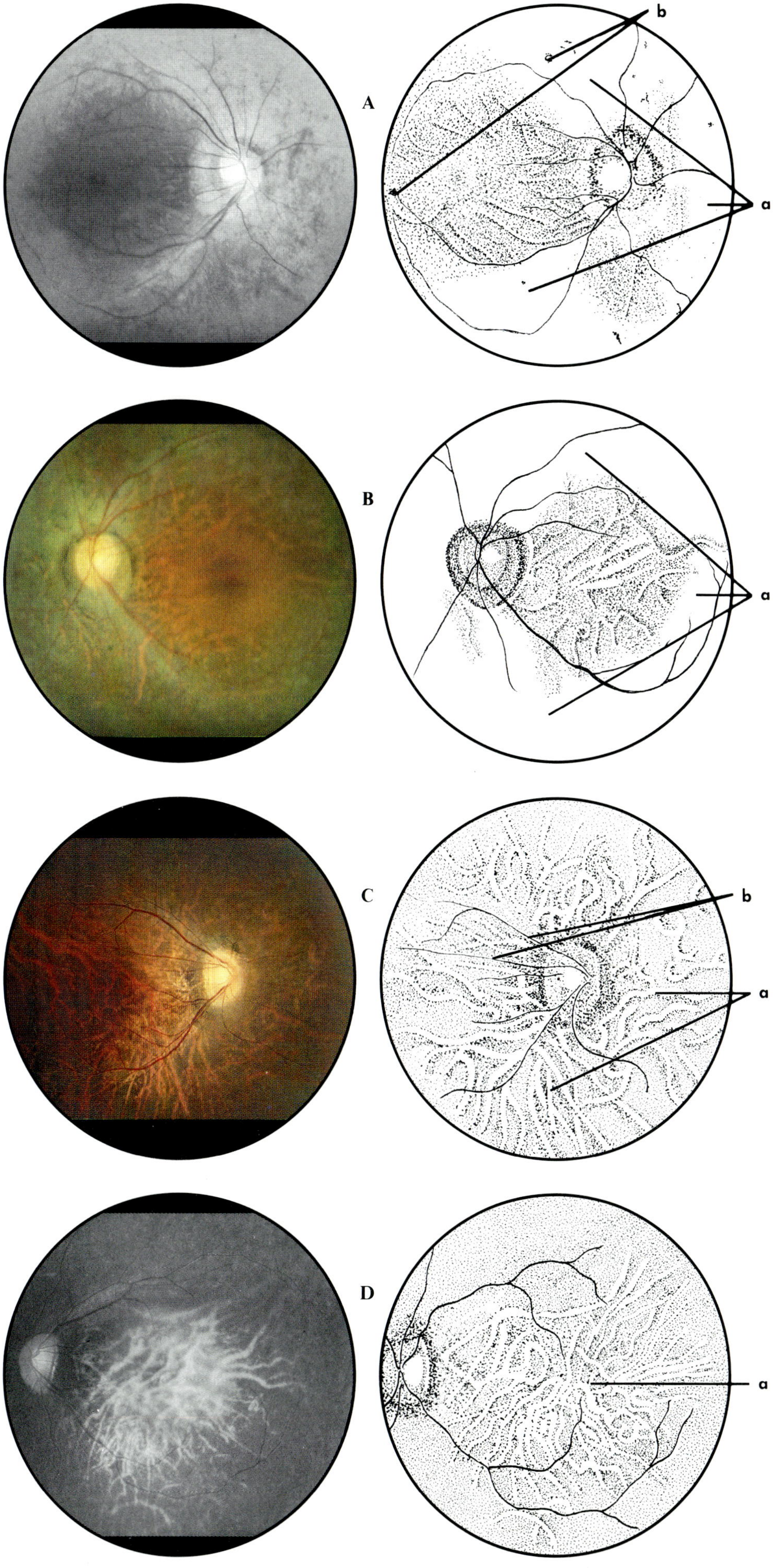

Figure 32
Retinitis Pigmentosa Sine Pigmento

A-B, A 32-year-old female with a history of nyctalopia for 14 years. She has visual field constriction, low myopia, and a nonrecordable ERG. Corrected visual acuity is 20/30 OD and 20/40 OS. No family members are affected. Fundus photographs (OD and OS) show large areas of RPE atrophy (a) sparing only the maculas. After 5 years of follow-up care, minimal pigmentary changes developed (b). The optic disc is pale, and the retinal vessels are narrow.

C-D, A 40-year-old female with progressive nyctalopia over 9 years; visual acuity is 20/30 OD and 20/20 OS. She has visual field constriction, abnormal dark adaptometry (absence of rod function), and a nonrecordable ERG. Fundus photographs show generalized RPE atrophy with visualization of choroidal vessels (a). No pigment clumping, mild pallor of optic discs, and narrow retinal vessels are seen (b). (**C-D,** courtesy of Steven Feldon, M.D.)

Sector Retinitis Pigmentosa FIGURE 33

KEY SYMPTOMS
Usually asymptomatic
Nyctalopia (rare)

KEY FINDINGS
Typical fundus changes, bone-spicule pigmentary retinopathy localized to one retinal sector
In some cases there is evidence of RPE abnormality localized to one retinal sector without pigment clumping
Usually bilateral and symmetric
Inferior nasal quadrants most often involved, producing superotemporal field defects
Vessels in the affected area often attenuated
The unaffected retina is normal in appearance and function
Slowly progressive and stationary forms occur
Usually a few vitreous cells and posterior vitreous detachment

INHERITANCE	ONSET	PROGRESSION	PROGNOSIS
Sporadic AD and AR	Before age 20	None or slow	Good; only 10% with less than 20/40

LABORATORY STUDIES
Visual Acuity	Usually normal
Refraction	Emmetropia or low myopia
Visual Fields	Defects correspond to affected areas
Color Vision	Normal
Dark Adaptation	Abnormal in affected areas for rods
ERG	Abnormal if affected area large
EOG	Probably normal
Fluorescein Angiogram	Affected areas show diffuse mottled hyperfluorescence resulting from RPE defects; choriocapillaris atrophy and attenuated vessels

TREATMENT
None

PATHOLOGY
Typical of retinitis pigmentosa in the affected areas with loss of receptors and RPE atrophy; also, histologic abnormalities in the normal appearing areas

SYNONYMS
Sector pigmentary retinal dystrophy
Sectorial retinitis pigmentosa

DIFFERENTIAL DIAGNOSIS
Focal onset of rod-cone dystrophy (AD) (p. 124)
Inflammatory process
Trauma
Vascular occlusion
Retinal detachment

REFERENCES
44, 130, 214, 244, 305

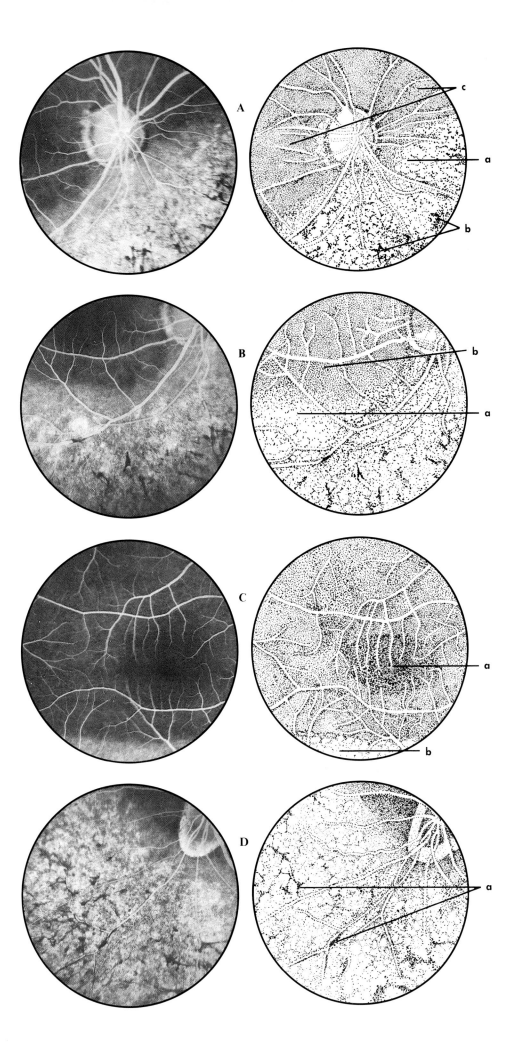

Figure 33
Sector Retinitis Pigmentosa

A 35-year-old asymptomatic male. Visual acuity is 20/20 OU, photopic and scotopic ERGs are reduced 20%, the EOG is normal, and visual fields show superotemporal defects. There is no history of affected family members.

A, Angiogram (OD) showing hyperfluorescence resulting from transmission defects in the inferonasal retina *(a)*; there are some spots of fluorescence blockage by pigment *(b)*. The superonasal and macular areas show normal fluorescence *(c)*.

B, Angiogram (OD) of the inferotemporal retina showing a sharp demarcation between affected *(a)* and nonaffected *(b)* retina.

C, Angiogram (OD) of the macular area showing the normal fluorescence at this level *(a)* and the hyperfluorescence of the inferior involved area *(b)*.

D, Angiogram (OS) of the inferonasal retina showing the symmetric and bilateral involvement. Note the pigment clumping *(a)*.

Unilateral Retinitis Pigmentosa FIGURE 34

KEY SYMPTOMS
Nyctalopia, unilateral
Frequently asymptomatic

KEY FINDINGS
The following criteria are those of François and Verriest for unilateral RP
Funduscopic and functional changes typical of a pigmentary retinopathy only in the affected eye
Absence of symptoms of a tapetoretinal degeneration and a normal ERG in the fellow eye
Sufficient period of observation (5 years) to rule out a delayed onset of pigmentary retinopathy in the unaffected eye
Exclusion of an inflammatory etiology in the affected eye
NOTE: Many authors deny that unilateral rod-cone dystrophy exists

INHERITANCE
Probably AD

ONSET
Third to fourth decade

PROGRESSION
Slow

PROGNOSIS
Less than 20/200 in affected eye

LABORATORY STUDIES
- **Visual Acuity**: 20/20 to hand motions in the affected eye only
- **Refraction**: Low myopia in the affected eye
- **Visual Fields**: Constricted in the affected eye only
- **Color Vision**: Normal to abnormal
- **Dark Adaptation**: Abnormal in the affected eye only
- **ERG**: Severely abnormal, affected eye only
- **EOG**: Severely abnormal, affected eye only
- **Fluorescein Angiogram**: Typical of retinitis pigmentosa, affected eye only; diffuse mottled hyperfluorescence; choriocapillaris atrophy, attenuated vessels

TREATMENT
None

PATHOLOGY
Typical of retinitis pigmentosa with loss of receptors; RPE atrophy and proliferation; vascular changes

SYNONYMS
Uniocular retinitis pigmentosa
Uniocular pigmentary retinopathy

DIFFERENTIAL DIAGNOSIS
Secondary pigmentary retinopathy (e.g., trauma, infection, retinal detachment, vascular occlusion)
AD retinitis pigmentosa with asymmetric onset (p. 124)

REFERENCES
60, 131, 197, 209, 287

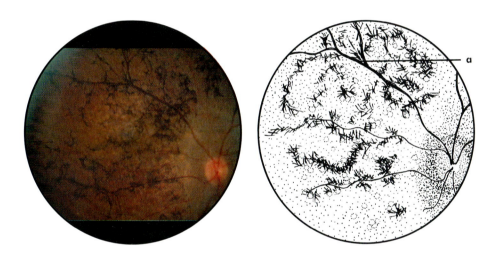

Figure 34
Unilateral Retinitis Pigmentosa

Establishing diagnosis of unilateral RP requires that the patient have all the typical features of RP in one eye only, accompanied by follow-up care lasting for at least 5 years. Fundus photograph (OS) showing the typical bone-spicule pattern of hyperpigmentation along the vessels *(a)* of classic RP, but affecting only OS.

Central Retinitis Pigmentosa (Inverse RP) FIGURE 35

KEY SYMPTOMS
Visual acuity reduction
Nyctalopia
Color vision abnormal

KEY FINDINGS
Macular pigment mottling and clumping with bone spicules, trabeculae, and black dots
Bone spicules are not seen in the fovea
RPE atrophy
Optic disc pallor and vessel attenuation develop later
Peripheral retina is normal early
Most cases called inverse retinitis pigmentosa are probably cone-rod degenerations
NOTE: Many authors deny the existence of central or inverse retinitis pigmentosa

INHERITANCE	ONSET	PROGRESSION	PROGNOSIS
AR	First to second decade	Slow	Poor

LABORATORY STUDIES
Visual Acuity	20/40 to 20/200
Refraction	Low myopia
Visual Fields	Central scotoma
Color Vision	Abnormal
Dark Adaptation	Normal
ERG	Normal or slightly reduced
EOG	Normal
Fluorescein Angiogram	Window defects and blocked fluorescence in the macula, normal periphery

TREATMENT	PATHOLOGY	SYNONYMS
None	Not described	Inverse retinitis pigmentosa

DIFFERENTIAL DIAGNOSIS
Rod-cone dystrophy (p. 124)
Central areolar choroidal dystrophy (p. 34)
Stargardt's disease (p. 92)

REFERENCES
129, 259

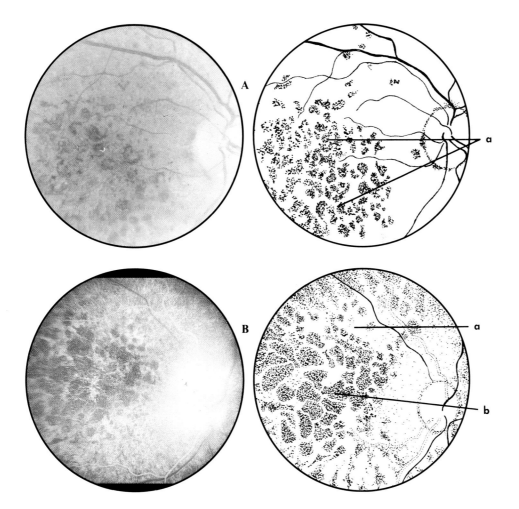

Figure 35

Central Retinitis Pigmentosa (Inverse RP)

A-B, A 34-year-old male with a 3-year history of loss of central vision. There is no family history of affected members. Visual acuity is 20/200 OU, and the ERG shows mild reduction in both photopic and scotopic responses.

A, Fundus photograph shows atypical, round pigment clumping principally affecting the central macula *(a)*. Pigment clumps are barely visible close to the temporal vessels and are absent in the periphery. The optic disc is pale, and the vessels show mild attenuation.

B, Angiogram in the arterial phase shows diffuse hyperfluorescence in the posterior pole resulting from transmission defects *(a)* and hypofluorescent central spots resulting from pigment clumps *(b)*.

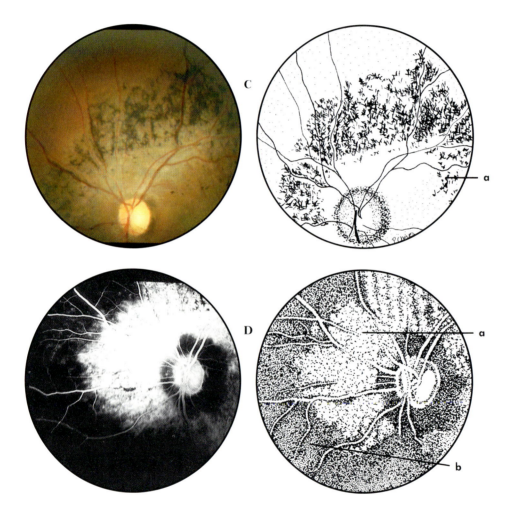

C, Fundus photograph (OS) showing the symmetry of bilateral involvement. In this eye there are some pigment clumps in the macular area *(a)*.

D, Angiogram (OS) showing an area of hyperfluorescence surrounding the optic disc *(a)* and the integrity of the RPE and retinal vessels corresponding to the clinically nonaffected areas *(b)*.

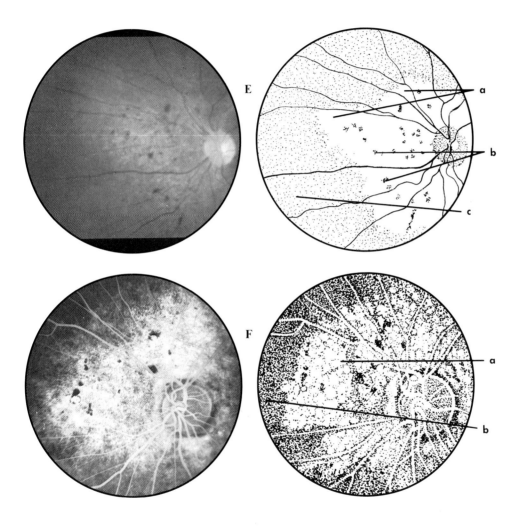

E-F, A 36-year-old female with a visual acuity of 20/30 OD and 20/60 OS and with a borderline normal ERG affecting photopic more than scotopic responses.

E, Fundus photograph (OS) showing the clinical area of RPE disturbance on the nasal side of the disc *(a);* some pigment clumps are present *(b).* The peripheral retina appears normal *(c).*

F, Angiogram showing hyperfluorescence in the area of RPE atrophy *(a)* and normal fluorescence around this lesion *(b).*

Retinitis Pigmentosa with Preserved Para-arteriolar Retinal Pigment Epithelium (PPRPE) FIGURE 37

KEY SYMPTOMS
Nyctalopia
Tunnel vision
Visual acuity reduction

KEY FINDINGS
Pigmentary changes: bone spicules in the midperiphery similar to that in retinitis pigmentosa; pigment clumps spread slowly toward the posterior pole
Preservation of para-arteriolar RPE is seen as a zone of normal retina next to and beneath arterioles
PPRPE is most easily seen in the midperiphery
PPRPE areas become abnormal late in the disease
All PPRPE patients are hyperopic, unlike myopic retinitis pigmentosa patients
Optic disc drusen and pallor are seen early
Vessel attenuation occurs late, unlike that occurring in typical retinitis pigmentosa
This disease is a variant of retinitis pigmentosa

INHERITANCE	ONSET	PROGRESSION	PROGNOSIS
AR	First decade	Rapid	Poor

LABORATORY STUDIES
Visual Acuity	20/20 to light perception
Refraction	Hyperopic
Visual Fields	Constricted with scotomas
Color Vision	Abnormal
Dark Adaptation	Abnormal
ERG	Severely abnormal to nonrecordable
EOG	Abnormal
Fluorescein Angiogram	Diffuse hyperfluorescence resulting from RPE atrophy, sparing the para-arteriolar retina; hypofluorescence resulting from pigment clumping

TREATMENT	PATHOLOGY	SYNONYMS
None	Not described	PPRPE

DIFFERENTIAL DIAGNOSIS
Retinitis pigmentosa (p. 124)
Pigmentary retinopathy (see Table 6, p. 118)
Progressive nyctalopia (see Table 7, p. 120)

REFERENCES
168

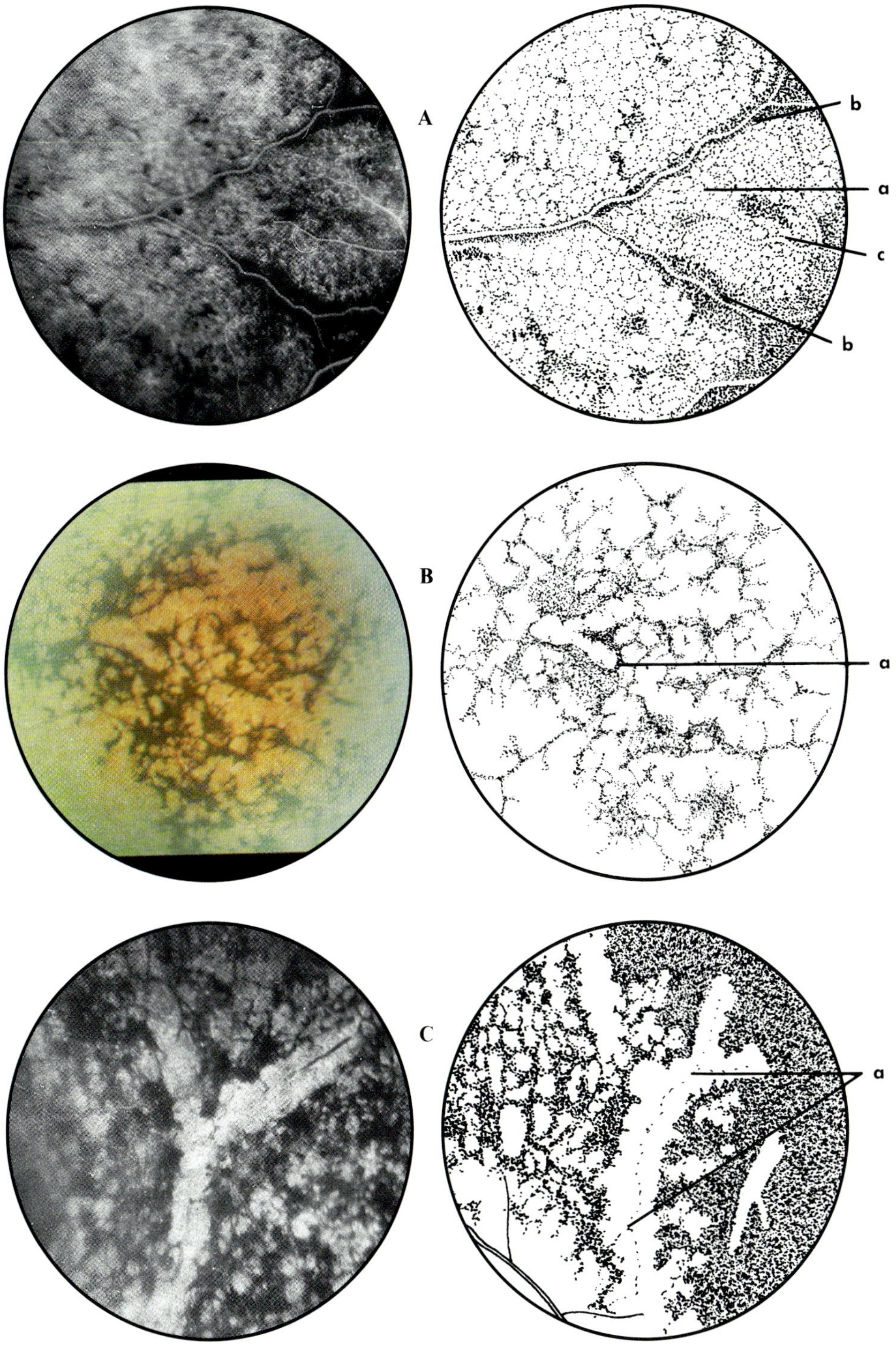

Figure 37
Retinitis Pigmentosa With PPRPE

A-C, Retinitis pigmentosa with PPRPE demonstrates late involvement of the RPE beneath the arterioles and late migration of pigment to the vessels. The RPE is also affected in advanced cases, but pigment clumping around the arterioles does not occur or occurs later in the disease.

A, Angiogram in venous phase showing diffuse hyperfluorescence by multiple transmission defects *(a)*, with hypofluorescence following the arterioles resulting from preservation of the RPE *(b)*. The RPE adjacent to the veins is affected *(c)*.

B, Fundus photograph showing a more advanced case with some pigment migration along the arterioles *(a)* and with involvement of the RPE beneath them.

C, Angiogram of advanced case with hyperfluorescence in the area corresponding to the arterioles showing RPE involvement but with minimal pigment migration.

… ROD-CONE DYSTROPHIES

Retinitis Punctata Albescens FIGURE 38

KEY SYMPTOMS
Nyctalopia
Progressive tunnel vision
Visual acuity reduction

KEY FINDINGS
Numerous small white dots scattered across the retina
Lesions are oval to round, often spare posterior pole
Lesions have a radial orientation in the midperiphery
Associated pigmentary retinopathy with optic disc pallor and vessel attenuation may resemble retinitis pigmentosa
Macular atrophy may develop late
Pigmentary changes less than those of retinitis pigmentosa
Progression, pigmentary changes, disc pallor, vessel narrowing, dark adaptometry, and ERG distinguish this disease from fundus albipunctatus

INHERITANCE	ONSET	PROGRESSION	PROGNOSIS
AR	First decade	Slow	Poor

LABORATORY STUDIES
Visual Acuity	20/20 to light perception
Visual Fields	Constricted and scotomas
Color Vision	Normal to abnormal
Dark Adaptation	Abnormal
ERG	Abnormal to nonrecordable
EOG	Abnormal
Fluorescein Angiogram	Dot lesions may show hyperfluorescence, multiple window defects, and areas of hypofluorescence resulting from RPE and choriocapillaris atrophy

TREATMENT
None

PATHOLOGY
RPE atrophy and pigment deposition; irregular distribution of melanin pigment in the RPE; this disease is probably a variant of retinitis pigmentosa

SYNONYMS
None in general use

DIFFERENTIAL DIAGNOSIS
Retinitis pigmentosa (p. 124)
Fundus albipunctatus (p. 184)
Flecked retina diseases (see Table 5, p. 114)

REFERENCES
95, 219, 220, 338, 364

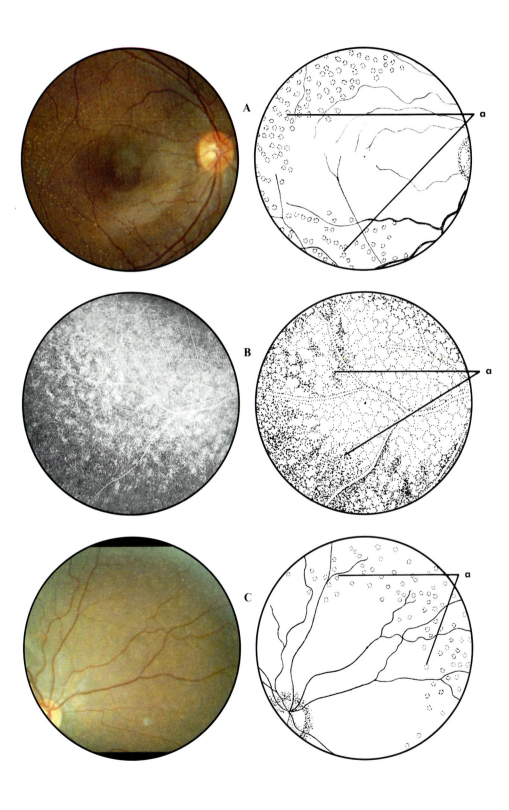

Figure 38
Retinitis Punctata Albescens

A-B, A 20-year-old female with progressive nyctalopia, a visual acuity of 20/20 OU, visual field constriction, ERG markedly abnormal, and dark adaptometry with abnormal rod adaptation and no recovery after 3 hours.

A, Fundus photograph shows multiple small white dots *(a)* surrounding the macular area, mild vessel attenuation, and a normal optic disc.

B, Angiogram in the midperiphery showing widespread transmission defects *(a)*.

C, Fundus photograph (OD) in the superonasal region of a patient with nyctalopia and a severely abnormal ERG. Note the widespread distribution of flecks *(a)* in the midperiphery. The vessels are mildly attenuated.

ROD-CONE DYSTROPHIES

Leber's Congenital Amaurosis FIGURE 39

KEY SYMPTOMS
Very low vision (first year)
Photophobia
Nystagmus

KEY FINDINGS
Searching or pendular nystagmus, strabismus
Enophthalmos
Oculodigital sign of Franceschetti (fists constantly pushed into the eyes)
Poorly reactive pupils
Fundus normal or abnormal: salt-and-pepper stippling of the retina; optic disc pallor with vessel attenuation; pigmentary retinopathy (second decade); macular colobomas with pigmented edges
Lens opacities (50% of patients), glaucoma, keratoconus
Neurologic disorders and mental retardation

INHERITANCE	ONSET	PROGRESSION	PROGNOSIS
AR (common)	AR—first year	Slow	Poor
AD (rare)	AD—first decade		

LABORATORY STUDIES

Visual Acuity	20/200 to light perception
Refraction	Usually hyperopia
Visual Fields	Difficult to test
Color Vision	Difficult to test
Dark Adaptation	Difficult to test
ERG	Severely abnormal to nonrecordable
EOG	Difficult to evaluate
Fluorescein Angiogram	Difficult to obtain because of nystagmus; photophobia and low vision

TREATMENT
None

PATHOLOGY
Loss of the outer segments of photoreceptors; retinal ganglion cell degeneration; optic atrophy; RPE usually normal

SYNONYMS
Amaurosis congenita
Heredoretinopathia congenitalis
Dysgenesis neuroepithelialis retinae
Hereditary retinal aplasia

DIFFERENTIAL DIAGNOSIS
Early retinitis pigmentosa (p. 124)
Cortical blindness
Optic atrophy

REFERENCES
124, 126, 181, 237, 254, 261, 292, 375

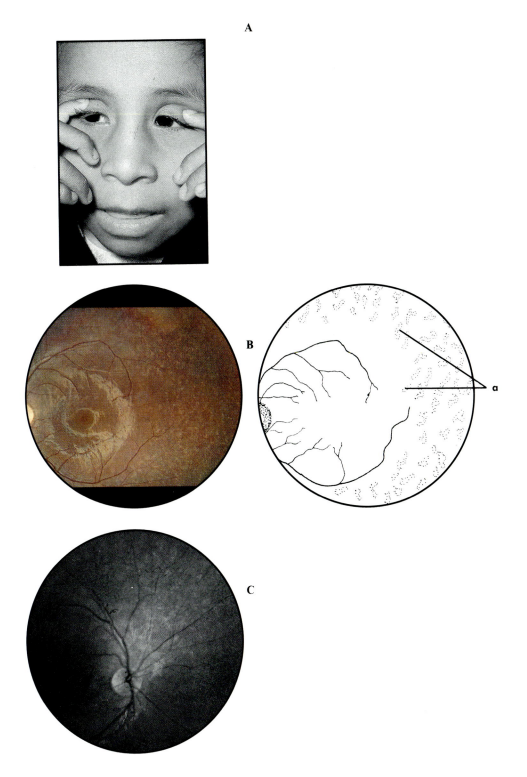

Figure 39

Leber's Congenital Amaurosis

A-C, A 10-year-old female with very low vision from birth, nystagmus, photophobia, and a family history of consanguinity (parents are first cousins). Three brothers are affected with the same condition. Visual acuity is light perception only, and the ERG is nonrecordable.

A, Note discrete enophthalmos and the oculodigital sign of Franceschetti.

B, Fundus photograph (OS) showing abnormal color, multiple RPE defects, salt-and-pepper appearance *(a),* and narrow vessels.

C, Fundus photograph (OD) of the superonasal region showing widespread pigmentary defects, narrow vessels, and a normal optic disc.

Pigmented Paravenous Chorioretinal Atrophy FIGURE 40

KEY SYMPTOMS
Usually asymptomatic
Visual acuity loss (rare)
Nyctalopia (rare)

KEY FINDINGS
This condition is bilateral and usually symmetric
Bone spicule pigmentation along one or more large veins
Pigmentation begins 1- to 7-disc diameters from the nerve head
A zone of RPE abnormality always extends beyond the area of pigmentation
Peripapillary atrophy seen in 75% of patients
Attenuated vessels seen in 50% of patients
Optic atrophy seen in 50% of patients
Associated strabismus is occasionally seen
Macular involvement is uncommon
Usually stationary, but progressive forms have been reported
This pattern of pigmentation has been observed after measles

INHERITANCE	ONSET	PROGRESSION	PROGNOSIS
Simplex, common; AD or X-L, rare	Probably congenital	Very slow or stationary	Good

LABORATORY STUDIES
Visual Acuity	20/20 to 20/40; worse if macula involved
Refraction	Emmetropia or hyperopia
Visual Fields	Scotomas radiate out from the blind spot
Color Vision	Normal
Dark Adaptation	Usually normal
ERG	Normal to subnormal
EOG	Normal to subnormal
Fluorescein Angiogram	Diffuse hyperfluorescence (window defects) in areas of RPE atrophy; veins normal; larger choroidal vessels seen; choriocapillaris atrophy

TREATMENT	PATHOLOGY	SYNONYMS
None	Not described	Pigmented paravenous retinochoroidal atrophy Paravenous degeneration Retinochoroiditis radiata

DIFFERENTIAL DIAGNOSIS
Wagner's vitreoretinal dystrophy (p. 214)
Retinitis pigmentosa (p. 124)
Pigmentary retinopathy (see Table 6, p. 118)
Progressive nyctalopia (see Table 7, p. 120)

REFERENCES
65, 127, 169, 179, 252, 264, 285

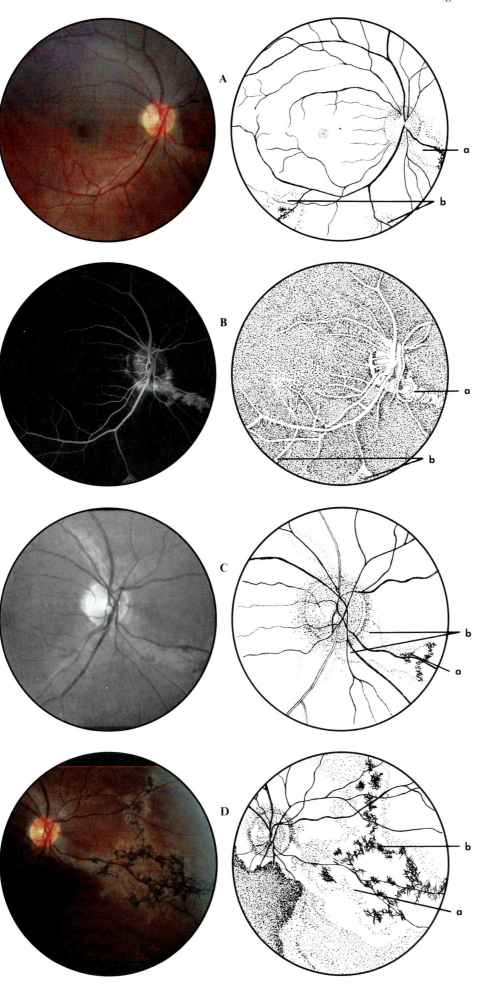

Figure 40

Pigmented Paravenous Chorioretinal Atrophy

A 23-year-old female with a visual acuity of 20/20 OU and unilateral paravenous chorioretinal atrophy. The ERG and EOG are normal.

A-B, Fundus photograph and fluorescein angiogram showing three areas of RPE disturbance, one surrounding the inferonasal vein *(a)* and two more along branches of the inferotemporal vein *(b)*. The angiogram shows these areas to be hyperfluorescent because of RPE atrophy *(a* and *b)*.

C, Magnified view of the nasal retina near the optic disc showing pigment clumping surrounding the inferonasal vein *(a)* and atrophic RPE extending to the optic disc *(b)*.

D, Inferonasal vein surrounded by paravenous chorioretinal atrophy *(a)* and pigment clumping *(b)*.

ROD-CONE DYSTROPHIES (RP-ASSOCIATED SYNDROMES)	Usher's syndrome Bardet-Biedl syndrome Kearns-Sayre syndrome Myotonic dystrophy of Steinert Refsum's disease Bassen-Kornzweig syndrome Olivopontocerebellar retinal degeneration

Several systemic diseases have been described with an associated retinal degeneration similar to that in retinitis pigmentosa. The more common are described here (see also Table 6, Pigmentary Retinopathy).

Congenital deafness, pigmentary retinopathy, and nyctalopia with a severely abnormal ERG constitute *Usher's syndrome*. There are several diseases with retinal degeneration and deafness (see Table 8). Usher's syndrome is relatively common.

Obesity, polydactyly, hypogenitalism, pigmentary retinopathy with an early macular lesion, nyctalopia, and sometimes nystagmus characterize *Bardet-Biedl syndrome,* a relatively common autosomal-recessive syndrome. When spastic paraplegia is also present, the syndrome is called Laurence-Moon syndrome.

Progressive external ophthalmoplegia, heart-block, and retinal degeneration are the common findings of *Kearns-Sayre syndrome*.

Myotonia, muscle weakness, hypogenitalism, progressive ophthalmoplegia, lens abnormalities, and retinal degeneration with macular reticular dystrophy suggest *myotonic dystrophy of Steinert*.

An atypical pigmentary retinopathy associated with multiple neurologic abnormalities, of which a neuropathy is most striking, suggests *Refsum's disease*.

The principal findings in *Bassen-Kornzweig syndrome* are neuromuscular and gastrointestinal abnormalities, vitamin A deficiency, pigmentary degeneration, and acanthocytosis.

Progressive cerebellar ataxia, pigmentary retinal degeneration, and an atrophic macular lesion are the principal findings in *olivopontocerebellar retinal degeneration*.

Table 8 RETINAL DEGENERATION AND DEAFNESS

Usher's syndrome is the name given to the association of retinitis pigmentosa and partial or complete congenital deafness. The disease is the result of the action of an autosomal-recessive pleiotropic gene. In addition to this specific association, there are a group of disorders with pigmentary retinopathy and deafness.

NAME	INHERITANCE	PRINCIPAL FINDINGS
Alport's syndrome	AD	Nephropathy, deafness, myopia, congenital cataract, aspherophakia, fundus changes, occasionally retinal detachment
Alström syndrome	AR	Pigmentary retinopathy, nystagmus, deafness, obesity, diabetes mellitus, nephropathy, acanthosis nigricans
Cockayne's syndrome	AR	Pigmentary retinopathy, optic atrophy, deafness, progeria, dwarfism, mental retardation
Dysplasia spondyloepiphysiana congenita	AD	Congenital high myopia associated with retinal degeneration and retinal detachment, dwarfism, mild deafness, cleft palate, cataract, congenital glaucoma
Flynn-Aird syndrome	AD	Pigmentary retinopathy, cataract, myopia, deafness, ataxia, peripheral neuritis, dementia, epilepsy, skin atrophy, baldness, dental caries, cystic bone changes
Friedreich's ataxia	AR	Retinal degeneration, optic atrophy, nystagmus, deafness, spinocerebellar dystrophy, dysarthria
Hallgren's syndrome	AR	(See Usher's syndrome, Merin classification, Type III, below)
Hurler syndrome (MPS-I)	AR	Early corneal clouding, gargoyle facies, deafness, mental retardation, dwarfism, skeletal abnormalities, hepatosplenomegaly, subnormal ERG, optic atrophy
Marshall's syndrome	AD (?)	Myopia, cataract, saddle nose, sensorineural hearing loss
Osteopetrosis (Albers-Schönberg disease)	AR	Defective resorption of immature bone, macrocephaly, progressive deafness, hepatosplenomegaly, anemia, retinal degeneration with abnormal ERG
Refsum's disease (heredopathia atactica polyneuritiformis)	AR	Pigmentary retinopathy, chronic polyneuritis, cerebellar signs, electrocardiographic changes, ichthyosis, accumulation of phytanic acid
Usher's syndrome (Merin classification)	AR	
Type I		Pigmentary retinopathy, congenital total deafness, no vestibular function
Type II		Pigmentary retinopathy, partial deafness, normal vestibular function
Type III (Hallgren's syndrome)		Pigmentary retinopathy, congenital deafness, vestibulo-cerebellar ataxia, psychoses
Type IV		Pigmentary retinopathy, congenital total deafness, mental retardation
Waardenburg syndrome	AD	Deafness, hypertelorism, blepharophimosis, heterochromia iridis, hyperplasia of eyebrows medially, white forelock, broad nasal root

Modified from Heckenlively JR: Retinitis pigmentosa, Philadelphia, 1988, J.B. Lippincott Co.

Usher's Syndrome FIGURE 41

KEY SYMPTOMS
Nyctalopia
Congenital deafness
Visual acuity reduction

KEY FINDINGS
Progressive pigmentary retinopathy similar to RP
Pale optic disc
Attenuation of retinal vessels
Posterior subcapsular cataract is common
Total or partial congenital deafness
Associated vestibular dysfunction occasionally seen
NOTE: See Table 8, p. 150, Retinal Degeneration and Deafness; some patients have mental deficiency and/or psychosis

INHERITANCE	ONSET	PROGRESSION	PROGNOSIS
AR	Congenital, with deafness	Slow	Poor

LABORATORY STUDIES
Visual Acuity	20/20 to light perception
Refraction	Low myopia
Visual Fields	Constricted with scotomas
Color Vision	Normal to abnormal
Dark Adaptation	Severely depressed rod function
ERG	Abnormal to nonrecordable
EOG	Severely abnormal
Fluorescein Angiogram	Diffuse mottled hyperfluorescence resulting from RPE atrophy; hypofluorescent areas; occasional areas of exposed choroidal vessels

TREATMENT	PATHOLOGY	SYNONYMS
None	Not reported	Pigmentary retinopathy with labyrinthine deafness

DIFFERENTIAL DIAGNOSIS	REFERENCES
Congenital deafness and pigmentary retinopathy of viral or other origin (see Table 8, p. 150)	16, 63, 248, 291

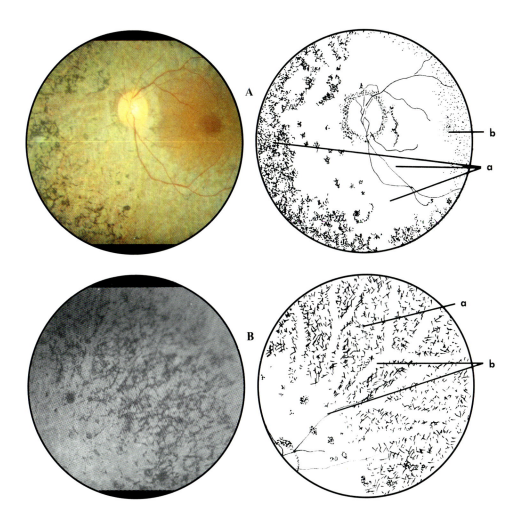

Figure 41
Usher's Syndrome

A 36-year-old female with congenital deafness and progressive nyctalopia, a visual acuity of 20/60 OU, visual field constriction, and a nonrecordable ERG.

A, Fundus photograph (OS) shows pigmentary retinal degeneration, a large area of RPE disturbance *(a)* sparing only the macular area, and atrophic pigmentary changes around the fovea *(b),* with optic disc pallor and vessel attenuation.

B, Fundus photograph (OD) of superonasal retina showing the bone-spicule pattern of pigmentary retinopathy *(a),* with severe attenuation of vessels *(b).*

Bardet-Biedl Syndrome FIGURE 42

KEY SYMPTOMS
Nyctalopia
Visual acuity reduction

KEY FINDINGS
Ocular Findings
Pigmentary retinopathy similar to RP
Some patients have marked symptoms with little or no pigmentary change evident in the fundus
Macular involvement is common early
Systemic Findings
Obesity of central type
Mental retardation
Polydactyly or syndactyly
Hypogenitalism
Less common findings are brachicephaly, short stature
Bardet-Biedl syndrome with spastic paraplegia and mental retardation is called Laurence-Moon syndrome

INHERITANCE	ONSET	PROGRESSION	PROGNOSIS
AR	First decade	Slow	Poor

LABORATORY STUDIES

Visual Acuity	Decreased
Refraction	Low myopia
Visual Fields	Constricted; central scotoma common
Color Vision	Normal early, then abnormal
Dark Adaptation	Abnormal rod function
ERG	Abnormal to nonrecordable
EOG	Abnormal
Fluorescein Angiogram	Typical of RP; diffuse hyperfluorescence resulting from multiple window defects

TREATMENT
None

PATHOLOGY
Diffuse retinal degeneration involving both rods and cones; RPE atrophy; pigment migration

SYNONYMS
Biedl-Bardet syndrome
Laurence-Moon-Bardet-Biedl syndrome

DIFFERENTIAL DIAGNOSIS
Retinitis pigmentosa (p. 124)
Laurence-Moon syndrome (p. 154)
Pigmentary retinopathy (see Table 6, p. 118)
Progressive nyctalopia (see Table 7, p. 120)

REFERENCES
1, 4, 33, 43, 49, 234

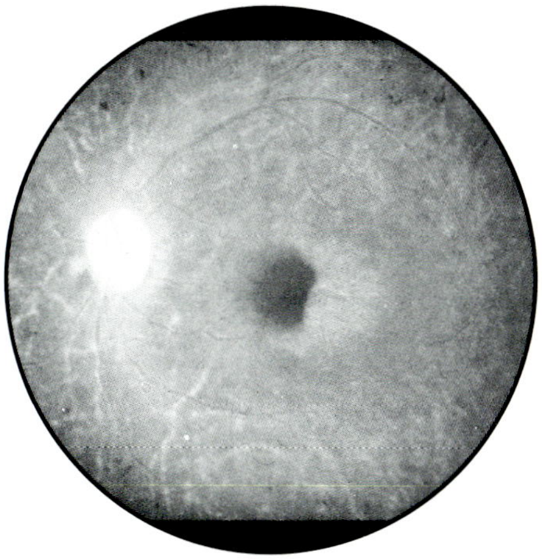

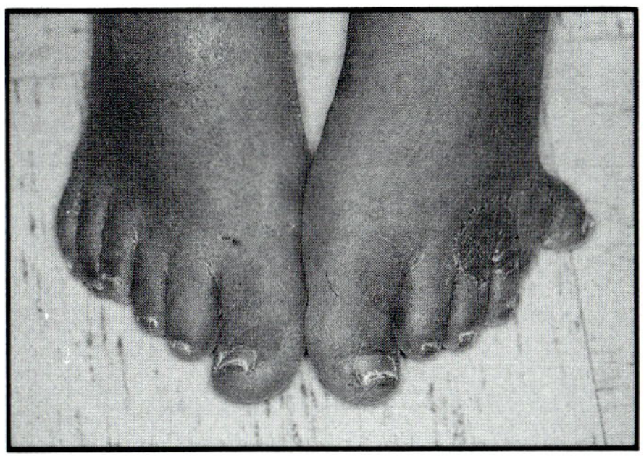

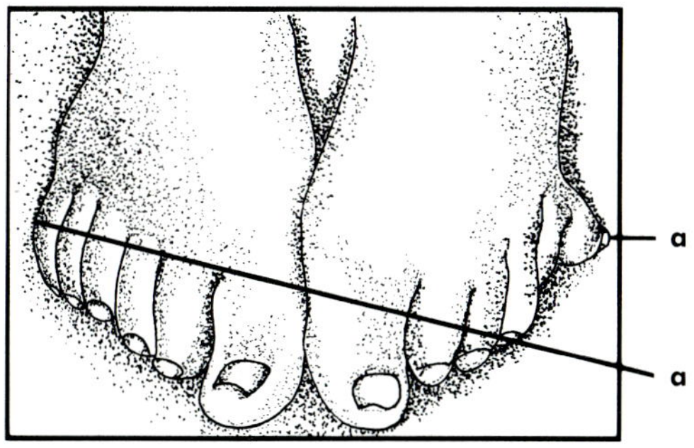

Figure 42
Bardet-Biedl Syndrome

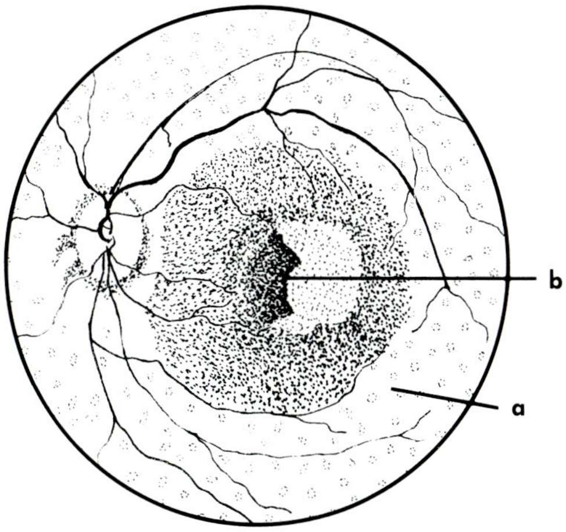

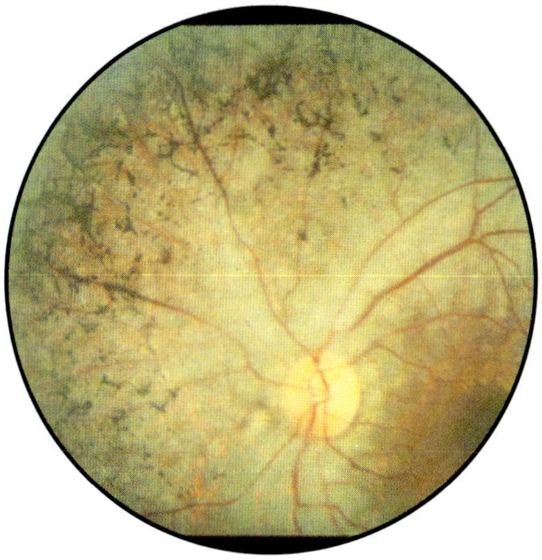

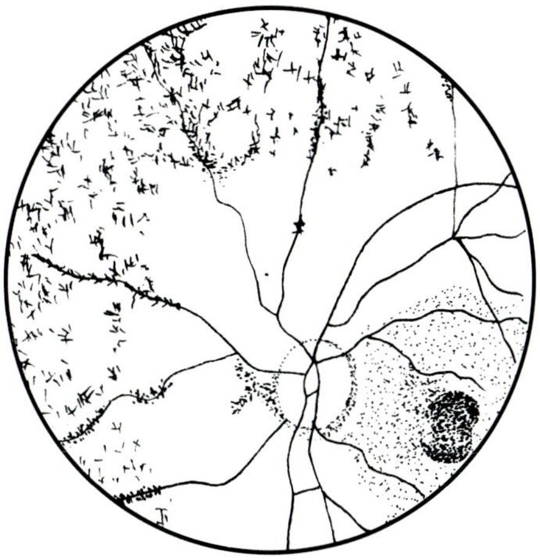

An 11-year-old male with nyctalopia, a corrected visual acuity of 20/100 OD to 20/200 OS, mild nystagmus, obesity, polydactyly, subnormal intelligence, and hypogenitalism. There is a family history of consanguinity (parents are first cousins), and one brother is affected with the same condition.

A, Fundus photograph (OS) showing an RPE abnormality *(a)* sparing only the macular area. A pigmented macular lesion is evident *(b)*, the optic disc is pale, and the retinal vessels are attenuated.

B, Fundus photograph (OS) of the superonasal retina showing pigmentary retinopathy similar to that in retinitis pigmentosa.

C, Photograph of the feet showing an extra toe *(a)* on both feet. Occasionally the polydactyly is not present in the hands, and examination of the toes can give the key for the diagnosis.

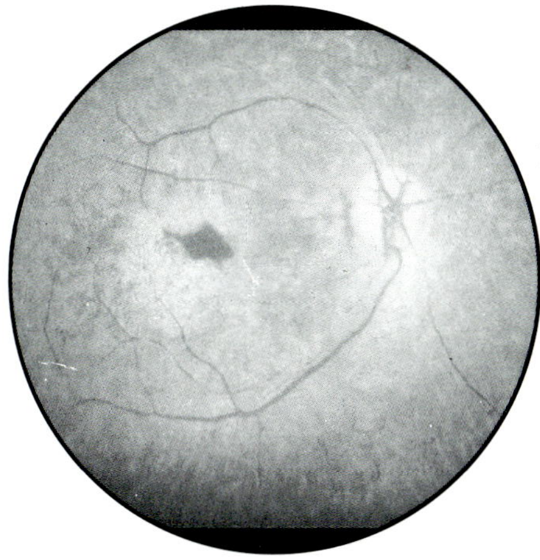

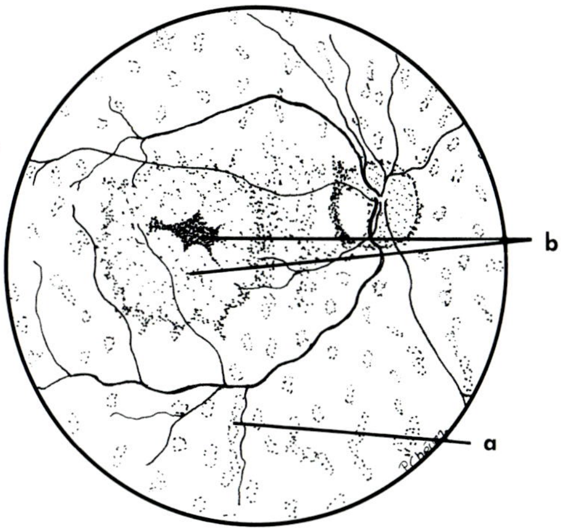

D, Fundus photograph (OD) of a 26-year-old male with Bardet-Biedl syndrome and a visual acuity of 20/400. The fundus shows multiple RPE defects *(a)* and a bull's-eye macular lesion. The retinal vessels are narrowed, and the optic disc is pale. The ERG was nonrecordable.

Kearns-Sayre Syndrome FIGURE 43

KEY SYMPTOMS
Nyctalopia (50% of patients)
Ptosis
Decrease in vision (late)

KEY FINDINGS
Myopathic external ophthalmoplegia with onset of ptosis in early childhood; pupils spared by ophthalmoplegia
Atypical retinal pigmentary degeneration (salt-and-pepper)
Cardiac conduction defect (heart-block)
Associated Manifestations
Corneal opacity, strabismus, deafness and vestibular dysfunction, elevated cerebrospinal fluid protein, widespread muscular dystrophy, short stature, hypogonadism, subnormal intelligence, cerebellar and corticospinal dysfunction, abnormal EEG, endocrine dysfunction, and nephropathy

INHERITANCE	ONSET	PROGRESSION	PROGNOSIS
None	First decade	Slow	Poor
AD (unusual)			

LABORATORY STUDIES
Visual Acuity	Mild reduction
Visual Fields	Constricted
Color Vision	Normal or abnormal
Dark Adaptation	Normal or abnormal
ERG	Subnormal to extinguished
EOG	Normal to subnormal
Fluorescein Angiogram	Mottled hyperfluorescence resulting from RPE defects with areas of hypofluorescence in the posterior pole

TREATMENT
None for muscular weakness; strabismus surgery and cardiac pacemaker for symptoms

PATHOLOGY
Mild loss of photoreceptors and RPE cells in the macular area; posterior pole more affected than periphery

SYNONYMS
Progressive external ophthalmoplegia with pigmentary retinopathy

DIFFERENTIAL DIAGNOSIS
Refsum's disease (p. 160)
Myasthenia gravis
Pigmentary retinopathy (see Table 6, p. 118)
Progressive nyctalopia (see Table 7, p. 120)
Bassen-Kornzweig syndrome (p. 162)

REFERENCES
13, 199, 200, 229

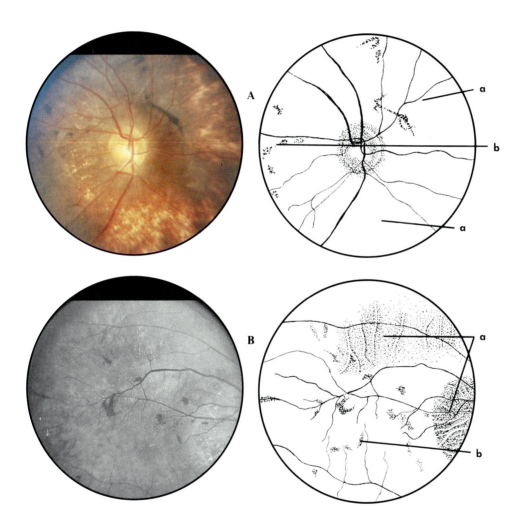

Figure 43

Kearns-Sayre Syndrome

A 30-year-old male with mental retardation, hearing deficit, chronic external ophthalmoplegia, and cardiac-block requiring a pacemaker. Visual acuity is 20/300 OD and 20/200 OS, and the ERG is nonrecordable. Muscle biopsy showed ragged red fibers.

A, Fundus photograph (OD) showing irregular areas of chorioretinal atrophy *(a)* surrounding a mildly pale optic disc, retinal vessel attenuation, and atypical pigmentary retinopathy *(b)*.

B, Macular region of the same eye showing a widespread RPE abnormality with some areas of chorioretinal atrophy and visualization of large choroidal vessels *(a)*. An atypical pigmentary retinopathy is present *(b)*. (Photographs **A-B,** courtesy of John Lean, M.D.)

Myotonic Dystrophy of Steinert FIGURE 44

KEY SYMPTOMS
Weakness and myotonia
Mildly decreased vision
Nyctalopia

KEY FINDINGS
Ocular
Ptosis and progressive ophthalmoplegia
Cataract with iridescent particles in lens cortex and posterior subcapsular cataract
Stellate pattern dystrophy of the fovea
Peripheral pigmentary retinopathy
Optic disc and vessels normal
Ocular hypotension (7mm Hg to 12mm Hg)
Neuromuscular
Myotonia, distal muscle weakness
Handshake is weak, and patient has difficulty opening his or her grip after shaking hands
Other Abnormalities
Frontal baldness, bradycardia, and heart-block
Testicular or ovarian atrophy and endocrinopathy

INHERITANCE	ONSET	PROGRESSION	PROGNOSIS
AD	Second to fourth decade	Very slow	Good (visual)

LABORATORY STUDIES
Visual Acuity	20/20 to 20/60
Visual Fields	Normal
Color Vision	Normal
Dark Adaptation	Normal to abnormal
ERG	Normal to abnormal
EOG	Usually normal
Fluorescein Angiogram	Hypofluorescence of central pigmented areas with hyperfluorescence of intervening areas of macula

TREATMENT	PATHOLOGY	SYNONYMS
None for visual symptoms except cataract extraction	RPE atrophy and pigment migration; photoreceptor degeneration in the midperiphery	Steinert's disease Myotonia dystrophica Myotonia atrophica

DIFFERENTIAL DIAGNOSIS	REFERENCES
Macular pattern RPE dystrophies (see Table 3, p. 13) Pigmentary retinopathy (see Table 6, p. 118)	28, 47, 64, 148, 236, 249

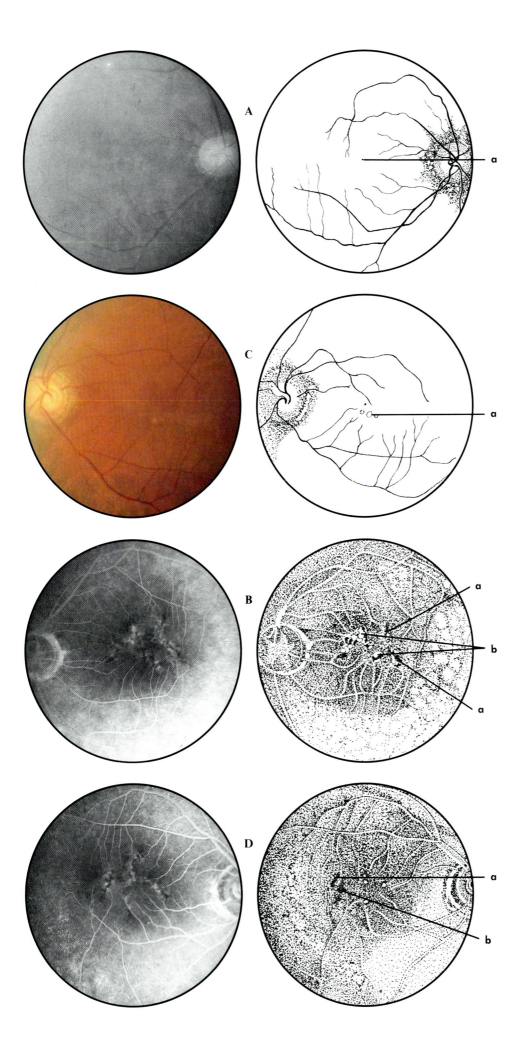

Figure 44
Myotonic Dystrophy of Steinert

A 30-year-old female with myotonic dystrophy with ptosis, mild lens opacities, and a stellate-pattern dystrophy of the fovea. Her visual acuity is 20/40 OU.

A and C, Fundus photographs (OD and OS) show minimal macular changes (a).

B and D, Fluorescein angiogram shows a patterned-type RPE dystrophy, with hypofluorescent crossing lines (a) surrounded by hyperfluorescence (b).

Refsum's Disease FIGURE 45

KEY SYMPTOMS
Nyctalopia
Distal sensory loss and weakness
Anosmia and deafness

KEY FINDINGS
Ocular
Atypical pigmentary retinopathy with optic disc pallor, vessel attenuation, and retinal mottling in a salt-and-pepper pattern and peripapillary sclerosis
Cases of a sine pigmento retinal dystrophy have been observed
Miosis and decreased pupillary reflexes
Acute open-angle glaucoma
Irregular thickening of Bowman's membrane; fibrovascular pannus
Posterior cortical and subcapsular cataract
Optic nerve atrophy (late)
Neurologic
Peripheral neuropathy, cerebellar ataxia progressing to quadriplegia, high cerebrospinal fluid protein concentrations without pleocytosis
Other
Dry scaly skin, psychosis, skeletal abnormalities, cardiomyopathy with abnormal EKG, ichthyosis

INHERITANCE	ONSET	PROGRESSION	PROGNOSIS
AR	First to fourth decade	Slow	Poor if no treatment

LABORATORY STUDIES
Visual Acuity	20/20 to 20/200 or less
Visual Fields	Constricted
Color Vision	Normal
Dark Adaptation	Abnormal rod function
ERG	Abnormal to nonrecordable
EOG	Abnormal
Fluorescein Angiogram	Diffuse mottled hyperfluorescence resulting from window defects and areas of blocked transmission

TREATMENT	PATHOLOGY	SYNONYMS
Strict elimination of phytol from diet (primarily leafy vegetables, butter, and animal fat)	Lipid deposits in RPE, iris, and trabecular meshwork; photoreceptor degeneration; defect in phytanic acid oxidase, which is needed to esterify vitamin A	Heredopathia atactica polyneuritiformis
Phytanic acid oxidase deficiency

DIFFERENTIAL DIAGNOSIS
Bassen-Kornzweig syndrome (p. 162)
Kearns-Sayre syndrome (p. 156)
Cockayne's syndrome
Chronic progressive external ophthalmoplegia
Pigmentary retinopathy (see Table 6, p. 118)

REFERENCES
17, 161, 306, 357, 376

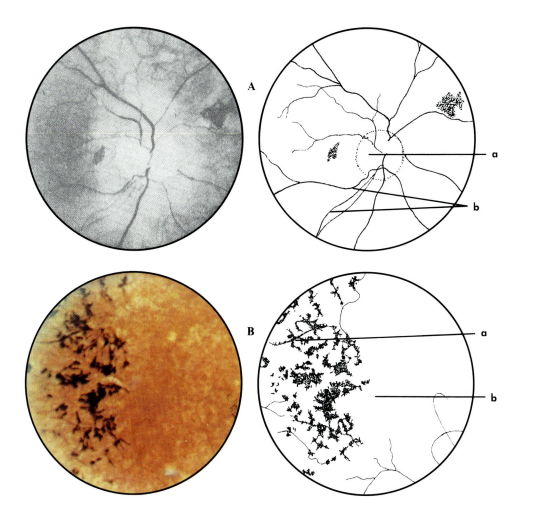

Figure 45
Refsum's Disease

A, Fundus photograph showing secondary optic atrophy *(a)* with a yellowish, pale disc and narrow vessels *(b)*.

B, Bone spicule retinal pigmentation at the equator *(a),* with mottled, atrophic RPE *(b)*. (**A-B,** reproduced and redrawn from Epstein RL: Inborn metabolic disorders and the eye. In Peyman GA, Sanders D, and Goldberg MI, editors: Principles and practice of ophthalmology, Philadelphia, 1980, WB Saunders Co.)

Bassen-Kornzweig Syndrome FIGURE 46

KEY SYMPTOMS
Nyctalopia
Neuromuscular disability
Dietary fat intolerance

KEY FINDINGS
Ocular
Ptosis, strabismus (exotropia), nystagmus
Pigmentary retinopathy similar to RP
Optic disc pallor; vessel attenuation
Peripapillary atrophy
Macular degeneration and fine granular pigmentation
Fundus may resemble that seen in fundus albipunctatus
Neurologic
Sensory neuropathy, posterior column signs
Cerebellar ataxia
Gastrointestinal
Dietary fat intolerance; vitamin A deficiency (secondary)
Laboratory Findings
Anemia, acanthocytosis, hypoproteinemia; absence of β-lipoproteins, α_2-lipoproteins, and chylomicrons; cholesterol lower than 100mg/100cc

INHERITANCE	ONSET	PROGRESSION	PROGNOSIS
AR	First decade	Slow	Poor

LABORATORY STUDIES
Visual Acuity	Normal to reduced
Refraction	Myopia (axial and lenticular)
Visual Fields	Constricted
Color Vision	Normal
Dark Adaptation	Abnormal rod function
ERG	Abnormal scotopic
EOG	Abnormal
Fluorescein Angiogram	Hyperfluorescence resulting from window defects from RPE atrophy, and hypofluorescence resulting from pigment clumps similar to those seen in RP

TREATMENT	PATHOLOGY	SYNONYMS
Massive doses of vitamin A will improve retinal function	Peripheral RPE atrophy; receptor degeneration; pigmentary retinopathy; sclerotic retinal vessels	Abetalipoproteinemia

DIFFERENTIAL DIAGNOSIS
Pigmentary retinopathy (see Table 6, p. 118)
Progressive nyctalopia (see Table 7, p. 120)

REFERENCES
15, 52, 141, 150, 210, 348, 363

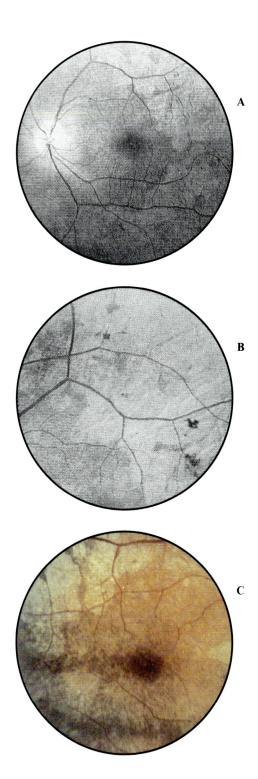

Figure 46
Bassen-Kornzweig Syndrome

A, Fundus photograph (OS) of a 35-year-old female complaining of decreased vision. The entire fundus is diffusely mottled. Note the extensive depigmentation surrounding the central area. This area has a white appearance with a sharply demarcated, serrated posterior border. There is mild arteriolar narrowing.

B, Fundus photograph (OS) of same patient taken 5 years later. The area of depigmentation has advanced centrally, and some of the formerly uninvolved areas have become depigmented. The choroidal vessels in the involved area look opaque.

C, Fundus photograph (OD) of the central area showing similar involvement. (**A-C,** reproduced and redrawn from Cogan DG, Rodrigues M, Chu FC, and Schaefer EJ: Ocular abnormalities in abetalipoproteinemia: a clinicopathologic correlation. Published courtesy of *Ophthalmology* 1984; 91:991-998.)

Olivopontocerebellar Retinal Degeneration FIGURE 47

KEY SYMPTOMS
Visual acuity reduction
Muscle spasticity and uncoordination

KEY FINDINGS
Ocular
Macular degeneration spreading to periphery
Areolar macular RPE atrophy with sharp border
Pigmentary changes, mottling, and granularity start in macula but progress to periphery
Pigment clumps in the posterior pole (late)
Progressive ophthalmoplegia, nystagmus, optic atrophy, and blindness
Neurologic
Progressive cerebellar ataxia with asynergia, dysmetria, and hyperreflexia
Progression to quadriplegia and mental deficiency

INHERITANCE	ONSET	PROGRESSION	PROGNOSIS
AD	First to third decade	Slow	Poor

LABORATORY STUDIES
Visual Acuity	20/80 to light perception
Visual Fields	Central scotoma early
Color Vision	Abnormal
Dark Adaptation	Normal to abnormal
ERG	Normal to abnormal
EOG	Normal to abnormal
Fluorescein Angiogram	Macular window defects early; central hypofluorescence late resulting from RPE and choriocapillary atrophy

TREATMENT
None

PATHOLOGY
RPE and photoreceptor atrophy; atrophy of pons and cerebellum
NOTE: Benign concentric annular macular dystrophy (Deutman) is probably the ocular expression of olivopontocerebellar atrophy

SYNONYMS
Olivopontocerebellar atrophy type III

DIFFERENTIAL DIAGNOSIS
Spinocerebellar degenerations
Choroidal atrophy (see Table 2, p. 19)

REFERENCES
82, 93, 163, 313, 314, 367

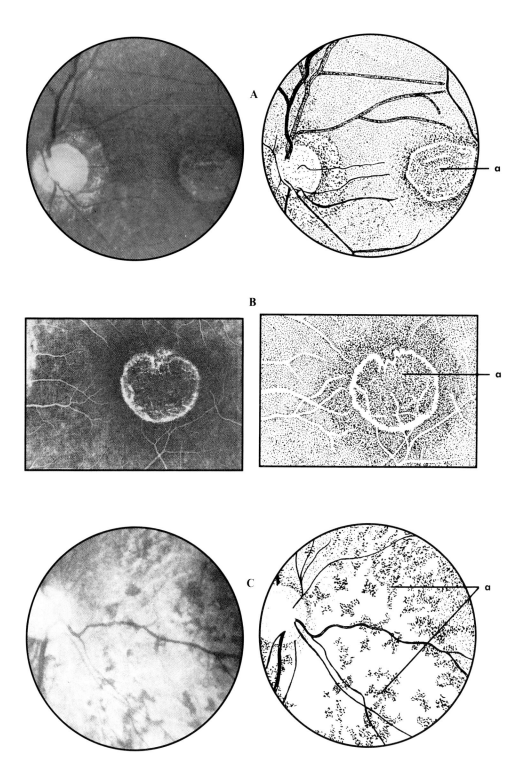

Figure 47
Olivopontocerebellar Retinal Degeneration

A 47-year-old male with ataxia for 10 years and decrease in vision for 1 year; a sister and a niece are also affected. His visual acuity is 20/200 OU, and the ERG and EOG are subnormal.

A, Fundus photograph shows a well-demarcated atrophic macular lesion *(a)* and a peripapillary chorioretinal degeneration.

B, Angiogram shows a well-demarcated lesion with loss of choriocapillaris *(a)* in the affected area.

C, Sister of the previous patient, with a visual acuity of 20/200. Fundus photograph demonstrates marked pigmentary degeneration *(a)* of the advanced stage. (**A-C,** reproduced and redrawn from Ryan SJ, and Smith RE: Retinopathy associated with hereditary olivopontocerebellar degeneration, Am J Ophthalmol 71:838, 1971. Published with permission from The American Journal of Ophthalmology. Copyright by the Ophthalmic Publishing Company.)

CONE AND CONE-ROD DEGENERATIONS

Cone dystrophy
Late-onset cone dystrophy with Mizuo phenomenon
Cone-rod degeneration

This group of cone and cone-rod degenerations is characterized by clinical and electrophysiologic findings (see Appendix A) which suggest that the first abnormality is in the cones. Some cases may progress to a generalized retinal degeneration. The common symptoms are decrease in central vision, abnormal color vision and photophobia, usually some degree of RPE atrophy in the macular area, and telangiectatic vessels in the temporal side of the optic disc. An abnormal sheen is seen in late-onset cone dystrophy with Mizuo phenomenon; pigmentary changes are seen in cone-rod degeneration.

Cone dystrophy seems to affect principally the cones. Photophobia, a decrease in central vision, and abnormal color vision are common. Some patients seek treatment for nystagmus. Occasionally, an area of RPE atrophy in the central macula with a bull's-eye pattern is seen. The photopic ERG is severely abnormal, but the scotopic ERG is close to normal.

The differential diagnosis includes the stationary cone disorders such as rod monochromatism and blue-cone monochromatism, but these disorders are congenital and nonprogressive. Stargardt's disease also must be considered in the differential diagnosis; however, the abnormalities in the fundus, angiographic changes, and the usually normal ERG distinguish the latter from the cone degenerations (see Table 9).

An X-linked disease affecting only males, *late-onset cone dystrophy with Mizuo phenomenon* is characterized by late onset, a tapetal-like sheen, Mizuo-Nakamura phenomenon, and an abnormal ERG.

Patients with *cone-rod degeneration* have a decrease in central vision, visual field constriction, pigmentary retinopathy, and (in late stages) nyctalopia with an ERG showing the cone response more severely affected than is the rod response.

Table 9 BULL'S-EYE MACULOPATHY

A bull's-eye is a central area of normal retina surrounded by a zone of depigmentation and pigment stippling. This lesion is more clearly visible with fluorescein angiography, showing a diffuse hyperfluorescence in the prearterial phase resulting from RPE defects (window defects) (see Figure 48, *A-D*).

NAME (CAUSE)	ONSET	PRINCIPAL FINDINGS	ERG	EOG	COLOR VISION	DARK ADAPTATION
Cone dystrophy	First and second decade	Decreased vision, abnormal color vision, nystagmus, photophobia, macular pigmentary changes, optic disc pale (temporal), optic disc telangiectasia, peripapillary atrophy	Photopic: abnormal Scotopic: normal	Usually normal	Abnormal	Normal—Abnormal
Stargardt's disease	First and second decade	Decrease in vision, abnormal color vision, fundus normal (early), bull's-eye (late), usually surrounded by flecks; beaten-bronze sheen, macular atrophy	Early: normal Late: normal—abnormal	Early: normal Late: normal—abnormal	Abnormal	Normal
Rod-cone dystrophy (RP)	First to third decade	Nyctalopia, constricted visual field, decreased vision (late), pigmentary retinopathy, optic disc pale, narrow vessels; posterior subcapsular cataract; in some patients, bull's-eye maculopathy	Abnormal	Abnormal	Normal—abnormal	Abnormal

Table 9 BULL'S-EYE MACULOPATHY—cont'd

NAME (CAUSE)	ONSET	PRINCIPAL FINDINGS	ERG	EOG	COLOR VISION	DARK ADAPTATION
Chloroquine toxicity	Usually with accumulated doses greater than 100 g	None or decreased vision and abnormal color vision; pigmentary changes in macula; bull's-eye maculopathy	Normal—abnormal	Normal—abnormal	Abnormal	Normal
Benign concentric annular macular dystrophy (bull's-eye)	Second decade	Asymptomatic or slight decrease in vision, bull's-eye, arteriolar attenuation; in some cases, drusenlike lesions	Normal—subnormal	Normal—abnormal	Abnormal	Normal—abnormal
Fenestrated sheen macular dystrophy	Second decade	Asymptomatic; yellowish refractile sheen with red fenestrations in the macula (early); annular zone of hypopigmentation of the RPE (bull's-eye) (late)	Normal—abnormal	Normal	Normal—abnormal	—
Bardet-Biedl syndrome (Laurence-Moon-Bardet-Biedl syndrome)	First decade	Obesity, pigmentary retinopathy, polydactyly, hypogenitalism, mental retardation, occasionally bull's-eye maculopathy	Abnormal	Abnormal	Normal—abnormal	Abnormal
Cohen syndrome	First decade	Obesity, hypotonia; facial, oral, and limb anomalies; short stature, mental deficiency; myopia and pigmentary retinopathy	Abnormal	Difficult to evaluate because of mental retardation		
Hallervorden-Spatz syndrome	First decade	Progressive rigidity of extremities, dysarthria, dementia, extrapyramidal signs	Probably normal	—	—	—
Fucosidosis mucolipidoses (mucopolysaccharidoses)	First decade	Severe mental retardation, normal renal function, dilated conjunctival vessels, angiokeratomas, deficiency of α-fucosidase	Probably normal	—	—	—
Sjögren-Larsson syndrome	First decade	Pigmentary retinal degeneration, ichthyosis, spasticity, short stature, mental retardation, speech defects, short fingers and toes	Probably abnormal	—	—	—
Sea-blue histiocyte disease (ophthalmoplegic dystonic lipidosis, juvenile dystonic lipidosis)	First decade	Splenomegaly, mild thrombocytopenia, numerous histiocytes containing cytoplasmic granules in the bone marrow (similar to Gaucher's disease and Niemann-Pick disease, type C); bull's-eye maculopathy reported	Probably normal	—	—	—
Neuronal ceroidlipofuscinosis (amaurotic idiocy)	First decade	Late infantile type (Jansky-Bielschowsky disease); see below for findings	Abnormal (b-wave reduced)	—	—	—
(Batten disease)	Second decade	Juvenile type (Batten-Spielmeyer-Vogt syndrome); the most common finding is a dark-red spot in the macula with peripheral retinal degeneration; in some cases, bull's-eye maculopathy				
Olivopontocerebellar degeneration (type III)	First to third decade	Decrease in vision, generalized weakness, pigmentary retinopathy, progressive cerebellar ataxia, quadriplegia, mental retardation, ophthalmoplegia; bull's-eye lesion reported	Normal—abnormal	Normal—abnormal	Abnormal	—
Areolar form of senile macular degeneration	Sixth decade	Metamorphopsia, decrease in vision, central scotoma, drusen, areas of RPE atrophy; lesion similar to bull's-eye maculopathy in some patients	Normal	Normal	Normal—abnormal	Normal

168 CONE AND CONE-ROD DEGENERATIONS

Cone Dystrophy FIGURE 48

KEY SYMPTOMS
Progressive visual loss
Abnormal color vision
Photophobia

KEY FINDINGS
Acquired nystagmus may be present
Only cone system is affected
Normal or near-normal fundi initially
Bull's-eye maculopathy develops later
Temporal optic disc pallor
Occasionally pigment clumping occurs in the macula
Occasionally geographic RPE atrophy in the macula
Symptoms are similar to those seen in rod monochromatism, but cone dystrophy is not congenital and is progressive, unlike rod monochromatism

INHERITANCE	ONSET	PROGRESSION	PROGNOSIS
Sporadic AD, AR	First to third decade	Slow	Poor

LABORATORY STUDIES
Visual Acuity	20/50 to 20/200
Refraction	Low myopia
Visual Fields	Central scotoma, normal periphery
Color Vision	Abnormal
Dark Adaptation	Abnormal cone, normal rod thresholds
ERG	Photopic abnormal, scotopic normal
EOG	Usually normal
Fluorescein Angiogram	Evidence of depigmentation in macula; bull's-eye pattern of hyperfluorescence surrounding a central nonfluorescent spot

TREATMENT	PATHOLOGY	SYNONYMS
None curative; dark glasses for photophobia	Unknown	Cone degeneration

DIFFERENTIAL DIAGNOSIS
Bull's-eye maculopathy (see Table 9, p. 166)
Abnormal color vision (see Table 11, p. 189)
Rod monochromatism (p. 192)

REFERENCES
21, 119, 149, 216, 217, 259, 286, 383

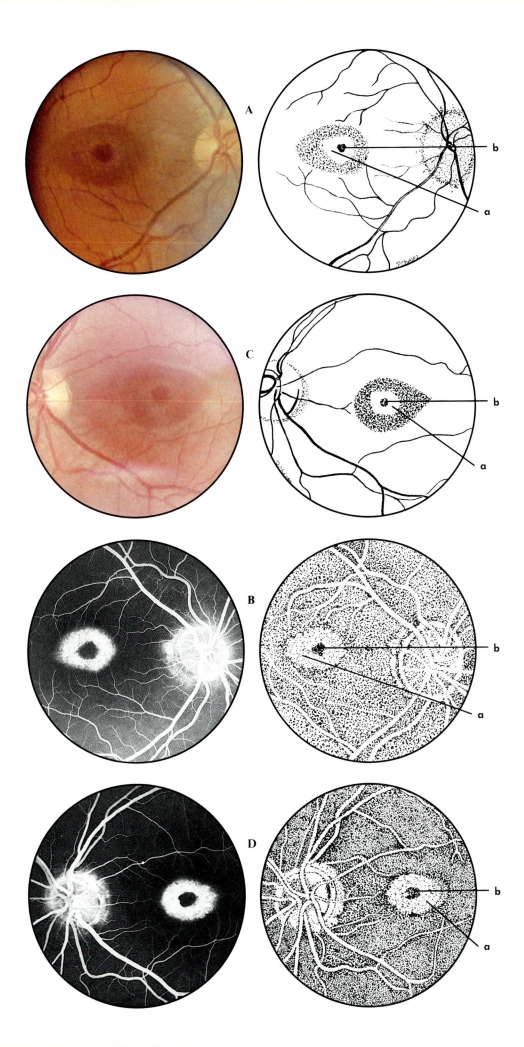

Figure 48
Cone Dystrophy

Typical bull's-eye macular lesion is seen in some cone dystrophies. This 25-year-old female had a 5-year history of photophobia, poor color vision, fine pendular nystagmus, a very abnormal photopic ERG, a normal scotopic ERG, and a normal EOG. Her corrected visual acuity is 20/80 OD and 20/100 OS. Her father and one uncle are affected with a similar condition.

A and C, Fundus photographs showing a zone of hypopigmentation *(a)* resulting from RPE atrophy surrounding a central, uninvolved spot of pigment epithelium *(b)*. These two areas are surrounded by a rim of normal appearing retina. There is also mild temporal pallor of the optic disc and mild attenuation of retinal arterioles.

B and D, Late venous-phase fluorescein angiogram showing a ring of hyperfluorescence *(a)* in the area of RPE atrophy and normal fluorescence in the central macula *(b)*, where the RPE appears to be normal. The lesion of the RPE is more easily seen with the angiogram.

Late-Onset Cone Dystrophy With Mizuo Phenomenon FIGURE 49

KEY SYMPTOMS
Asymptomatic early
Visual acuity reduction
Color vision defect
Photophobia

KEY FINDINGS
Male propositus
Greenish-golden tapetal-like sheen in large areas of the fundus
Sheen varies with the angle of view with indirect ophthalmoscopy
Sheen changes to orange-red with 3 hours dark adaptation (Mizuo phenomenon)
Sheen present from childhood, but visual acuity decrease occurs later
Bull's-eye maculopathy occasionally seen
Temporal pallor of the optic nerve head occasionally seen
After age 40, lesion may resemble macular degeneration
Female carriers also have a mild tapetal-like sheen and abnormalities of the ERG and cone adaptation

INHERITANCE	ONSET	PROGRESSION	PROGNOSIS
X-L	Symptoms in third decade	Slow	Visual acuity of <20/200 by age 40 to 50

LABORATORY STUDIES
Visual Acuity	20/30 to hand motions
Refraction	Myopia
Visual Fields	Peripheral normal; central scotoma late
Color Vision	Abnormal
Dark Adaptation	Cone threshold elevated, rods slightly abnormal
ERG	Photopic abnormal to nonrecordable
EOG	Normal to abnormal
Fluorescein Angiogram	Not published

TREATMENT
None

PATHOLOGY
Not known; similar sheen in Oguchi's disease is associated with deposition of a layer of lipofuscin granules on the RPE

SYNONYMS
X-linked recessive cone dystrophy with tapetal-like sheen and Mizuo-Nakamura phenomenon of Heckenlively and Weleber

DIFFERENTIAL DIAGNOSIS
Autosomal dominant cone dystrophy (p. 168)
Oguchi's disease (p. 180)
Blue cone monochromatism (p. 194)
Cone-rod degeneration (p. 172)

REFERENCES
173

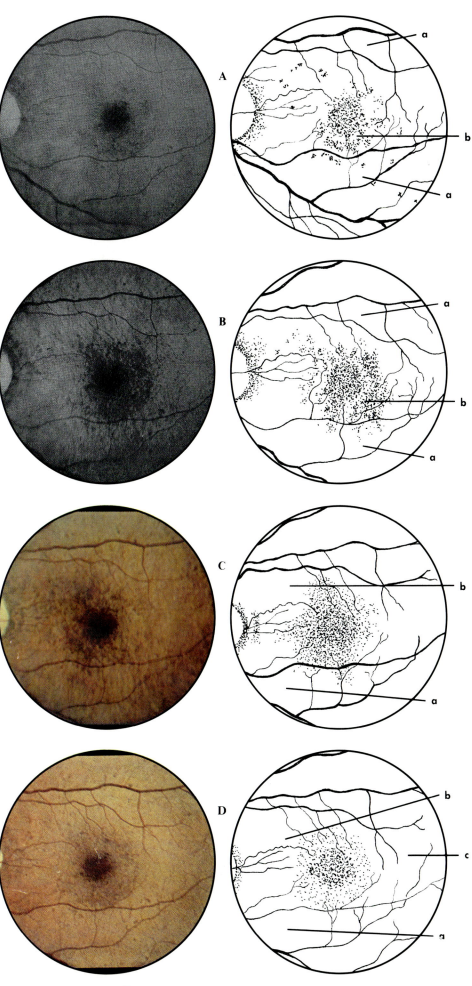

Figure 49
Late-Onset Cone Dystrophy
With Mizuo Phenomenon

A 54-year-old male with a corrected visual acuity of 20/70 OS and better vision in the dark. Two half brothers by the same mother and two other fathers were also affected.

A-B, Posterior pole of left eye in light-adapted state, with only slightly different viewing angle, demonstrating variability of sheen *(a)* and more granular, or topographic, appearance *(b)*. Sheen looks more confluent, and hyperpigmented dots appear more distinct *(a)* in **B.**

C, Baseline photograph. Compare with **D** to see the Mizuo-Nakamura phenomenon in this eye. After 3 hours of dark adaptation, the greenish-yellow sheen is greatly reduced *(a)*, with increased visibility of choroidal structures *(b)* and a generalized reddish-orange hue to the fundus *(c)*. (**A-D,** reproduced and redrawn from Heckenlively JR, and Weleber RG: X-linked recessive cone dystrophy with tapetal-like sheen: a newly recognized entity with Mizuo-Nakamura phenomenon, Arch Ophthalmol 104:1322, 1986. Copyright 1986, American Medical Association.)

Cone-Rod Degeneration FIGURE 50

KEY SYMPTOMS
Visual acuity loss
Color vision abnormal
Photophobia
Nyctalopia (late)

KEY FINDINGS
The fundus may be normal early
Probably the first abnormalities are the disc changes: temporal disc atrophy, temporal peripapillary atrophy, disc nerve fiber swelling, and telangiectasia of disc vessels
Hypopigmentation and/or hyperpigmentation in macula
50% of the patients develop pigmentary changes in the midperiphery similar to those seen in RP (late)
Bull's-eye maculopathy (rare)
The rod-cone and cone-rod degenerations constitute a spectrum of manifestations and diseases varying from primarily rod to primarily cone loss, but always involving both eventually

INHERITANCE	ONSET	PROGRESSION	PROGNOSIS
AR, AD, X-L	First to third decade	Slow	Poor

LABORATORY STUDIES
Visual Acuity	20/25 to <20/400
Refraction	Low myopia
Visual Fields	Constricted and scotomas
Color Vision	Abnormal
Dark Adaptation	Abnormal cones early, abnormal rods late
ERG	Abnormal—photopic more abnormal than scotopic
EOG	Abnormal usually
Fluorescein Angiogram	Diffuse hyperfluorescence in macula and midperiphery resulting from window defects

TREATMENT
None

PATHOLOGY
Loss of photoreceptors in macula and midperiphery and diffuse atrophy of the RPE with pigment migration

SYNONYMS
Cone-rod dystrophy

DIFFERENTIAL DIAGNOSIS
Retinitis pigmentosa (rod-cone) (p. 124)
Retinitis pigmentosa sine pigmento (p. 128)
Congenital optic atrophy

REFERENCES
20, 21, 110, 119, 149, 171, 216, 217, 259

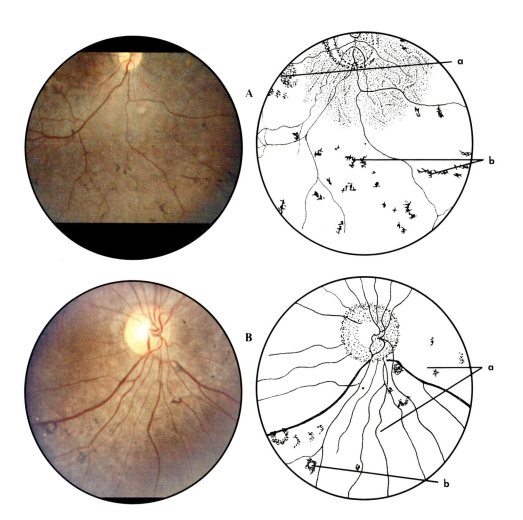

Figure 50
Cone-rod Degeneration

A 33-year-old male with decreased central vision of 5 years' duration. His visual acuity is 20/200 OU. He developed nyctalopia 2 years after onset. The ERG was abnormal, with cone responses more affected than were rod responses. There is no pertinent family history.

A, Fundus photograph (OD) of the retina inferior to the optic disc shows a slightly pale optic disc, a bull's-eye macular lesion, macular pigment clumping *(a)*, and some midperipheral pigment clumping *(b)* with attenuated vessels.

B, Fundus photograph (OD) of a 33-year old female with a visual acuity of 20/160 OU and a history of decreased acuity since the age of 25. The photopic ERG is severely abnormal, and the scotopic ERG is moderately abnormal. Color vision is severely abnormal. The family history is not pertinent. The fundus shows RPE mottling extending from the macula to the periphery *(a)*, attenuated vessels, some pigment clumps *(b)*, and mild pallor of the optic disc.

Congenital Stationary Night Blindness With Normal Fundus FIGURE 51

KEY SYMPTOMS
Nyctalopia
Normal vision or mild acuity reduction

KEY FINDINGS
The fundus is normal or shows only myopic changes
X-linked inheritance
Usually high myopia, nystagmus, and decreased vision
Two types are found by electrophysiologic testing
Type I (Riggs, Nougaret)
Abnormality in photoreceptor; both a- and b-wave reduced in scotopic ERG
Type II (Schubert-Bornschein)
Abnormality in bipolar cell layer; scotopic b-wave reduced; scotopic a-wave normal (see Figure 86, Appendix A)

INHERITANCE	ONSET	PROGRESSION	PROGNOSIS
AR, AD, X-L	Congenital	None or little	AR or AD: Good XL: 20/200

LABORATORY STUDIES
Visual Acuity	AD: 20/20; AR: 20/80; X-L: 20/200
Refraction	AD: hyperopia; AR: low myopia; X-L: high myopia
Visual Fields	Usually normal
Color Vision	Normal
Dark Adaptation	I: no rod function; II: rod function depressed (see Appendix B)
ERG	See Key Findings
EOG	I: abnormal; II: normal
Fluorescein Angiogram	Normal

TREATMENT	PATHOLOGY	SYNONYMS
None	Retinal structure normal except minimal abnormalities of photoreceptors	CSNB

DIFFERENTIAL DIAGNOSIS
Congenital stationary night blindness (CSNB) (see Table 10, p. 176)

REFERENCES
3, 9, 53, 57, 58, 132, 172, 176, 184, 192, 223, 227, 253, 307, 324, 375

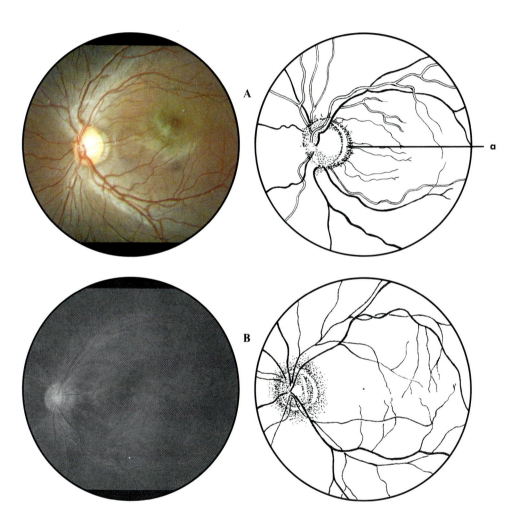

Figure 51
Congenital Stationary Night Blindness with Normal Fundus

A, Fundus photograph of a 17-year-old female with nonprogressive nyctalopia since birth, a corrected visual acuity of 20/20 OU, and a refractive error of −2.50 OU. The scotopic ERG b-wave is severely abnormal, the photopic ERG is normal, and the EOG is normal. She has abnormal dark adaptometry (elevated rod threshold) and normal photopic visual fields. There is no pertinent family history. Optic disc, vessels, and macula are normal. The pigment crescent on the temporal rim of the optic disc *(a)* is a normal variation.

B, Fundus photograph of an 11-year-old male with stationary nyctalopia since birth and normal visual acuity. The photopic ERG is normal, and the scotopic ERG is abnormal. The EOG is normal. Dark adaptometry shows abnormal rod function. There is no pertinent family history. The fundus appears to be normal.

Oguchi's Disease FIGURE 52

KEY SYMPTOMS
Stationary nyctalopia

KEY FINDINGS
Light Adapted

Fundus has a yellow-gray sheen from optic disc to equator that obscures distinction of arteries and veins

Dark Adapted

After 2 to 3 hours, fundus appears normal (Mizuo phenomenon); 30 to 60 minutes of light adaptation causes abnormal appearance

The three types of Oguchi's disease seen are based on the presence of the Mizuo phenomenon and dark adaptation results

Mizuo phenomenon present (type I); partial (type II, A); absent (type II, B)

Dark adaptation recovers to normal rod thresholds after several hours (type I); does not recover (type II, A, type II, B)

This disease is most common in Asians

INHERITANCE	ONSET	PROGRESSION	PROGNOSIS
AR	Congenital	None	Good

LABORATORY STUDIES

Visual Acuity	20/20 to 20/40
Visual Fields	Normal
Color Vision	Normal
Dark Adaptation	Abnormal rod function or delayed adaptation (see Figure 113, Appendix B)
ERG	Normal photopic; abnormal scotopic
EOG	Normal
Fluorescein Angiogram	Diffuse hyperfluorescence without leakage in light-adapted retina

TREATMENT	PATHOLOGY	SYNONYMS
None	Cones appear to be more numerous than normal; an amorphous material is seen between the receptors and the RPE	None in general use

DIFFERENTIAL DIAGNOSIS
Congenital stationary night blindness (CSNB) (see Table 10, p. 176)

REFERENCES
54, 56, 277, 377, 381

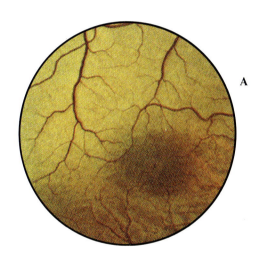

Figure 52
Oguchi's Disease

A, Fundus photograph (OD) in the light-adapted state showing the abnormal greenish-golden coloration typical of this condition. Note that the vessels look dark, with little difference between arteries and veins.

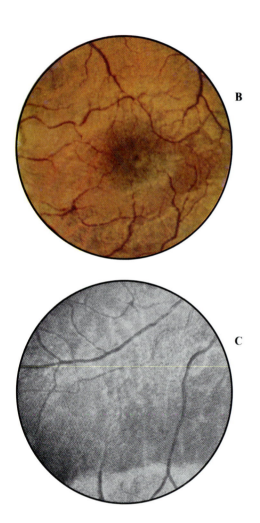

B, Fundus photograph (OD) of the same area after 4 hours of dark adaptation; the changes represent the Mizuo phenomenon, and the fundus looks more normal.

C, Fundus photograph (OD) in the midperipheral region showing a reddish-brown appearance.

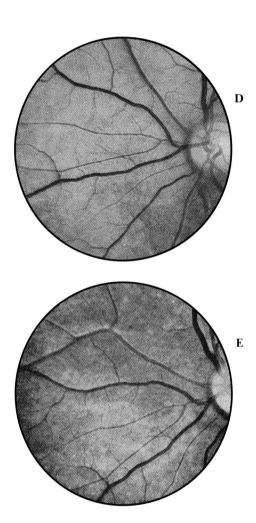

D, Fundus photograph (OS) of the nasal retina in a light-adapted state showing abnormal coloration.

E, Fundus photograph (OS), same region as in **D,** but after 4 hours of dark adaptation. The changes show the Mizuo phenomenon. (**A-E,** reproduced and redrawn from Winn S, Tasman W, Spaeth G, McDonald PR, and Justice J, Jr.: Oguchi's disease in Negroes, Arch Ophthalmol 81:503, 1969. Copyright 1969, American Medical Association.)

Fundus Albipunctatus FIGURE 53

KEY SYMPTOMS
Stationary nyctalopia or asymptomatic

KEY FINDINGS
Uniform, dull white round dots in the midperiphery and paramacula at the level of the RPE
Dots or flecks rare in fovea or parafovea
Flecks, too small to be seen by indirect ophthalmoscopy; may have a radial orientation in the midperiphery
Flecks occasionally change in shape or disappear with time
Macular atrophy is sometimes seen
Optic nerve and vessels are normal
Retinitis punctata albescens may occur in the same family, but this is a progressive disease and is less common than is fundus albipunctatus

INHERITANCE	ONSET	PROGRESSION	PROGNOSIS
AR	Congenital	None	Good

LABORATORY STUDIES
Visual Acuity	Usually 20/20
Visual Fields	Normal
Color Vision	Normal
Dark Adaptation	Markedly delayed rod adaptation (1 to 3 hours)
ERG	Abnormal, becomes normal with prolonged dark adaptation (3 hours)
EOG	Normal or abnormal
Fluorescein Angiogram	Multiple, small window defects in the midperiphery

TREATMENT	PATHOLOGY	SYNONYMS
None	Not known	Stationary albipunctate degeneration

DIFFERENTIAL DIAGNOSIS
Retinitis punctata albescens (p. 144)
Flecked retina diseases (see Table 5, p. 114)
Congenital stationary night blindness (CSNB) (see Table 10, p. 176)
Vitamin A deficiency (p. 240)

REFERENCES
108, 144, 220, 238

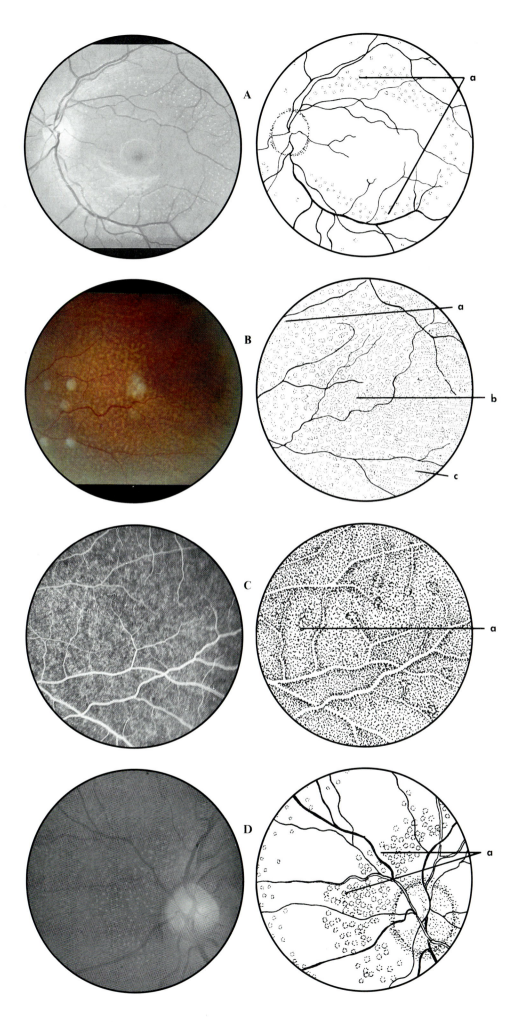

Figure 53
Fundus Albipunctatus

A 12-year-old male with nyctalopia since birth, a visual acuity of 20/20 OU, normal visual fields, and an ERG with a subnormal b-wave that becomes normal after prolonged dark adaptation. He has dark adaptometry with an elevated rod threshold that becomes normal after 3 hours.

A, Fundus photograph (OS) showing multiple, small, round white dots in the posterior pole *(a)*. The macular area is spared, and the optic disc and vessels are normal.

B, Fundus photograph (OS), superotemporal quadrant, showing a larger concentration of dots. In this particular case, there are three types of flecks: white punctiform flecks in the macular area *(a)*, yellowish-white pisiform or linear flecks in the midperiphery *(b)*, and grayish-white linear flecks with a radial orientation in the periphery *(c)*.

C, Angiogram of a patient with fundus albipunctatus showing multiple small transmission defects *(a)*.(**C,** courtesy of Horacio Ponce, M.D.)

D, Fundus photograph showing multiple yellow-white dots surrounding the posterior pole *(a)* and in the midperiphery. The retinal vessels and the optic disc are normal.

Flecked Retina of Kandori   FIGURE 54

KEY SYMPTOMS
Nyctalopia

KEY FINDINGS
Peripheral retinal flecks, irregular, dirty yellow, sharply defined, primarily equatorial
Flecks vary in size up to 1.5-disc diameters
Retina around flecks slightly brown
Normal optic disc and vessels
No macular or pigmentary changes
NOTE: This disease closely resembles CSNB except for the flecks, which are identical to those of grouped albinotic spots of the RPE

INHERITANCE	ONSET	PROGRESSION	PROGNOSIS
Probably AR	Congenital	None	Good

LABORATORY STUDIES
Visual Acuity	20/20
Visual Fields	Normal
Color Vision	Normal
Dark Adaptation	Delayed rod adaptation (40 minutes)
ERG	Scotopic b-wave normal only after prolonged dark adaptation
EOG	Normal
Fluorescein Angiogram	Hyperfluorescence corresponding to flecks during arterial phase

TREATMENT	PATHOLOGY	SYNONYMS
None	Not described	None in general use

DIFFERENTIAL DIAGNOSIS
Congenital stationary night blindness (CSNB) (see Table 10, p. 176)
Flecked retina (see Table 5, p. 114)
Congenital grouped albinotic spots (p. 106)

REFERENCES
194, 195, 196, 197

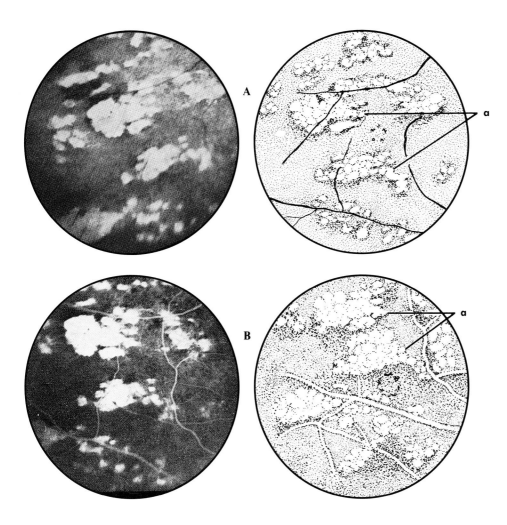

Figure 54

Flecked Retina of Kandori

A, Fundus photograph showing numerous deep-seated, dirty yellow, sharply defined flecks of varying sizes in the midperipheral region *(a)*.

B, Late-phase angiogram of the same eye showing persistence of the fluorescent lesions without change in size *(a)*. (**A-B,** reproduced and redrawn from Kandori F, Tamai A, Kurimoto S, and Fukunaga K: Fleck retina, Am J Ophthalmol 73:673, 1972. Published with permission from The American Journal of Ophthalmology. Copyright by the Ophthalmic Publishing Company.)

CONE SYSTEM DISORDERS (STATIONARY CONE DISORDERS)	Rod monochromatism Cone monochromatism Central cone monochromatism Blue cone monochromatism Dichromatism (protanopia, deuteranopia, tritanopia) Trichromatism (protanomaly, deuteranomaly, tritanomaly)

The organization of cone system disorders is presented in Flowchart 6. They are attended by prominent nystagmus and photophobia. The diagnostic import of these common findings and symptoms is presented in Flowcharts 7 and 8.

Cone system disorders are characterized by nonprogressive cone abnormalities, with onset at birth and with abnormal color vision (see Table 11). Two of these diseases, rod monochromatism and blue cone monochromatism, are of special interest because of low central vision, nystagmus, and photophobia.

The remaining diseases in this group are considered only in Table 11.

Rod monochromatism, also called *achromatopsia,* is an autosomal-recessive disease that manifests in one of two forms: (1) the complete form, with virtually no color sense and a visual acuity of 20/200, and (2) the incomplete form, with some color sense and better visual acuity. The fundus may be normal or show minimal macular changes in both forms. The photopic ERG is absent or severely abnormal, and the scotopic ERG is usually normal. The Sloan achromatopsia test is positive only in the complete form. The differential diagnosis is with blue cone monochromatism and cone dystrophy. The latter is distinguished by onset after birth and progression.

Blue cone monochromatism is an X-linked disease affecting only males and manifesting with the same symptoms as does rod monochromatism. The Sloan achromatopsia test and Berson arrow test are negative (see Appendix B).

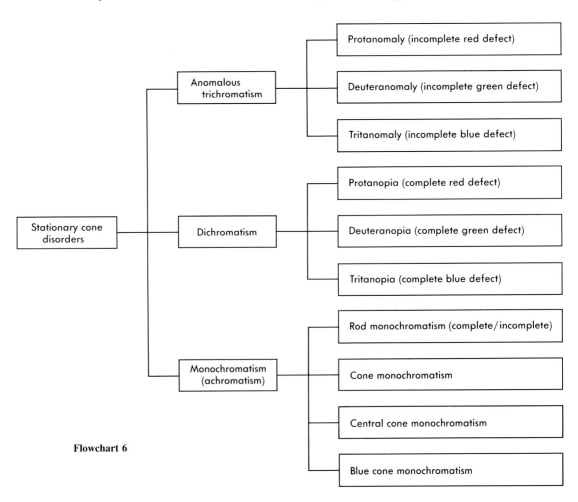

Flowchart 6

Table 11 STATIONARY CONE DEFECTS (STATIONARY COLOR VISION DEFECTS)

Stationary cone defects include all of the nonprogressive color vision abnormalities with onset from birth and with normal or decreased vision. The differences from the cone dystrophies are congenital onset and nonprogression. This group is divided according to the trichromatic theory of color vision, using the words protanomaly/protanopia, deuteranomaly/deuteranopia, and tritanomaly/tritanopia.
- *Protos* (red), *deuteros* (green), and *tritanos* (blue) defects.
- *Anomaly* is the partial absence of one color sense.
- *Anopia* is the total absence of one color sense.
- *Protan, deutan,* or *tritan* is used if the degree of abnormality is not known.

Trichromats require all three primary colors properly mixed to match a test color. Dichromats match a test color using a mixture of only two primary colors. Monochromats match all test colors using varying degrees of brightness of any primary (see Appendix B).

NAME	INHERITANCE	PRINCIPAL FINDINGS
Group: Anomalous Trichromatism		In this group, patients match colors with all three primary pigments but use different proportions of each to make matches. Patients are usually asymptomatic with normal vision, and the diagnosis is made by color testing with an anomaloscope.
Protanomaly (1%)	X-L	Red deficiency
Deuteranomaly (5%)	X-L	Green deficiency
Tritanomaly (very rare)		Blue deficiency
Group: Dichromatism		In this group, patients match colors using only two colors. Visual acuity is normal, and the patients manifest "color confusion." This group includes the common red/green color blindness.
Protanopia (1%)	X-L	Red mechanism absent (red/green confusion)
Deuteranopia (1%)	X-L	Green mechanism absent (red/green confusion)
Tritanopia (0.005%)	AD	Blue mechanism absent (blue/yellow confusion)
Group: Monochromatism		
Rod monochromatism (achromatism)	AR	Complete type: visual acuity is 20/200 Incomplete type: visual acuity is 20/40 to 20/100 Complete: virtual absence of color vision (Sloan test) Incomplete: abnormal color vision Photophobia, nystagmus, usually normal fundus with decreased foveal reflex; ERG photopic abnormal, ERG scotopic normal; photophobia and nystagmus may be minimal in the incomplete type, or may diminish after the second decade
Cone monochromatism (atypical monochromatism)	Unknown	Visual acuity is 20/20 Severely abnormal color vision, no photophobia, no nystagmus, fundus normal, postreceptor abnormality showing a normal photopic and scotopic ERG
Central cone monochromatism	AR	Visual acuity is 20/200 Only the macular cones are affected; photophobia, nystagmus; color vision mildly affected; normal photopic and scotopic ERG; close to normal flicker frequency
Blue cone monochromatism (atypical incomplete rod monochromatism)	X-L	Visual acuity is 20/60 to 20/200 No photophobia, minimal nystagmus, blue cones are minimally involved or not at all; abnormal photopic ERG, normal scotopic ERG; female carriers may show psychophysical and electrophysiologic abnormalities

190 REVIEW OF DISEASES

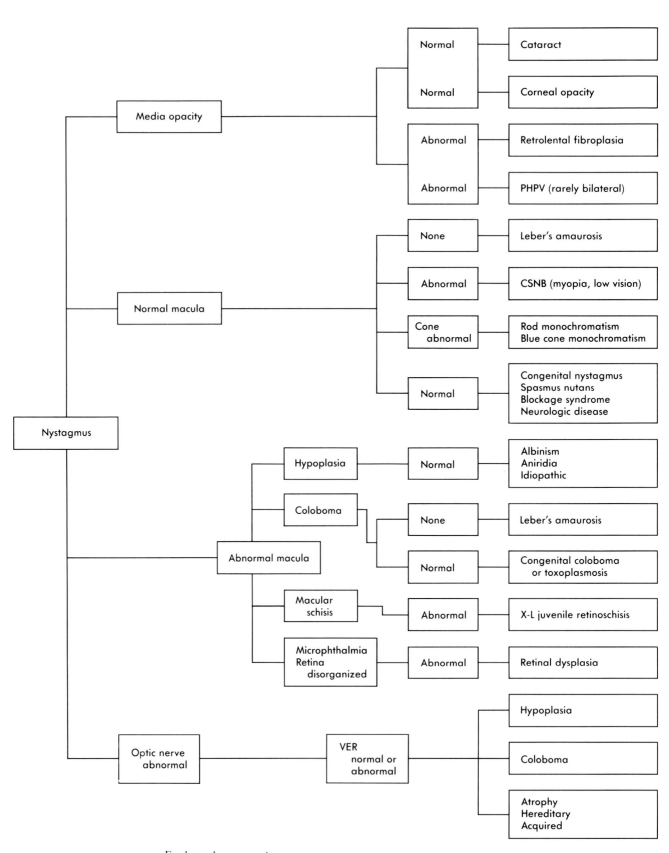

For legend see opposite page.

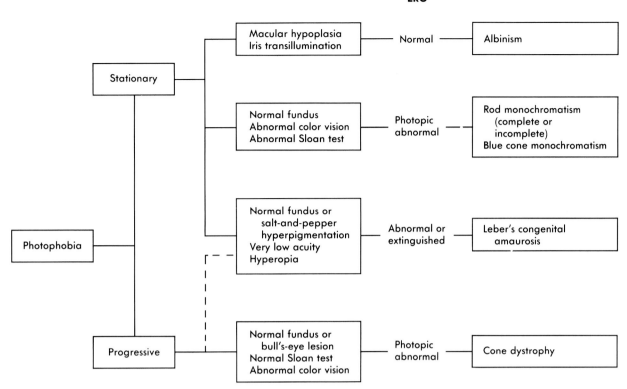

Flowchart 8
Photophobia

Photophobia associated with low vision and nystagmus in the first decade should be classified as progressive, which suggests a dystrophy, or as stationary, which indicates a congenital defect.

Progressive disability with a normal fundus or a bull's-eye macular lesion and defective color vision strongly suggests a cone dystrophy, in which case the photopic ERG but not the scotopic ERG will be abnormal.

Stationary photophobia suggests three conditions easily distinguished by the ERG: albinism, with a normal ERG, rod (or blue cone) monochromatism, with an abnormal cone ERG, or Leber's amaurosis, with a severely abnormal or extinguished ERG. In rare instances, Leber's amaurosis may not be fully expressed at birth and visual function may deteriorate over a period of a few years, suggesting progression. However, these children have a severe impairment at birth, whereas children with dystrophies show normal function at birth.

Flowchart 7
Nystagmus

Deprivation of visual fixation early in life results in nystagmus. The deprivation can be the result of bilateral opacity of the lens or cornea or of abnormality of the macula or optic nerve. If the problem is simply media opacity, there is no associated retinal degeneration and the ERG is normal. Abnormality of the ERG in the presence of media opacities can occur in cases of retrolental fibroplasia and bilateral primary hypoplastic posterior vitreous (PHPV).

In the absence of media opacity or macular abnormality, four conditions should be considered on the basis of ERG findings. A normal ERG indicates a nonretinal problem such as congenital nystagmus. A severely abnormal or extinguished ERG suggests Leber's amaurosis. An abnormal rod ERG with myopia suggests CSNB, and an abnormal cone ERG (associated with photophobia and nystagmus) suggests rod or blue cone monochromatism.

If the principal finding is macular abnormality, five conditions must be considered. Macular hypoplasia with a normal ERG suggests albinism, aniridia, or idiopathic macular hypoplasia; a coloboma suggests Leber's amaurosis if the ERG is abnormal or congenital coloboma or perhaps toxoplasmosis if the ERG is normal. Macular schisis indicates X-linked retinoschisis, and a poorly developed retina with an abnormal ERG suggests retinal dysplasia.

Nystagmus resulting from optic nerve abnormality may be associated with hypoplasia, coloboma, or atrophy.

Rod Monochromatism FIGURE 55

KEY SYMPTOMS
Abnormal color vision
Low vision from birth
Photophobia

KEY FINDINGS
Nystagmus of pendular type, congenital
Photophobia, extreme, with hemeralopia (day blindness)
Normal fundus, pigment changes rare in macula
Decreased foveal reflex
Incomplete Form
Visual acuity is 20/60 to 20/100; nystagmus and photophobia mild or absent and may decrease with age
Complete Form
Visual acuity is 20/200

INHERITANCE	ONSET	PROGRESSION	PROGNOSIS
AR	Congenital	None	Incomplete: good
			Complete: poor

LABORATORY STUDIES
Visual Acuity	20/60 to 20/200
Visual Fields	Central scotoma
Color Vision	Absent: Sloan achromatopsia test in complete form (see Appendix B, p. 261)
Dark Adaptation	No cone function; rods normal (see Figure 112, Appendix B)
ERG	Abnormal photopic; normal scotopic
EOG	Normal
Fluorescein Angiogram	Normal

TREATMENT
None curative; use of dark glasses for photophobia

PATHOLOGY
Rods are normal; cones are markedly deficient (5% to 10% of normal); foveal cones are abnormal

SYNONYMS
Achromatopsia, complete and incomplete

DIFFERENTIAL DIAGNOSIS
Blue cone monochromatism (see Table 11, p. 189)
Cone dystrophy (p. 168)

REFERENCES
8, 10, 26, 295, 297, 326, 335, 336, 340, 341, 342

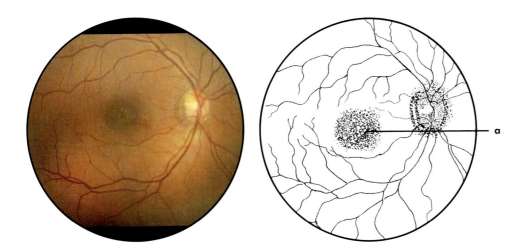

Figure 55
Rod Monochromatism

A 25-year-old female with a history of poor vision all her life, extreme photophobia, mild nystagmus, and color blindness. There is no pertinent family history. Her corrected visual acuity is 20/200 OU. The ERG showed absent photopic and normal scotopic response. The Sloan achromatopsia test was positive.

Fundus photograph shows granular pigmentation in the macula *(a)*. The remainder of the fundus is normal.

Blue Cone Monochromatism FIGURE 56

KEY SYMPTOMS
Low vision from birth
Photophobia

KEY FINDINGS
Only males affected
Nystagmus
Fundus usually normal or minimal foveal granularity
The disease resembles rod monochromatism, which can be distinguished by spectral sensitivity tests and ERG responses
Maximum sensitivity of blue cone monochromat is 440nm (deep blue); maximum sensitivity of rod monochromat is 504nm (blue green)
Use Sloan achromatopsia test (see Appendix B)
Cone monochromat has a small photopic ERG response; rod monochromat (complete) has virtually no such response

INHERITANCE	ONSET	PROGRESSION	PROGNOSIS
X-L	Congenital	None	20/100 to 20/200

LABORATORY STUDIES
Visual Acuity	20/100 to 20/200
Refraction	Myopia
Visual Fields	Central scotoma
Color Vision	Abnormal—deutanlike axis
Dark Adaptation	Normal
ERG	Photopic reduced; scotopic normal
EOG	Normal
Fluorescein Angiogram	Normal

TREATMENT
Dark glasses are helpful for photophobia

PATHOLOGY
The findings suggest absence of a functioning red and green cone mechanism and normal blue cones

SYNONYMS
Blue monocone monochromatism

DIFFERENTIAL DIAGNOSIS
Rod monochromatism (p. 192)
Stationary color vision defects (see Table 11, p. 189)
Cone dystrophy (p. 168)

REFERENCES
8, 24, 26, 35, 296, 297, 340

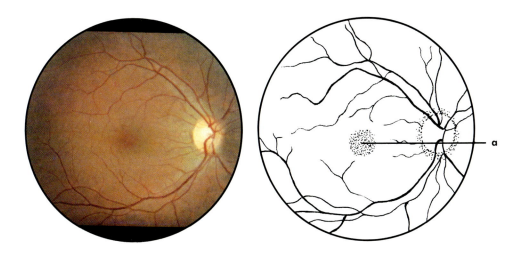

Figure 56

Blue Cone Monochromatism

A 21-year-old male with a history of poor vision since birth, photophobia, nystagmus, and abnormal color vision. His corrected visual acuity is 20/200 OU. He had a negative Sloan achromatopsia test, a severely abnormal photopic ERG, a normal scotopic ERG, and a normal EOG. Two brothers are affected with the same condition.

Fundus photograph shows an abnormal fundus reflex with minimal pigmentary changes (a). The optic disc and vessels are normal.

Abnormalities of the Inner Retina

INNER RETINAL DISEASES

The inner retina includes the inner nuclear, inner plexiform, ganglion cell, and nerve fiber layers.

INNER RETINAL DISEASES

Dominant cystoid macular dystrophy
Familial foveal retinoschisis
Gangliosidosis (Tay-Sachs disease)

Inner retinal diseases are a heterogenous group of diseases, some of which could well be classified into other groups. Their common characteristic is abnormality of the inner retinal layers, which in some cases may extend to other layers.

Dominant cystoid macular dystrophy is characterized by clinical and angiographic cystoid macular edema and a decrease in central vision. Some patients also have a peripheral pigmentary retinopathy and vitreous abnormalities.

Familial foveal retinoschisis is a rare disease manifesting with a retinoschisis in the fovea identical to that seen in X-linked juvenile retinoschisis. Familial foveal retinoschisis differs in that females are affected and peripheral retinoschisis is absent.

Gangliosidosis (ganglion cell dystrophies) is a large group of systemic disorders with incidental involvement of the retina. In some of the diseases, a typical cherry-red spot is seen in the fovea resulting from accumulation of abnormal material in the ganglion cell layer of the parafovea. Detailed consideration of gangliosidosis is beyond the scope of this text. Only one illustrative example, Tay-Sachs disease (familial amaurotic idiocy) is given.

Other ganglion cell dystrophies with cherry-red spots include Niemann-Pick disease, Sandhoff disease, G_{M1} gangliosidosis, and metachromatic leukodystrophy. Ganglion cell dystrophies with different findings are juvenile Tay-Sachs disease (Bielschowsky-Jansky disease), Batten-Mayou disease, Batten disease, and sea-blue histiocyte syndrome.

Familial Foveal Retinoschisis FIGURE 58

KEY SYMPTOMS
Visual acuity reduction
Abnormal color vision
Metamorphopsia

KEY FINDINGS
Radial folds of fovea identical to those seen in juvenile retinoschisis; retina splits into inner and outer layers
Multiple tiny, round, radially distributed microcysts
No peripheral retinoschisis
Vessels, RPE, optic disc, and vitreous are normal
NOTE: In X-L juvenile retinoschisis the retinal periphery and vitreous are abnormal, unlike that seen in this disease

INHERITANCE	ONSET	PROGRESSION	PROGNOSIS
AR	First decade	Very slow	Usually good

LABORATORY STUDIES
Visual Acuity	20/25 to 20/30
Refraction	Low hyperopia
Visual Fields	Irregular central scotoma
Color Vision	Abnormal
Dark Adaptation	Normal to subnormal
ERG	Normal
EOG	Normal
Fluorescein Angiogram	Normal or foveal hyperfluorescence

TREATMENT	PATHOLOGY	SYNONYMS
None	Not described	None in general use

DIFFERENTIAL DIAGNOSIS	REFERENCES
X-linked juvenile retinoschisis (p. 210)	233

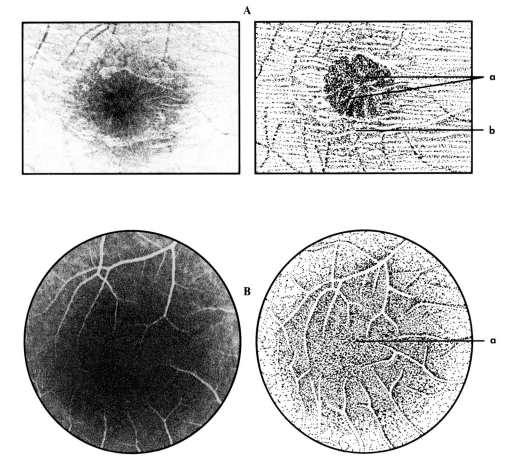

Figure 58
Familial Foveal Retinoschisis

A, Monochromatic fundus photograph (OD) of fovea. Note intraretinal spokelike septae *(a)*, the microcysts between them, and the fine corrugation of reflexes *(b)* from surrounding retinal surfaces.

B, Angiogram (OD) of fovea showing normal fluorescence *(a)*. (**A-B,** reproduced and redrawn with permission from Lewis RA, Lee GB, Martonyi CL, Barnett JM, and Falls HF: Familial foveal retinoschisis, Arch Ophthalmol 95:1190, 1977. Copyright 1977, American Medical Association.)

Gangliosidosis (Tay-Sachs Disease) FIGURE 59

KEY SYMPTOMS
Asymptomatic early
Psychomotor retardation
Apathy

KEY FINDINGS
More common in patients of Jewish descent
Early onset with psychomotor deterioration, apathy, hypotony, exaggerated startle reflex, macrocephaly (second year), and seizures
Later decerebrate rigidity, spasticity, generalized paralysis, froglike position, ineffective swallowing, and death before age 4

Ocular Findings
Cherry-red spot in the fovea (95%)
Optic atrophy, nystagmus, strabismus
Blindness by age 2, with pupil reaction to light often retained

INHERITANCE	ONSET	PROGRESSION	PROGNOSIS
AR	First 6 months	Rapid	Death before age 4

LABORATORY STUDIES
Visual Acuity	Progressive loss to blindness
Visual Fields	Difficult to assess
Color Vision	Difficult to assess
Dark Adaptation	Difficult to assess
ERG	Usually normal, may be abnormal late
EOG	Difficult to record
Fluorescein Angiogram	Not described

TREATMENT
None

PATHOLOGY
Vacuolization of ganglion cells; accumulation of G_{M2} ganglioside; deficiency of hexosaminidase A; carriers can be detected by enzyme assay

SYNONYMS
Infantile familial idiocy

DIFFERENTIAL DIAGNOSIS
Ganglion cell dystrophies and other lipidoses

REFERENCES
70, 74, 343

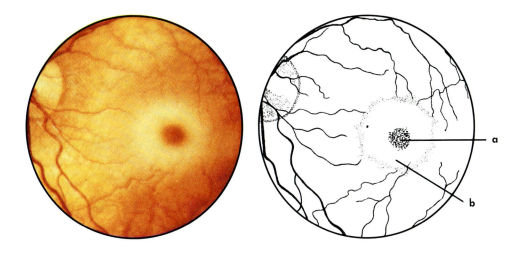

Figure 59

Gangliosidosis (Tay-Sachs Disease)

Fundus photograph (OS) showing the typical macular cherry-red spot. This appearance results from the accumulation of lipids in the ganglion cells, which are most abundant in the macula (except in the fovea). The fovea (a) has a normal coloration, but looks reddish by contrast to the surrounding affected retina (b). (Photograph reproduced and redrawn from Gil-Gibernau JJ: El fondo del ojo en el nino, Barcelona, 1982, Espaxs.)

Vitreoretinal Abnormalities

VITREORETINAL DYSTROPHIES

VITREORETINAL DYSTROPHIES

X-linked juvenile retinoschisis
Goldmann-Favre vitreoretinal dystrophy
Wagner's vitreoretinal dystrophy
Stickler's arthroophthalmopathy
Snowflake vitreoretinal degeneration
Familial exudative vitreoretinopathy
Autosomal dominant vitreoretinochoroidopathy

The vitreoretinal dystrophies are a mixed group of diseases that involve different retinal layers but have abnormality of the vitreous in common. Retinal detachment is relatively common in several of the diseases.

The common inheritance pattern of these diseases is autosomal dominant, with two exceptions: juvenile retinoschisis is X-linked, and Goldmann-Favre dystrophy is autosomal recessive. Some of them (e.g., juvenile retinoschisis, Goldmann-Favre dystrophy) have characteristic electrophysiologic findings (see Table 12 and Appendix A).

X-linked juvenile retinoschisis is a relatively common vitreoretinal dystrophy affecting only males and is characterized by central retinoschisis, a decrease in central vision, peripheral retinoschisis (50% of the patients), vitreous veils and strands, and an abnormal ERG b-wave. Unlike those carriers of X-linked dystrophies, the female carriers of juvenile retinoschisis cannot be detected.

Goldmann-Favre vitreoretinal dystrophy, a rare disease, is characterized by retinoschisis, pigmentary retinal degeneration with nyctalopia, and a severely abnormal ERG.

Wagner's vitreoretinal dystrophy is relatively common and manifests with myopia, vitreous degeneration, and large areas of lattice degeneration. Other symptoms can include pigmentary retinopathy, vessel sheathing, and inverse optic disc. Electrophysiology may be normal to abnormal.

Stickler's arthroophthalmopathy is relatively common and is related to Wagner's vitreoretinal dystrophy but includes systemic abnormalities such as Pierre Robin anomaly, flattened facies, and arthropathy.

Snowflake vitreoretinal degeneration, a rare disease, is characterized by vitreous degeneration, white with pressure, small, peripheral, yellow-white spots, and chorioretinal atrophy. The ERG is also abnormal.

Familial exudative vitreoretinopathy is a relatively common disease characterized by vitreous traction, dragged disc, retinal and subretinal exudates, abnormal peripheral vessels, and retinal detachment. The penetrance and expressivity are variable in the same family; the ERG is variable.

Autosomal dominant vitreoretinochoroidopathy is a rare disease characterized by myopia, vitreous degeneration and hemorrhage, cystoid macular edema, and peripheral pigmentary degeneration between the vortex veins and the ora serrata. ERG is normal to abnormal.

Table 12 VITREORETINAL DYSTROPHIES

NAME	INHERITANCE	FINDINGS	ERG	EOG
Juvenile retinoschisis	X-L	Only in males; decrease in vision, foveal retinoschisis (radiate plication), peripheral retinoschisis in 50%, vitreous veils, vitreous hemorrhage, foveal atrophy; retinal detachment rare	Scotopic b-wave reduced	Normal
Goldmann-Favre vitreoretinal dystrophy	AR	Nyctalopia, central and peripheral retinoschisis, vitreous strands and veils, peripheral pigmentary retinopathy, cataracts, retinal detachment	Severely abnormal to nonrecordable	Abnormal
Wagner's vitreoretinal dystrophy	AD	Vitreous optically empty, preretinal avascular membrane, myopia, retinal breaks and holes, lattice degeneration, cataract, inverse optic disc, macula normal, retinal pigmentation, retinal detachment	b-wave reduced	Normal
Stickler's arthroophthalmopathy	AD	Myopia, cataract, vitreous optically empty, pigmentary retinopathy, Pierre Robin syndrome (micrognathia, cleft palate, and glossoptosis), arthritis, spondyloepiphyseal dysplasia	Subnormal b-wave	Normal
Snowflake vitreoretinal degeneration	AD	White with pressure with small, peripheral, yellow-white crystalline spots, vitreous degeneration, sheathing of retinal vessels, small areas of chorioretinal atrophy, pigmentary retinopathy	Scotopic b-wave reduced	Normal or subnormal
Familial exudative vitreoretinopathy	AD	Posterior vitreous detachment, vitreous traction, white with and without pressure, dragged disc, temporal retinal exudation, retinal detachment	Normal to abnormal	Normal to abnormal
Autosomal dominant vitreoretinochoroidopathy	AD	Myopia, pigmented vitreous cells, fibrillar condensation, vitreous hemorrhage, peripheral pigmentary degeneration, arteriolar narrowing, cystoid macular edema	Normal to abnormal	Probably normal

Other Wagnerlike syndromes
  Hereditary arthroophthalmopathy with Weill-Marchesani-like habitus
  Kniest disease
  Diastrophic variant
  Spondyloepiphyseal dysplasia congenita
  Short stature, type undetermined
	AD	Common to all: short stature, severe myopia, vitreous veils, perivascular lattice, occasional retinal detachment and cataract	Subnormal	Normal

X-Linked Juvenile Retinoschisis FIGURE 60

KEY SYMPTOMS
Visual acuity reduction (first decade)

KEY FINDINGS
Male propositus

Retinoschisis implies splitting of the neurosensory retina; this occurs between the nerve fiber and ganglion cell layers and may resemble a detachment; pathognomonic if the fovea is involved

Fifty percent of patients have only foveal involvement; this is described as a radiate plication formed by small folds of the inner retina

Peripheral retinoschisis (50%) is most common inferotemporally; the inner lamina may be elevated with sclerotic sheaths and also with new vessels, which may bleed; retinal detachment is uncommon (5% to 22%)

Peripheral schisis may extend from fovea to ora (rare)

Holes occur in the inner lamina (75%) and outer lamina (13%)

Posterior vitreous detachment, degeneration, veils and strands

Pigmentary retinopathy or macular atrophy may occur late

Rare

Strabismus, nystagmus, cataracts, and pseudopapillitis

INHERITANCE	ONSET	PROGRESSION	PROGNOSIS
X-L	Probably congenital	Slow	Poor

LABORATORY STUDIES

Visual Acuity	20/100 to 20/400
Refraction	Hyperopia with astigmatism
Visual Fields	Central and peripheral scotomas
Color Vision	Abnormal; tritan or deutan defects common
Dark Adaptation	Slightly abnormal
ERG	Reduced scotopic b-wave; normal a-wave
EOG	Normal
Fluorescein Angiogram	Normal early; central hyperfluorescence with macular atrophy and leakage from new peripheral vessels late

TREATMENT
None or prophylactic scleral buckling and cryopexy; retinal surgery for detachment

PATHOLOGY
Retinal split between the nerve fiber layer and the ganglion cell layer

SYNONYMS
Congenital vascular veils
Congenital cystic detachment
Congenital retinoschisis

DIFFERENTIAL DIAGNOSIS
Vitreoretinal dystrophies (see Table 12, p. 209)
Senile retinoschisis
Familial retinoschisis
Retinal detachment
Stargardt's disease (p. 92)

REFERENCES
48, 59, 71, 162, 182, 191, 267, 280, 290, 302, 361, 382

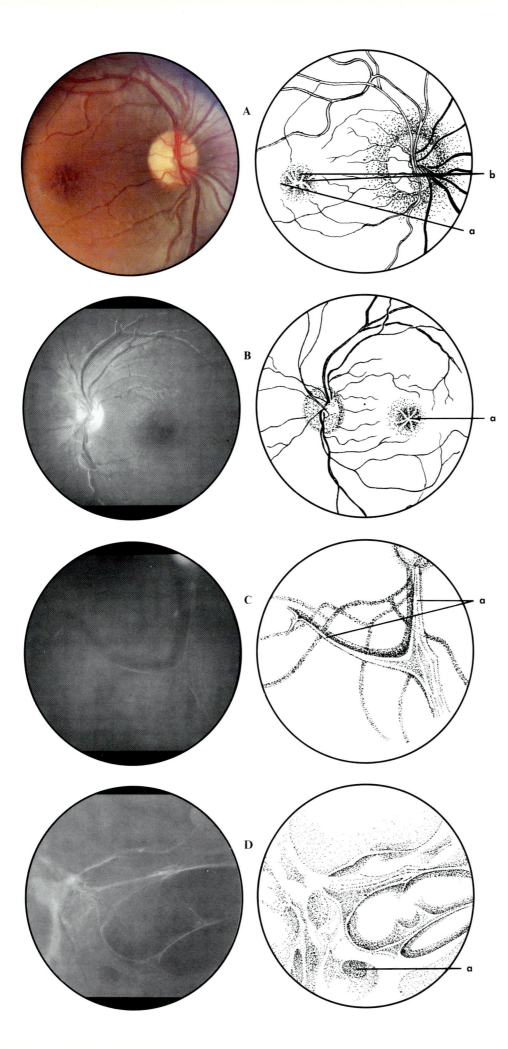

Figure 60
X-Linked Juvenile Retinoschisis

A 12-year-old male with a visual acuity of 20/200 OU and mild nystagmus; ERG shows subnormal b-waves. One brother is affected with the same condition.

A, Fundus photograph (OD) shows the typical macular lesion *(a)* with radiating retinal cysts (macular schisis) *(b)*. No peripheral retinoschisis is present.

An 11-year-old male with a visual acuity 20/200 OU. He has two brothers who are affected with the same condition.

B, Fundus photograph (OS) showing macular retinoschisis *(a)*. Optic disc and vessels are normal.

C, Fundus photograph (OD) of the inferonasal retina shows vitreous veils *(a)* from the optic disc.

D, Inferotemporal retina (OD) showing the area of peripheral schisis with large holes *(a)*.

Goldmann-Favre Vitreoretinal Dystrophy FIGURE 61

KEY SYMPTOMS
Nyctalopia
Visual acuity reduction

KEY FINDINGS
Central and peripheral retinoschisis, usually located in inferotemporal quadrants (see juvenile retinoschisis)
Posterior vitreous detachment
Vitreous degeneration, strands and veils
Preretinal membranes
Peripheral pigmentary retinopathy similar to retinitis pigmentosa; the pigmented lesions may be round
Pale optic disc with attenuated vessels
Complicated cataracts (posterior subcapsular)
Retinal detachment is common
Opaque dendritic-like peripheral retinal vessels
Cystoid macular edema

INHERITANCE	ONSET	PROGRESSION	PROGNOSIS
AR	First decade	Slow	Poor

LABORATORY STUDIES

Visual Acuity	20/30 to light perception
Refraction	Usually low myopia
Visual Fields	Central and peripheral defects
Color Vision	Abnormal
Dark Adaptation	Severely abnormal
ERG	Abnormal to nonrecordable
EOG	Abnormal
Fluorescein Angiogram	Normal macular fluorescence, perifoveal vessels may leak; marked leakage from peripheral retinal vessels; midperipheral hyperfluorescence

TREATMENT
Cataract extraction may be necessary; retinal surgery; prophylactic treatment for retinal detachment

PATHOLOGY
Degeneration of RPE and sensory retina; thickened retinal vessels; preretinal glial membrane

SYNONYMS
Favre's microfibrillar vitreoretinal degeneration
Hyaloideotapetoretinal degeneration

DIFFERENTIAL DIAGNOSIS
X-Linked juvenile retinoschisis (p. 210)
Vitreoretinal dystrophies (see Table 12, p. 209)
Pigmentary retinopathy (see Table 6, p. 118)
Progressive nyctalopia (see Table 7, p. 120)

REFERENCES
59, 103, 118, 180, 267, 290

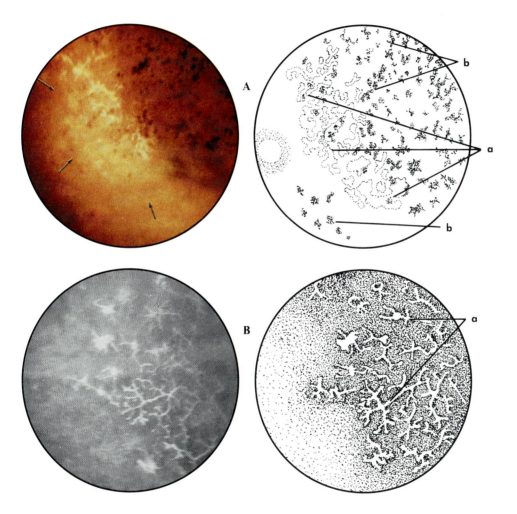

Figure 61
Goldmann-Favre Vitreoretinal Dystrophy

A, Fundus photograph (OD) showing highly raised retinoschisis in temporal periphery *(a)*. Pigment clumping is also apparent *(b)*.

B, Fundus photograph showing opaque, dendritic appearance of peripheral vessels *(a)*. (**A-B,** reproduced and redrawn from Fishman GA, Jampol LM, and Goldberg MF: Diagnostic features of the Favre-Goldmann syndrome, Br J Ophthalmol 60:345, 1976.)

Wagner's Vitreoretinal Dystrophy FIGURE 62

KEY SYMPTOMS
Visual acuity reduction
Symptoms caused by myopia

KEY FINDINGS
Posterior vitreous detachment; optically empty vitreous
Linear preretinal membrane around equator with avascular preretinal membranes elsewhere
Lattice degeneration and white without pressure
Retinal detachment common; 75% have retinal holes
Myopia in 85%; cataracts common after age 20
Inverse, pale optic disc; meridional folds
Pigmentary retinopathy along the vessels; vessel attenuation and sheathing
Glaucoma may occur
Macula not usually affected

INHERITANCE	ONSET	PROGRESSION	PROGNOSIS
AD	First decade	Slow	Good

LABORATORY STUDIES
Visual Acuity	Close to normal with correction
Refraction	Moderate to high myopia
Visual Fields	Normal or constricted
Color Vision	Normal
Dark Adaptation	Normal
ERG	Subnormal rod b-wave
EOG	Normal to abnormal
Fluorescein Angiogram	Equatorial hyperfluorescence (RPE atrophy); macular fluorescence normal; poor filling of choriocapillaris; retinal vessel occlusion in periphery

TREATMENT
Cataract extraction; retinal detachment treatment

PATHOLOGY
Retina
Thin with photoreceptor degeneration and with thickened vessels; RPE, choriocapillaris atrophy
Vitreous
Liquefaction, preretinal membranes

SYNONYMS
Wagner's disease

DIFFERENTIAL DIAGNOSIS
Goldmann-Favre vitreoretinal dystrophy (p. 212)
X-Linked juvenile retinoschisis (p. 210)
High myopia (AD) (p. 56)
Vitreoretinal dystrophies (see Table 12, p. 209)

REFERENCES
59, 177

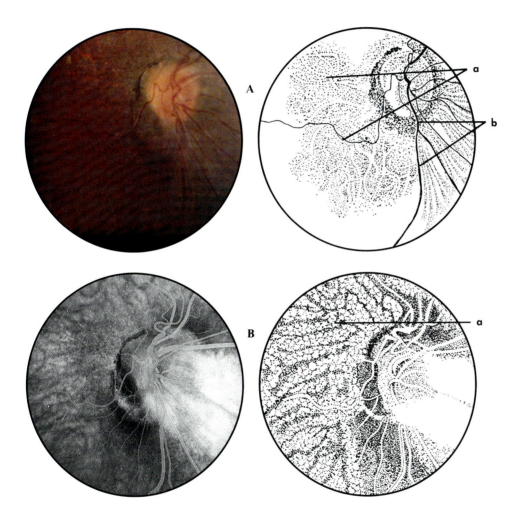

Figure 62

Wagner's Vitreoretinal Dystrophy

A 12-year-old male with high myopia and vitreoretinal degeneration. Several other family members are also affected.

A, Fundus photograph showing inverse pale optic disc and diffuse chorioretinal degeneration *(a);* vessel attenuation and sheathing *(b)* are also present.

B, Angiogram show hyperfluorescence in the areas of chorioretinal atrophy *(a).* (**A-B,** courtesy of Hugo Quiroz, M.D.)

Stickler's Arthroophthalmopathy FIGURE 63

KEY SYMPTOMS
Visual acuity reduction

KEY FINDINGS
Ocular Abnormalities
High myopia, cataract, glaucoma, retinal detachment
Optically empty vitreous, vitreous degeneration
Pigmentary retinopathy, lattice degeneration
Orofacial Abnormalities
Pierre Robin malformation: cleft palate, glossoptosis, and micrognathia
Flattened facies, dental abnormalities, maxillary hypoplasia
Skeletal Abnormalities
Arthropathy
Spondyloepiphyseal dysplasia, long limbs, hypotonia
Joint hyperextensibility and enlargement

INHERITANCE	ONSET	PROGRESSION	PROGNOSIS
AD	First decade	Slow	Poor

LABORATORY STUDIES
Visual Acuity	Close to normal with correction
Refraction	High myopia
Visual Fields	Usually normal
Color Vision	Normal
Dark Adaptation	Usually normal
ERG	Subnormal b-wave caused by myopia
EOG	Normal
Fluorescein Angiogram	Myopic changes include choroidal and retinal atrophy; poor filling of choriocapillaris; retinal vessel occlusion in the periphery

TREATMENT	PATHOLOGY	SYNONYMS
Specific for complications	Not described	Stickler's syndrome

DIFFERENTIAL DIAGNOSIS
Wagner's vitreoretinal dystrophy (p. 214)
Vitreoretinal dystrophies (see Table 12, p. 209)
Marfan syndrome
Ehlers-Danlos syndrome
Turner's syndrome

REFERENCES
37, 208, 245, 349

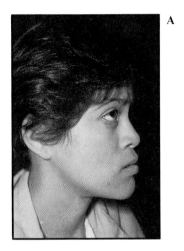

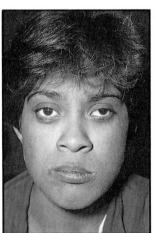

Figure 63

Stickler's Arthroophthalmopathy

A-B, Concurrent photographs of a 19-year-old female with a history of retinal detachment OS at the age of 14 and OD at the age of 19, when the detachment was successfully repaired. Visual acuity is 20/40 OD and 20/400 OS with mild lens opacity. Refraction is −9.00 diopters OD and −11.00 diopters OS. She has an exotropic strabismus. The patient has midfacial flattening, saddle nose, facial asymmetry, and maxillary hypoplasia with an arched palate. She has one brother who has cataracts and retinal detachment.

218 VITREORETINAL DYSTROPHIES

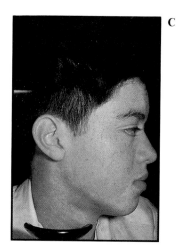

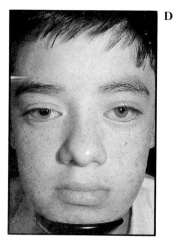

C-D, Photographs of a 17-year-old male with vitreoretinal degeneration and a history of retinal detachment OS. He has a flattened face, mandibular hypoplasia, and strabismus.

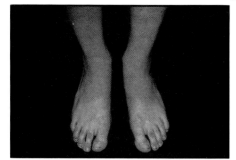
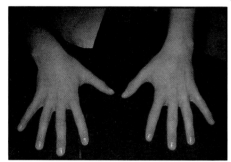
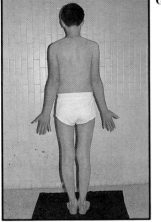
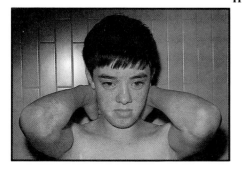

E-F, Marfanoid habitus with arachnodactyly is shown.

G-H, Scoliosis, joint deformities, and osteoarthritis are shown.

Snowflake Vitreoretinal Degeneration FIGURE 64

KEY SYMPTOMS
Visual acuity reduction

KEY FINDINGS
Stage I
Extensive white with pressure around periphery in young patients (<15); scattered yellow-white spots; vitreous degeneration
Stage II
Snowflake degeneration—areas of small yellow-white refractile dots that extend to the periphery
Stage III
Peripheral vascular sheathing and pigmentation
Stage IV
Progressive pigmentation and disappearance of vessels in periphery; pigment clumping interspersed with small areas of chorioretinal atrophy; fewer snowflakes; neovascularization
Other Abnormalities
Retinal detachment; cataracts (late)

INHERITANCE	ONSET	PROGRESSION	PROGNOSIS
AD	First to second decade	Slow	Good unless retinal detachment occurs

LABORATORY STUDIES
Visual Acuity	20/20 to 20/200: rare light perception
Refraction	Low myopia
Visual Fields	Upper field depression common
Color Vision	Normal to abnormal
Dark Adaptation	Elevated rod threshold
ERG	Scotopic b-wave reduced
EOG	Normal to subnormal
Fluorescein Angiogram	Areas of nonperfusion and spots of leakage from abnormal capillaries

TREATMENT	PATHOLOGY	SYNONYMS
None; prophylactic laser photocoagulation	Not known	None in general use

DIFFERENTIAL DIAGNOSIS
Vitreoretinal dystrophies (see Table 12, p. 209)

REFERENCES
178, 183, 299

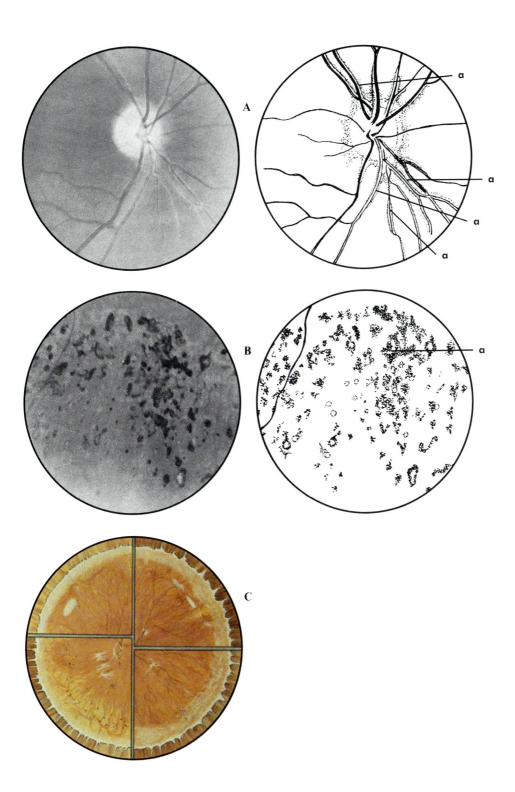

Figure 64
Snowflake Vitreoretinal Degeneration

A, Fundus photograph (OD) of a 44-year-old male. Retinal arteries and veins show sheathing near the optic disc *(a)*.

B, Fundus photograph of the same patient shows clumps of pigment near the equator *(a)*. If a scleral depressor is used, snowflakes are observed in this area. Most of the snowflakes are so tiny that they are not clearly visible as individual dots in this picture. Fundus changes represent stages III and IV.

C, Fundus drawings at different stages of the disease. Top left, stage I: marked white with pressure (WWP) is all around the extreme fundus periphery. A separate area of WWP is found between the ora and equator. Top right, stage II: snowflake degeneration is apparent. Minute discrete yellow-white dots that resemble snowflakes appear in the areas of WWP. Surface of the affected retina is slightly elevated, and elevation is craterlike in some places. Snowflakes also appear along retinal vessels. Chalky white clusters of short, needlelike structures are seen in an equatorial area in the 2 o'clock position. Faint vitreous opacity appears near the posterior pole. Bottom right, stage III: this drawing shows sheathing of retinal vessels, chorioretinal pigmentation, and fibrillar vitreous condensation. Bottom left, stage IV: stage is characterized by increased pigmentation and the disappearance of retinal vessels. Retinal vessels cannot be traced as far as the equator. Note sheathing of the vessels near the disc and focal chorioretinal atrophy. The whole retina looks atrophic. Swirling vitreous strands float in the vitreous cavity. (**A-C,** reproduced and redrawn from Hirose T, Lee KY, and Schepens CL: Snowflake degeneration in hereditary vitreoretinal degeneration, Am J Ophthalmol 77:143, 1974. Published with permission from The American Journal of Ophthalmology. Copyright by the Ophthalmic Publishing Company.)

Familial Exudative Vitreoretinopathy FIGURE 65

KEY SYMPTOMS
Asymptomatic or visual acuity reduction
Strabismus

KEY FINDINGS
Three stages (Gow and Oliver)
Stage 1
Asymptomatic and good vision; posterior vitreous detachment; retinal traction, white with or without pressure, and peripheral cystoid degeneration
Stage 2
Temporal vessels tortuous; subretinal exudate and temporal fibrovascular scar; dragged disc; ectopic macula
Stage 3
Retinal detachment, secondary cataracts, band keratopathy, iris atrophy, posterior synechiae, and secondary neovascular glaucoma
Also Reported
Vitreous hemorrhage; peripheral avascular areas; progression usually stops at any stage at age 20

INHERITANCE	ONSET	PROGRESSION	PROGNOSIS
AD	First and second decade	Slow	Good to poor

LABORATORY STUDIES
Visual Acuity	20/20 to light perception
Refraction	80% of patients are myopic
Visual Fields	Constricted
Color Vision	Normal to abnormal
Dark Adaptation	Normal
ERG	Usually normal
EOG	Usually normal
Fluorescein Angiogram	Tortuous vessels, macular leakage, some vessels stretched out, avascular near equator, leaking neovascularization, and macular edema

TREATMENT
Photocoagulation and cryopexy of some lesions

PATHOLOGY
Retinal detachment, acellular vitreous membrane, telangiectatic blood vessels with thick walls, and exudates

SYNONYMS
Criswick-Schepens syndrome

DIFFERENTIAL DIAGNOSIS
Retrolental fibroplasia
Congenital retinal folds
Vitreoretinal dystrophies (see Table 12, p. 209)
Uveitis
Coats' disease
Eales' disease
Toxocara
Persistent hypoplastic posterior vitreous

REFERENCES
38, 41, 50, 78, 151, 269, 337, 351, 355

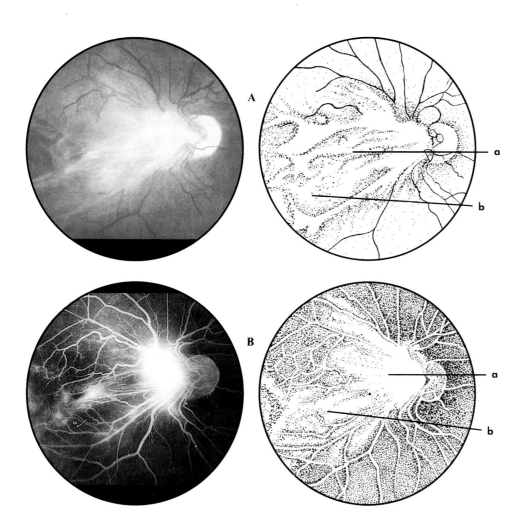

Figure 65

Familial Exudative Vitreoretinopathy

A 19-year-old female with a 10-year history of decreased vision OD. One sister is also affected.

A, Fundus photograph (OD) shows traction on the retina to the temporal side *(a)*, with a falciform fold that extends toward the temporal retina through the macula. There is a shallow retinal detachment *(b)* between the macula and the temporal periphery.

B, Angiogram shows hyperfluorescence of the temporal side of the optic disc *(a)* and distortion of the retinal vessels in the macular area *(b)*.

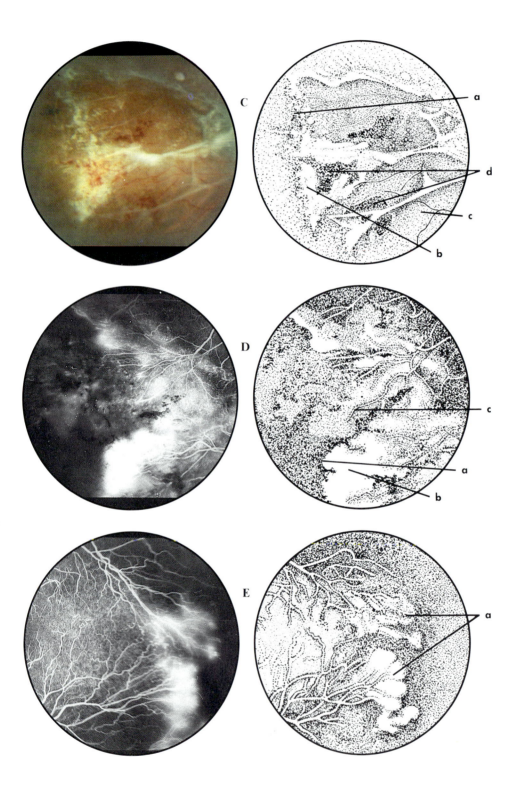

C, Fundus photograph of the temporal retina showing a well-demarcated line *(a)* with subretinal yellow exudates *(b)*, shallow tractional retinal detachment *(c)*, and some intraretinal and subretinal hemorrhage *(d)*.

D, Angiogram shows abrupt cessation of the choriocapillaris in the temporal periphery *(a)*, with leakage *(b)* and some shunts *(c)*.

E, Angiogram (OS) showing diffuse dye leakage from the retinal vessels in the temporal periphery *(a)*. No vessels are seen beyond this line.

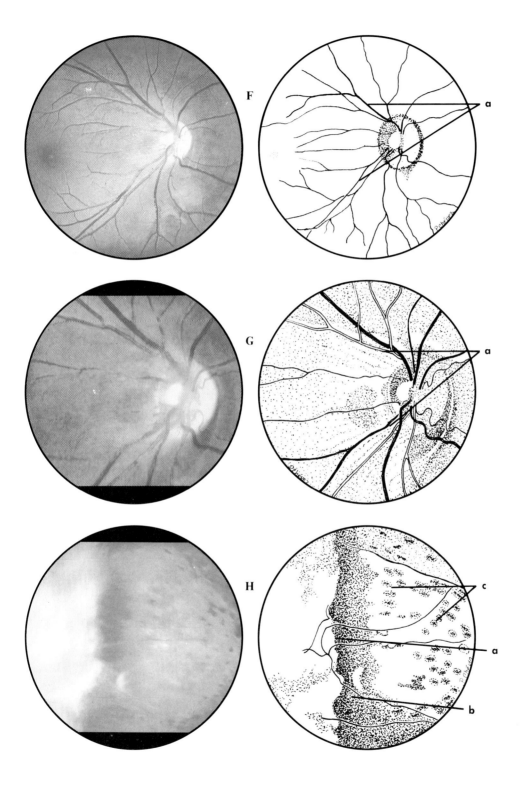

F-G, Fundus photographs of a 17-year-old female who has 2 family members with retinal detachment. The photographs show dragging of the vessels *(a)*.

G, Enlargement of **F** showing the optic disc in greater detail. Note dragged vessels *(a)*.

H, Fundus photograph of the temporal periphery showing a well-demarcated line *(a)*, with fibrovascular proliferation and hemorrhages. There is a shallow retinal detachment inferiorly *(b)*. Photocoagulation scars are visible in the temporal retina *(c)*.

Autosomal Dominant Vitreoretinochoroidopathy FIGURE 66

KEY SYMPTOMS
Asymptomatic (early)
Mild decrease in vision (late)
(Note absence of nyctalopia)

KEY FINDINGS
Coarse pigmentary retinopathy; 360 degrees, extends from the vortex veins to the ora serrata
Superficial punctate yellow-white opacities in pigmented areas
Arteriolar narrowing and occlusion
Microaneurysms and neovascularization in nonischemic areas
Cystoid macular edema
Choroidal atrophy may be seen in some cases
Vitreous changes include fibrillar condensation, opacities, pigmented cells, and hemorrhages
Presenile cortical and subcortical cataract

INHERITANCE	ONSET	PROGRESSION	PROGNOSIS
AD	First decade	Slow	Good to 20/100

LABORATORY STUDIES
Visual Acuity	20/20 to 20/100
Refraction	Emmetropia to low myopia
Visual Fields	Normal to mild constriction
Color Vision	Not described
Dark Adaptation	Not described
ERG	Normal early; slight abnormality late
EOG	Usually normal
Fluorescein Angiogram	Window defects in the periphery with multiple foci of blocked fluorescence; cystoid macular edema is common

TREATMENT	PATHOLOGY	SYNONYMS
None	Not described	None in general use

DIFFERENTIAL DIAGNOSIS
Vitreoretinal dystrophies (see Table 12, p. 209)

REFERENCES
38, 198

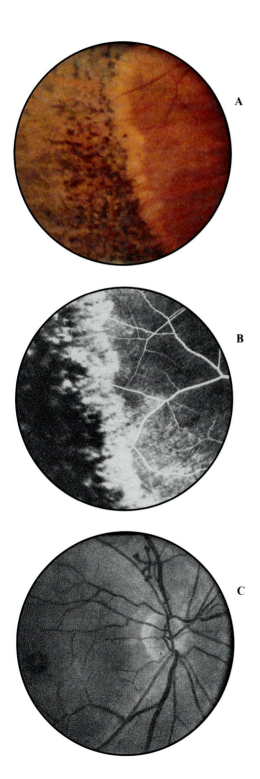

Figure 66
Autosomal Dominant Vitreoretinochoroidopathy

A, Fundus photograph showing diffuse pigmentation between the equator and the ora serrata. Note the discrete posterior boundary with an annular band of hypopigmentation. The retinal vessels are occluded inside the dystrophic zone.

B, Angiogram showing closure of the retinal vessels in the hypofluorescent hypopigmented zone. Hyperfluorescence is present along the central margin of the dystrophic zone.

C, Fundus photograph (OD) of a 7-year-old male showing preretinal neovascularization adjacent to the optic disc. (**A-C,** reproduced and redrawn from Kaufman SJ, Goldberg MF, Orth DH, Fishman GA, Tessler H, and Mizuno K: Autosomal dominant vitreoretinochoroidopathy, Arch Ophthalmol 100:272, 1982. Copyright 1982, American Medical Association.)

Other Causes of Retinal Diseases

CONGENITAL INFECTIONS
TOXIC RETINOPATHIES
NUTRITIONAL DISEASE

Other causes of retinal diseases are included because some of these diseases may result in a secondary retinal degeneration similar to that in the retinal and choroidal dystrophies. Descriptions of these diseases are provided to facilitate differential diagnosis.

Congenital Luetic (Syphilis) Chorioretinitis   FIGURE 67

KEY SYMPTOMS
Asymptomatic or mild visual loss
Photophobia (corneal involvement)

KEY FINDINGS
Variable picture; syphilis is the "great imitator"
Pigmentary retinopathy similar to retinitis pigmentosa
Salt-and-pepper changes in the midperiphery
Optic disc pallor and narrowing of vessels
Areas of chorioretinal atrophy along vessels in some cases
Ocular abnormalities may not be evident at birth but are usually apparent by the age of 6
Interstitial keratitis may occur later (ages 6 to 25)
Early systemic findings in the newborn include dermatitis, hepatosplenomegaly, meningitis, and osteochondritis
Late sequelae include frontal boss, saddle nose, Hutchinson's teeth, deafness, cataracts, and glaucoma

INHERITANCE	ONSET	PROGRESSION	PROGNOSIS
Congenital	Before age 6	Rapid (early)	Good for vision

LABORATORY STUDIES

Visual Acuity	Normal, unless macula or cornea involved
Visual Fields	Scotomas corresponding to the lesions
Color Vision	Normal
Dark Adaptation	Normal
ERG	Usually normal
EOG	Usually normal
Fluorescein Angiogram	Multiple choroidal and RPE defects with variable hyperfluorescence

TREATMENT	PATHOLOGY	SYNONYMS
Penicillin	RPE and choroidal atrophy, with RPE migration and dehiscence of Bruch's membrane	None in general use

DIFFERENTIAL DIAGNOSIS
Pigmentary retinopathy (see Table 6, p. 118)
Progressive nyctalopia (see Table 7, p. 120)

REFERENCES
18, 312, 320

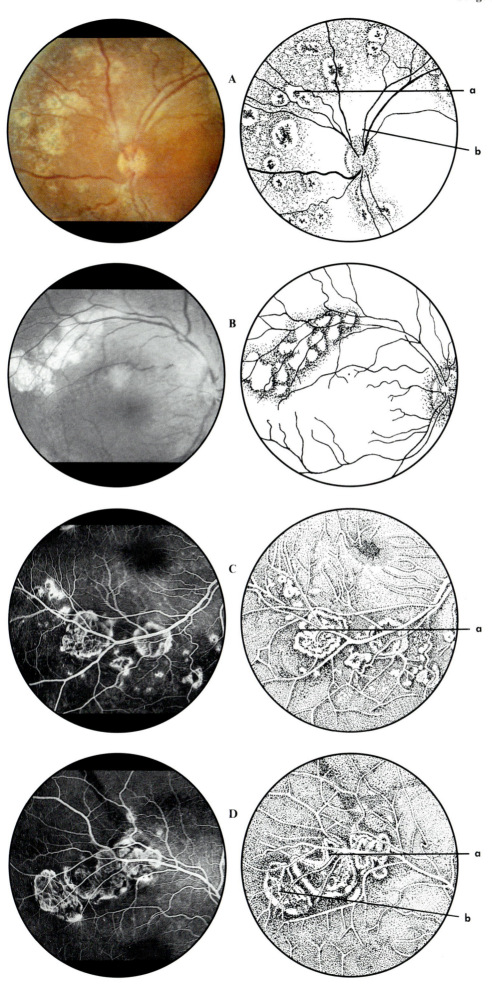

Figure 67
Congenital Luetic (Syphilis) Chorioretinitis

A 9-year-old male with congenital syphilis whose mother acquired the infection in the first trimester of pregnancy. His visual acuity is 20/30 OU. The ERG and EOG are normal.

A, Fundus photograph (OS) shows multiple pigmentary changes in the nasal retina *(a)* and an area of RPE disturbance *(b)* that extends to the optic nerve.

B, Fundus photograph (OD) of the macular area showing some areas of RPE and choroidal atrophy along the temporal vessels. The optic nerve is normal, and there is no vessel attenuation.

C-D, Angiogram (OD) of the superior and inferior temporal vessels showing a well-demarcated area of atrophy *(a)* with loss of choriocapillaris. Large choroidal vessels remain in some lesions *(b)*.

Congenital Rubella Retinitis FIGURE 68

KEY SYMPTOMS
Asymptomatic or mild visual acuity reduction

KEY FINDINGS
Maternal infection acquired in the first trimester of pregnancy
Salt-and-pepper mottling of the RPE in the posterior pole
Bilateral in 80%; may progress in early childhood
Pigment mottling becomes less prominent in adulthood
Other findings include cataracts, glaucoma, microphthalmos, depigmented iris, deafness, and congenital heart disease

INHERITANCE	ONSET	PROGRESSION	PROGNOSIS
None	Congenital	Usually none	Good for vision

LABORATORY STUDIES
Visual Acuity	20/20 to 20/50
Visual Fields	Normal
Color Vision	Normal
Dark Adaptation	Normal
ERG	Normal
EOG	Usually normal
Fluorescein Angiogram	Shows mottled hyperfluorescence caused by loss of RPE

TREATMENT	PATHOLOGY	SYNONYMS
None	Focal areas of atrophy of the RPE; the macular area is more affected; retina and choroid are unaffected	None in general use

DIFFERENTIAL DIAGNOSIS
Dystrophies of the RPE (p. 60)
Carrier state of X-L dystrophies
Toxic retinopathies (pp. 236, 238)

REFERENCES
2, 42, 175, 380

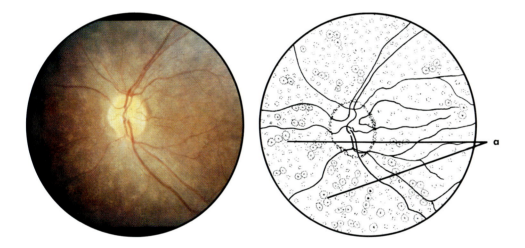

Figure 68

Congenital Rubella Retinitis

Fundus photograph (OS) of a 13-year-old male with a history of congenital rubella. His symptoms are deafness, cardiac defects, dental abnormalities, cataracts, and nystagmus. The photograph shows mottling of the fundus with a salt-and-pepper pattern *(a)*. There is also mild pallor of the optic disc.

Phenothiazine Retinopathy FIGURE 69

KEY SYMPTOMS
Decreased "brownish" vision
Nyctalopia
Color vision defect

KEY FINDINGS
Pigmentation of skin, conjunctiva, cornea, and lens
Fundus shows widespread fine granularity and clumping of pigment caused by RPE changes
Some patients have pigmentary changes with RPE and choriocapillaris atrophy
Toxicity may develop in 3 to 8 weeks with as little as 800 mg of phenothiazine
Phenothiazine derivatives are accumulated in the pigment granules of the RPE and uvea, so toxicity may progress after the medication is discontinued
Severe cases may simulate chorioretinal diseases such as gyrate atrophy or choroideremia
Vessel attenuation is seen late in the disease

INHERITANCE	ONSET	PROGRESSION	PROGNOSIS
None	Variable	Rapid	Good if medication is discontinued

LABORATORY STUDIES
Visual Acuity	Decreased
Visual Fields	Constricted, central scotoma
Color Vision	Abnormal; tritan defect common
Dark Adaptation	Delayed rod adaptation
ERG	Abnormal to nonrecordable
EOG	Abnormal
Fluorescein Angiogram	Mottled hyperfluorescence caused by RPE atrophy; areas of hypofluorescence

TREATMENT	PATHOLOGY	SYNONYMS
Stop medication	Widespread RPE and photoreceptor atrophy; RPE proliferation and lipofuscin accumulation	Thioridazine retinopathy Mellaril® toxicity

DIFFERENTIAL DIAGNOSIS
Pigmentary retinopathy (see Table 6, p. 118)

REFERENCES
73, 81, 211, 247, 300, 366

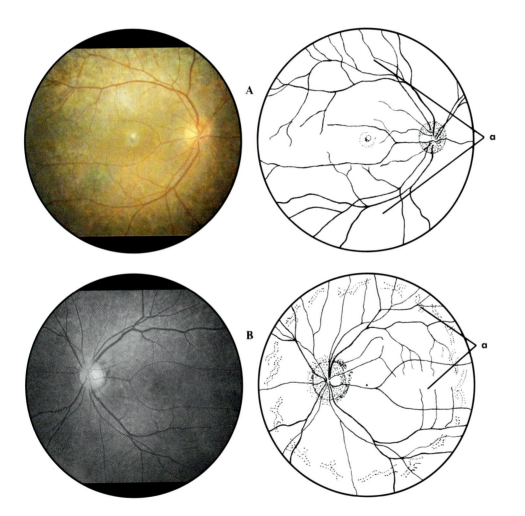

Figure 69
Phenothiazine Retinopathy

A 41-year-old female, asymptomatic, with a visual acuity of 20/25 OU, who has a 2-year history of ingesting high doses of phenothiazine. The scotopic ERG is abnormal, the photopic ERG is normal, and the EOG is subnormal.

A-B, Fundus photographs (OD and OS) showing abnormal coloration of the fundus, widespread defects of the RPE, and characteristic mottling *(a)*. Optic disc and retinal vessels are normal. (**A-B,** courtesy of John Lean, M.D.)

Chloroquine Retinopathy FIGURE 70

KEY SYMPTOMS
Asymptomatic (early) or color vision abnormal
Visual acuity reduction (late)

KEY FINDINGS
Fundus is normal early; later there is macular mottling, loss of foveal reflex, and parafoveal ring of RPE atrophy with paracentral scotoma
Bull's-eye maculopathy develops later
Pigmentary retinopathy, with a pale optic disc and attenuated vessels, develops late
Chloroquine is accumulated in the RPE and is slowly excreted; damage may progress after cessation of treatment in advanced cases
Retinal toxicity occurs with accumulated doses of 100 grams or more
Other reported abnormalities are diminished corneal sensitivity, subepithelial pigmentation, poliosis and extraocular muscle palsies

INHERITANCE	ONSET	PROGRESSION	PROGNOSIS
None	Variable	Rapid or slow	Good in early stages; poor later on

LABORATORY STUDIES
Visual Acuity	Decreased
Visual Fields	Central, paracentral, and ring scotomas
Color Vision	Abnormal
Dark Adaptation	Usually normal
ERG	Abnormal (see Figure 82, Appendix A)
EOG	Normal to abnormal (see Figure 91, Appendix A)
Fluorescein Angiogram	Normal early; bull's-eye pattern of hyperfluorescence later

TREATMENT	PATHOLOGY	SYNONYMS
Stop medication	Degeneration of the RPE with migration into the retina; degeneration of sensory retina and ganglion cells	Chloroquine toxicity Hydroxychloroquine toxicity

DIFFERENTIAL DIAGNOSIS
Pigmentary retinopathy (see Table 6, p. 118)
Bull's-eye maculopathy (see Table 9, p. 166)

REFERENCES
6, 45, 79, 170, 174, 304, 318, 369

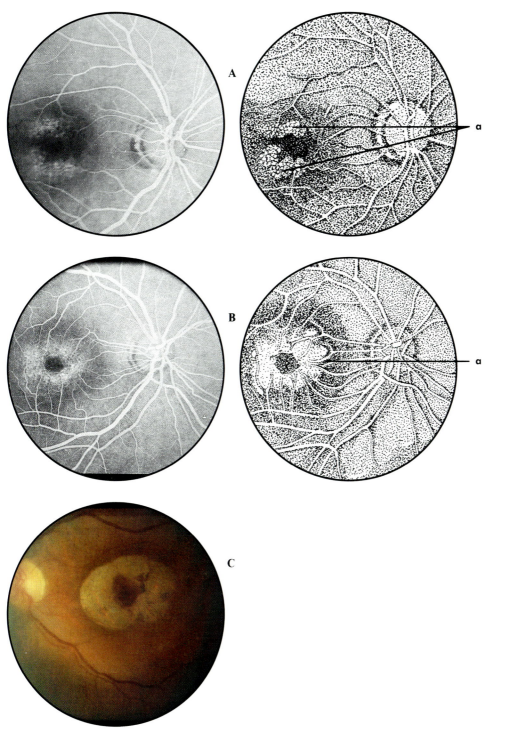

Figure 70
Chloroquine Retinopathy

A, Angiogram (OD) of a 42-year-old female with rheumatoid arthritis who was treated with chloroquine for several years. Hyperfluorescent area is seen surrounding the central macula *(a)*. This case probably represents an early macular toxicity.

B, Angiogram (OD) of a 53-year-old female treated with chloroquine for lupus erythematosus. A bull's-eye macular lesion *(a)* is evident in the angiogram.

C, Fundus photograph (OS) showing an advanced macular lesion. This patient received several years of treatment with chloroquine for juvenile rheumatoid arthritis. (**C,** courtesy of Peter Liggett, M.D.)

Metallosis Bulbi (Metallic Intraocular Foreign Bodies) FIGURE 71

KEY SYMPTOMS
Visual acuity reduction
Nyctalopia (occasionally)
Tunnel vision (occasionally)

KEY FINDINGS
Siderosis
Retained ferrous intraocular foreign body
Retinal toxicity begins within days or years
Rust spots on iris, cornea, or lens may occur
Pigmentary retinopathy, cataracts, retinal detachment, glaucoma, and vitreous liquefaction may contribute to visual loss
Chalcosis
Intraocular metallic copper
Large bodies may cause acute chalcosis with hypopyon
Kayser-Fleischer ring; corneal pigmentation
Sunflower anterior capsular cataract
Disease progression is similar to that of siderosis, but prognosis is much better

INHERITANCE	ONSET	PROGRESSION	PROGNOSIS
None	Days to years	Variable	Good to poor

LABORATORY STUDIES
- **Visual Acuity**: 20/40 to light perception
- **Visual Fields**: May be constricted
- **Color Vision**: Normal to abnormal
- **Dark Adaptation**: Normal to abnormal rod function
- **ERG**: Abnormal: b-wave reduction (see Figure 82, Appendix A)
- **EOG**: Usually abnormal (may be normal)

TREATMENT
Remove intraocular foreign body if toxicity is documented

PATHOLOGY
RPE atrophy and proliferation with extensive retinal degeneration or necrosis is possible but is usually not uniform; some areas are spared

SYNONYMS
Chalcosis
Siderosis

DIFFERENTIAL DIAGNOSIS
Pigmentary retinopathy (see Table 6, p. 118)
Progressive nyctalopia (see Table 7, p. 120)
Proliferative vitreoretinopathy

REFERENCES
5, 68, 207, 323, 327

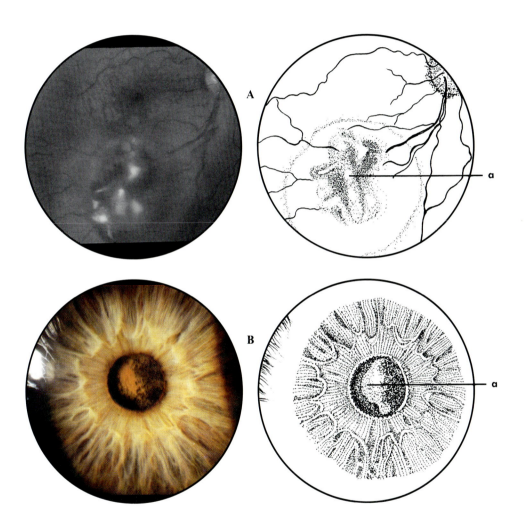

Figure 71
Metallosis Bulbi (Metallic Intraocular Foreign Bodies)

An intraocular metallic foreign body can produce a toxic reaction that is localized to the retina or that affects several tissues in the eye.

A, Fundus photograph taken shortly after the introduction of a metallic foreign body into the eye. Localized hemorrhage and edema *(a)* are present. If surgery is not performed soon after the accident, the patient should be monitored with the ERG and EOG to detect toxicity of the retina. If the ERG or EOG shows progressive loss, surgical removal of the foreign body is necessary.

B, Fundus photograph showing advanced siderosis bulbi with lens deposits of metal ions *(a)*.

NUTRITIONAL DISEASE

Vitamin A Deficiency Retinopathy FIGURE 72

KEY SYMPTOMS
Nyctalopia
Tunnel vision

KEY FINDINGS
Vitamin A deficiency can be secondary to inadequate dietary intake (malnutrition syndrome) or malabsorption states (celiac sprue, jejunal bypass surgery)
Conjunctival and corneal xerosis (Bitot's spots and superficial punctate keratopathy)
Multiple flecks at the level of the RPE; these lesions are yellow-white, small, irregular, and similar to drusen
The funduscopic appearance has been called *fundus xerophthalmicus*
After vitamin A treatment, there may be a reversal of the symptoms and lesions

INHERITANCE	ONSET	PROGRESSION	PROGNOSIS
None	Variable	Rapid	Good with treatment

LABORATORY STUDIES
Visual Acuity	Not affected
Visual Fields	Constricted
Color Vision	Normal
Dark Adaptation	Abnormal rod function
ERG	Scotopic severely abnormal; photopic abnormal
EOG	Probably normal
Fluorescein Angiogram	Fundus lesions may show hyperfluorescence at the level of the RPE

TREATMENT
Vitamin A

PATHOLOGY
In animals there is disorganization of rod outer segments and loss of photoreceptors

SYNONYMS
Fundus xerophthalmicus
Uyemura's syndrome

DIFFERENTIAL DIAGNOSIS
Flecked retina diseases (see Table 5, p. 114)
Progressive nyctalopia (see Table 7, p. 120)

REFERENCES
52, 167, 231, 344, 356

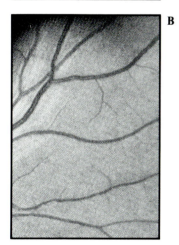

Figure 72
Vitamin A Deficiency Retinopathy

A-B, Fundus photographs (OD) from a 25-year-old female with panocular xerophthalmia.

A, Photograph shows a sharp transition between normal and abnormal retina.

B, Photograph shows the same area 1½ months later, after treatment with vitamin A. Depigmented lesions have largely disappeared. (**A-B,** reproduced and redrawn from Sommer A, Tjakrasudjatma S, Djunaedi E, and Green R: Vitamin A–responsive panocular xerophthalmia in a healthy adult, Arch Ophthalmol 96:1630, 1978. Copyright 1978, American Medical Association.)

Part III APPENDICES

Review of Electrophysiologic Tests
Review of Psychophysical Tests

Appendix A   REVIEW OF ELECTROPHYSIOLOGIC TESTS

The electroretinogram (ERG) and the electrooculogram (EOG) are essential, objective tests of retinal function without which many retinal diseases could not by identified with certainty. The tests are now widely available, and experience with the tests is required in all ophthalmology residency training programs. The visual-evoked response (VER) is less useful in diagnosing retinal disease, but it is essential in evaluating impairment of the optic nerve. The VER and ERG are particularly useful in the early distinction between congenital optic atrophy and Leber's amaurosis. The VER is absent in both, but the ERG is normal in the former.

The following pages present a brief overview of the basis and utility of these tests. An understanding of the usefulness of the ERG and EOG requires recognition of their important limitations. The tests represent *total* retinal function. Focal abnormalities are associated with normal test results. When retinal involvement approaches 30% to 40% the tests become more abnormal, so progressing abnormality can be used to document progressing retinal involvement. Many retinal diseases are global but initially give normal test results when the disease is minimal. Again, progressing test abnormality may signify disease progression. Finally, abnormal test results indicate involvement of a large percentage of the retinal area, even though the retina may show only focal abnormality. Thus the abnormal EOG in Best's disease reflects abnormality of the RPE of the entire retina.

The ERG is a flash-evoked potential recorded from the cornea with a contact lens electrode and topical anesthesia. It provides an objective measure of total retinal function and can be recorded at any age. Standard recordings take about 30 minutes and should include pupillary dilation. The ERG should be used to confirm the diagnosis of any retinal degeneration, toxic retinopathy, metallosis, or generalized retinal dysfunction. It is not useful in focal disease (Figure 73).

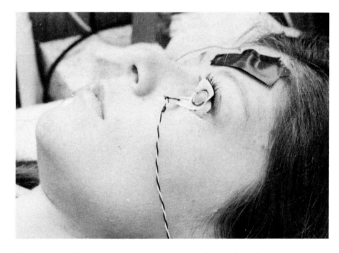

Figure 73. Burian-Allen contact lens electrode. The frosted lens provides Ganzfeld stimulation.

ERG waveform consists of an initial negative wave (a-wave) followed by a larger positive wave (b-wave). Small wavelets surmounting the b-wave are called oscillatory potentials. The time from the flash to the onset of the response is called its latency. The time from the flash to the peak of a response is called its peak delay. Latency and peak delay may be prolonged in a diseased retina. The amplitude is measured baseline to trough (a-wave) or a-wave trough to b-wave peak (b-wave, Figure 74).

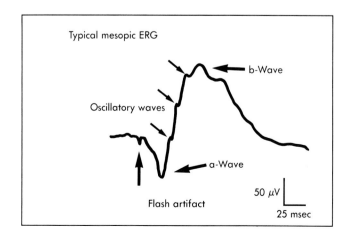

Figure 74. Mesopic ERG recorded with a high-intensity flash from a dark-adapted eye.

Generators of the ERG are (1) the receptors that produce a cornea-negative slow potential called the *late receptor potential*, or *PIII*, and (2) the postsynaptic cells of the inner plexiform layer, including Müller cells, which generate a delayed cornea-positive potential called *PII*. These two potentials of opposite polarity are added together to produce the biphasic ERG. Oscillatory potentials are added to the b-wave by elements of inner retina. *Ganglion cells do not contribute to the ERG* (Figure 75).

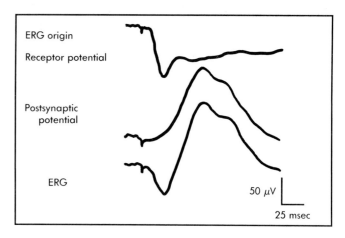

Figure 75. The ERG recorded at the cornea is the sum of a negative receptor potential and a positive wave generated by Müller cells.

Rod and cone ERGs are easily distinguished by their waveforms, which vary according to whether rods only (scotopic), rods and cones (mesopic), or cones only (photopic) are activated (Figure 76):

Dim flash + dark adaptation = scotopic ERG
Bright flash + dark adaptation = mesopic ERG
Bright flash + light adaptation = photopic ERG

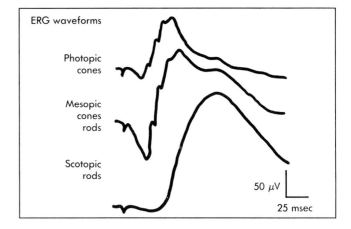

Figure 76. The ERG waveform varies according to whether the stimulus conditions excite rods and/or cones.

ERG evaluation: Providing the entire retina is stimulated, the amplitude of the ERG is proportional to the total area of functional retina. Amplitude reduction without alteration of waveform suggests a focal abnormality such as an area of retinal detachment or atrophy with the remaining retina being normal. A 50% detachment reduces amplitude by 50%. Generalized abnormalities that reduce amplitude are always associated with an abnormal waveform such as slowing and loss of b-wave (Figure 77).

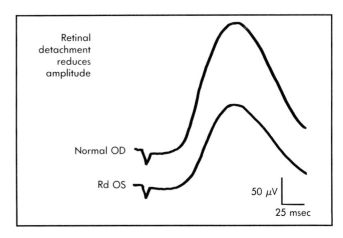

Figure 77. ERG of a patient with 50% retinal detachment (Rd) OS. Note that the amplitude is reduced, but the waveform is normal.

Slowing of the ERG waveform is typical of retinal degenerations and toxicities. It is particularly significant in early tapetoretinal degenerations and may be seen in carriers of these conditions (retinitis pigmentosa and choroideremia). Waveforms may appear slowed if retinal illumination by the flash is inadequate, thus several intensities of stimulation should always be used (Figure 78). Abnormality of ERG waveform always indicates generalized retinal abnormality.

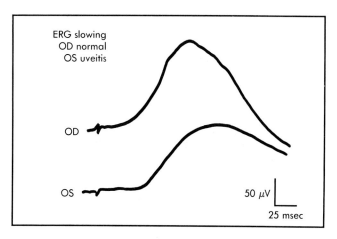

Figure 78. ERGs from a patient with uveitis OS. Note the loss of amplitude and the increased peak delay of b-wave OS.

b-Wave reduction or loss may occur without loss of the receptor potential in conditions affecting the inner retina and in various degenerations and toxicities. The resulting ERG is referred to as *negative*. Negative ERGs are often seen in CSNB, diabetic retinopathy, and retinoschisis, as well as in the retinal degenerations (Figure 79).

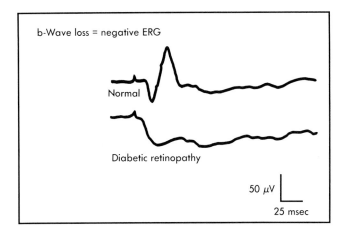

Figure 79. ERG of a patient with severe diabetic retinopathy. The b-wave is lost because of inner retinal ischemia.

CAUTION: **With high-intensity stimulation** such as is used for the bright-flash ERG, the a-wave becomes very large and may submerge the b-wave. The normal bright-flash ERG, however, is very fast and does not resemble the negative ERG, which is always slowed, even when evoked by a bright flash. ERG latency also decreases with intensity in a normal eye, and this serves to distinguish normal from abnormal bright-flash ERGs (Figure 80).

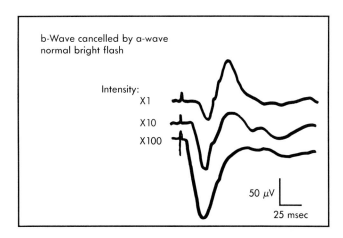

Figure 80. The ERG evoked by a very bright flash is normally negative because of a large a-wave. Note that latency is very short.

Oscillatory potentials are small wavelets on the b-wave best evoked with mesopic stimulation *(a)*. The wavelets can be emphasized with appropriate filtering *(b)*. Loss of wavelets occurs in diseases such as diabetic retinopathy that are characterized by inner retinal ischemia *(c)*. However, these diseases are sometimes patchy in retinal involvement, so loss of oscillatory potentials is not seen in all such patients. Also, some normal subjects have negligible oscillatory potentials (Figure 81).

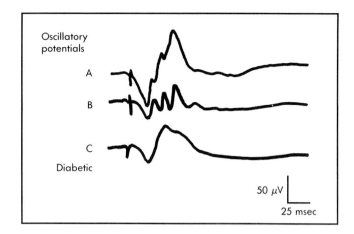

Figure 81. ERGs showing a normal photopic response *(a)* also recorded to show the oscillatory potentials *(b)*, which are lacking in diabetic retinopathy *(c)*.

Retinal toxicity resulting from conditions such as metallosis or drugs (e.g., chloroquine) usually causes depression of the b-wave, slowing, and a shift of the ERG to negative. If retinal involvement is patchy, however, loss of amplitude can occur without the other changes, simulating retinal detachment. It is not unusual for the ERG abnormalities to reverse following removal of a foreign body or cessation of therapy. Toxicity usually also results in an abnormal EOG (Figure 82).

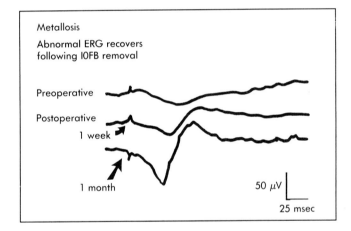

Figure 82. ERGs from a patient with metallosis recorded before and after the removal of a ferrous intraocular foreign body. Good function was recovered.

Bright-flash ERG is evoked with a photographic flash about 100,000 times brighter than the standard ERG flash. It is used in patients with dense opacities or vitreous hemorrhage. For the test to be most successful, a saturated response must be obtained; that is, using still brighter flashes does not increase the response amplitude. The amplitude and waveform of the saturated response then accurately reveal the status of the total retina. Of course, the response does not reflect macular function (Figure 83).

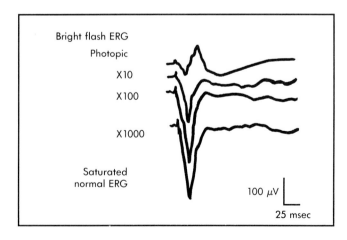

Figure 83. ERGs evoked with progressively more intense flashes. The b-wave is overcome by the a-wave. Latencies become shorter.

Focal ERG: It is possible to evoke an ERG with a small spot of light centered on the macula. This is best done with a modified nonmydriatic fundus camera, with which the fundus is visualized by infrared light during testing. This ensures that the stimulus is directed onto the macula during the many repetitions of the test. The test is useful in evaluating macular involvement in patients with a retinal degeneration but normal acuity or with reduced acuity of unexplained origin (Figure 84).

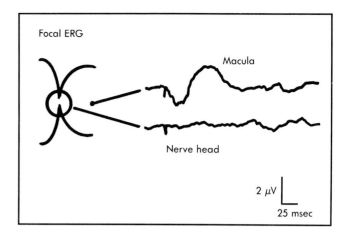

Figure 84. ERGs evoked with a 5-degree spot centered on the macula. No response is obtained when the spot is centered on the nerve head.

Focal pathology: The standard ERG is normal in macular degeneration unless the disease process extends well beyond the macula, as in advanced Stargardt's disease. This occurs because the macula generates only about 1% of the ERG, a contribution too small to be detected. Generally, disease processes involving less than about 15% of the retina cannot be detected by the ERG. Because ganglion cells do not contribute to the ERG, it is normal in optic atrophy. The ERG is also normal with drusen of the retina or nerve head (Figure 85).

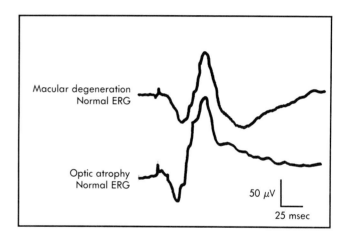

Figure 85. ERGs recorded from a patient with macular degeneration and a patient with a traumatic section of the optic nerve (lower trace) 3 years before recording.

CSNB can be classified on the basis of ERG pattern. CSNB type I is characterized by a negative mesopic ERG that is peculiar in that it is not slowed and has a rather square waveform. CSNB type II is associated with reduction of both a- and b-waves. The photopic b-wave in CSNB type I may be relatively normal. In both types of CSNB the scotopic ERG is severely depressed or absent. Those cases in which the scotopic ERG is still present are called *incomplete* (Figure 86).

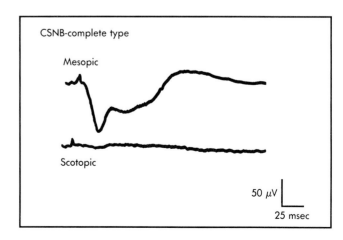

Figure 86. ERGs recorded from a patient with CSNB. Absence of the scotopic ERG indicates the complete type.

Cone degenerations, achromatopsia, rod monochromatism: These conditions are characterized by a severely depressed or absent photopic ERG and a normal scotopic ERG. Testing with colored light may reveal relative preservation of one cone mechanism in some patients. The ERG will be abnormal only if the disease process involves the entire retina. Abnormality of scotopic responses, even if slight, indicates a cone-rod degeneration with a substantially different prognosis (Figure 87).

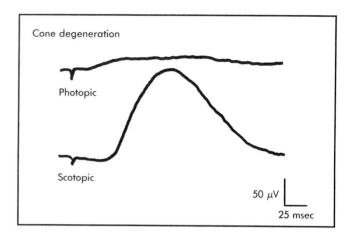

Figure 87. ERGs from a patient with a cone degeneration. Rod function (scotopic ERG) is normal.

Tapetoretinal degeneration, choroideremia, retinitis pigmentosa, rod-cone degeneration: These progressive retinal degenerations are associated with ERG abnormality early in onset. The abnormality is typically loss of rod function in excess of cone function, but both photopic and scotopic ERGs are abnormal (Figure 88). ERG abnormality may be seen in carriers and is often found in patients before the onset of symptoms. ERG responses may be unrecordable, although some visual function remains.

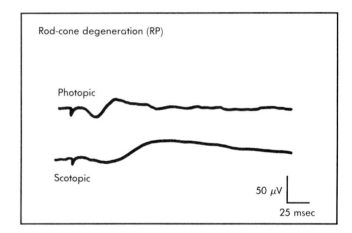

Figure 88. ERGs from a patient with a rod-cone degeneration. Both scotopic and photopic ERGs are abnormal.

The EOG is a recording of the corneofundal potential. Metabolic activity of the retinal pigment epithelium and the photoreceptors generates a steady transretinal voltage that causes the cornea to be about 10 mv positive with respect to the back of the eye. This corneofundal potential decreases during dark adaptation and increases during light adaptation. It is evaluated indirectly by noting the voltage between periorbital electrodes during eye movement (Figure 89).

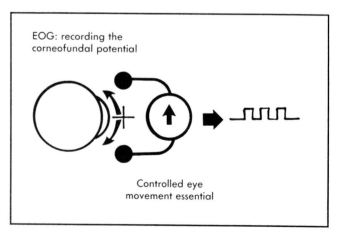

Figure 89. A diagram of EOG generation. The positive cornea causes the periorbital electrodes to become positive as the cornea nears the electrodes.

The light-dark ratio of the EOG is calculated by dividing the minimum value obtained during dark adaptation into the maximum value obtained during light adaptation. A ratio of 2.0 ± 0.4 is normal. Values of 1.5 or less are almost always abnormal. The test requires patient cooperation and standard light adaptation; thus it is not appropriate for small children or those who cannot be adequately light adapted. Normal values are never artifactual, but abnormal values may be so (Figure 90).

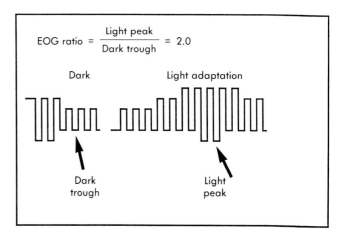

Figure 90. A diagram of an EOG recording: 15 minutes dark adapted and 15 minutes light adapted. The method of EOG ratio calculation is shown.

Retinal degeneration, regardless of cause, is associated with an abnormal EOG *if* the receptors or RPE are involved in the disease process. The EOG is occasionally abnormal when the ERG is borderline in retinal toxicity resulting from metallosis or chloroquine. Abnormal EOGs may be found in carriers of retinitis pigmentosa or choroideremia. Generally, the EOG should be recorded from any patient capable of the test and for whom an ERG is indicated (Figure 91).

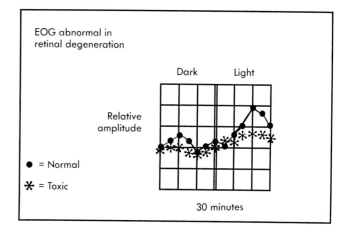

Figure 91. A graph of typical normal and abnormal EOGs. The latter is from a patient with chloroquine retinopathy. The EOG ratio is 1.3.

Vitelliform dystrophy (Best's disease) is associated with an abnormal EOG and a normal ERG. This dissociation is also seen in butterfly dystrophy and pattern dystrophy of Marmor and Byers. The diagnosis of adult-onset Best's disease should not be made without an EOG because some patients with late-onset vitelliform degeneration have normal EOGs. Also, cases of adult-onset Best's disease will be missed unless EOGs are recorded from patients with atypical macular degeneration (Figure 92).

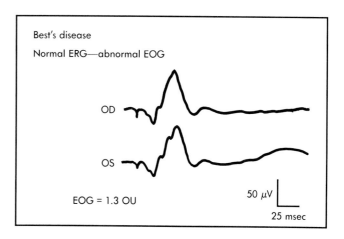

Figure 92. ERGs from a patient with Best's disease are normal, but the EOG ratio was 1.3 OU.

Flash visual-evoked response, or **VER,** is an electrical response recorded from the scalp overlying the occipital or visual cortex, evoked by a bright flash of light. A substantial part of the retina and central visual pathways must be intact for the response to be normal. The VER is very variable among individuals but is symmetric between the two eyes of the same individual. It is a useful objective test of visual function in infants and of the optic nerve and tract in adults (Figure 93).

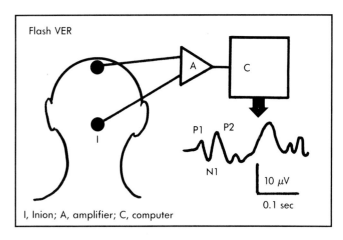

Figure 93. The method for flash VER recording. Primary response components P1, N1, and P2 are less variable than are the later secondary components.

VER waveform is complex and varies sufficiently among individuals so that subtle changes with disease may not be detected. However, a pathologic condition in one pathway can be recognized by comparing results with a normal VER evoked by stimulation of the fellow eye. A typical flash VER has an M shape with alternating positive and negative waves labelled *P1, N1, P2,* and *N2*. This primary response is followed by even more variable secondary waves. Abnormality of the VER results from either a retinal or a central nervous system (CNS) pathologic condition (Figure 94).

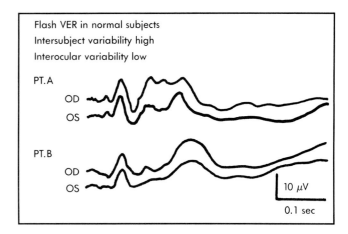

Figure 94. Flash VERs of two normal subjects. Intersubject variation is large, whereas interocular variation is small.

Lesions of the optic nerve or tract severely reduce or eliminate the VER. Normally the responses from stimulation of the two eyes are symmetric to within 10%; larger differences indicate a unilateral pathologic condition. Absence of the VER in a blind infant with a normal ERG is diagnostic of optic atrophy. In Leber's amaurosis, the ERG is abnormal. Compressive lesions, vascular accidents, and optic neuritis can also cause asymmetry of the VER (Figure 95).

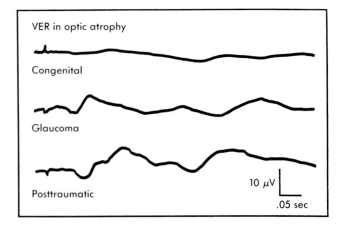

Figure 95. VERs of patients with optic atrophy. Note the loss of amplitude and simplification of waveform.

Amblyopia ex anopsia is often associated with loss of amplitude and slowing of responses in the affected eye. Thus the flash VER can be used to detect amblyopia in infants and children too young for subjective tests. The VER can also be used to monitor for the effects of eye patching. Changes associated with amblyopia are reversible as the dysfunction reverses. However, the test is not very sensitive, and substantial dysfunction often exists by the time the test is abnormal (Figure 96).

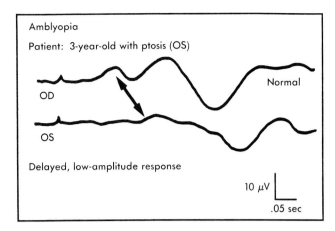

Figure 96. VER of a patient with amblyopia resulting from congenital ptosis. Note the loss of amplitude and slowing.

The pattern VER is recorded from the scalp, as is the flash VER, but the stimulus is an alternating checkerboard pattern of varying sized checks. A prominent feature of the response is a positive wave with a peak delay of about 100 msec, called *P100*, that shows very little variability among individuals. The pattern VER provides an indication of acuity in that the response is absent if the pattern is not resolved. The response is normal in functional amblyopia and in malingerers (Figure 97).

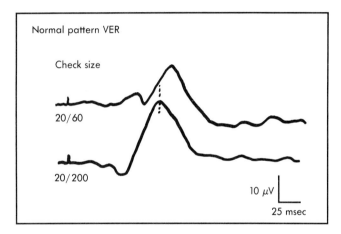

Figure 97. A normal pattern VER evoked by small and large checks. Note the shorter delay of the P100 wave with the larger checks.

Optic neuritis is associated with a characteristic delay of P100 in over 90% of patients. The delay persists, even though functional recovery of vision may have occurred. Often a delay is found in the apparently normal fellow eye of such patients (Figure 98). Tests for P100 should involve several check sizes to obtain the shortest peak delays. Generally, peak delays are longer with smaller check sizes (Figure 97). The pattern VER is often of lower amplitude in an amblyopic eye.

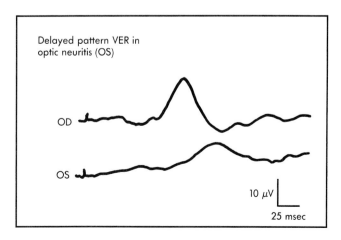

Figure 98. VERs of a patient with a history of optic neuritis OS. Note the delay of P100 OS compared with that of OD.

The pattern VER can be recorded only if the image is cast on the retina. Subject cooperation is required, and the response may be absent or delayed in a subject who refuses to maintain gaze on the pattern. Thus a normal response is possibly more significant than the absence of a response, particularly if the patient is not fully cooperative. The smallest pattern to evoke a response in a normal subject has an angular subtense equivalent to a Snellen acuity of about 20/60 (Figure 99).

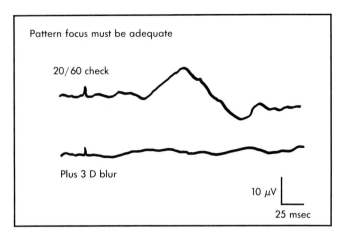

Figure 99. Pattern VERs evoked with the proper refraction and with a 3 diopter blur, which abolishes the response.

Retinal disease can cause the pattern VER to be abnormal. The patient in Figure 100 manifested severe uveitis and a visual acuity of counting fingers. The ERG was abnormal, and the flash and pattern VER were nonrecordable. After treatment and recovery the ERG returned to normal and visual acuity returned to 20/40. However, the pattern VER showed a delayed P100, suggesting that this patient had an associated optic neuritis that was masked by the uveitis.

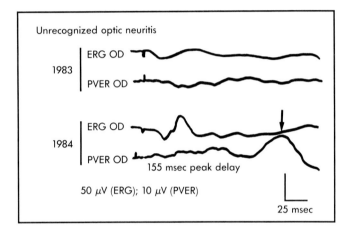

Figure 100. Pattern VERs of a patient with uveitis and unrecognized optic neuritis, which became evident because of a delayed P100 after recovery from the uveitis.

Appendix B   REVIEW OF PSYCHOPHYSICAL TESTS

This section includes brief discussions of the following tests:

Color vision tests
Dark adaptometry tests
Macular function tests
Laboratory tests
Visual field tests

This appendix provides an overview of the basis of each test and some of its technical limitations. Forms of the tests not generally used in the office are described because these tests are usually done in central laboratories and the procedures may not be familiar to the practicing clinician. Each of the tests has a well-defined role to play in the diagnostic process. Indeed, many of the diseases described in this text cannot be differentiated without using the tests presented here.

Although many of the tests require special equipment, the tests are not difficult to administer and the equipment is not so expensive that office use is impractical.

COLOR VISION AND TESTING
Mechanisms of Normal Color Vision

Normal color vision is trichromatic with three cone types, each cone most sensitive to either reddish, greenish, or bluish light. Each cone type responds to virtually all colors if the light is sufficiently intense. Normal color vision depends on the relative activity of all three color mechanisms and provides normal observers with over 200 different color sensations.[297]

Abnormalities

Color vision abnormalities can be classified as being either congenital or acquired.

Congenital color vision defects are stationary defects that are present at birth and do not change over time. These defects affect a specific color mechanism, which effects characteristic results on color vision tests. Both eyes are affected equally, and generally there are no additional ocular complaints, except in cases of rod or cone monochromatism (see Table 11), p. 189.

Acquired color vision defects are not present at birth, progress over time, and are not associated with a specific color mechanism.[30,77] Therefore, test results do not present a typical pattern; different tests may implicate different color mechanisms, and test object size may also affect the results. As the abnormality progresses, the color defect may change (i.e., going from a blue/yellow defect to a nonspecific defect). Acquired defects are usually associated with other ocular abnormalities such as visual acuity loss and may not affect the two eyes equally. Acquired defects may be secondary to retinal or optic nerve disease or may result from a change in the transparency of the ocular media.[19]

Types of Color Vision Defects

The anomalous trichromatic color defect is one in which all three color mechanisms are functional, but one mechanism is weak. The abnormality may be mild, moderate, or severe and usually affects the red or green color mechanism.

The dichromatic color defect is one in which one color mechanism, usually red or green, is nonfunctioning. The defect probably occurs at a level above the cones themselves, as the photopic ERGs are normal unless a secondary disease process is present.

In blue monocone monochromatism both the green and red color mechanisms are nonfunctioning. The only color mechanism that functions normally is the blue color mechanism. There is severe color blindness associated with reduced visual acuity. The macula is dominated by red and green cones, and the fovea has only these two cone types, the loss of which causes a central scotoma. The patient also complains of mild photophobia and has mild nystagmus. Because there are relatively few blue cones in the retina, the photopic ERGs are virtually nonrecordable. The scotopic ERGs are normal.

In complete rod monochromatism the patient has no functioning cones. The patient has no color perception and complains of reduced visual acuity, nystagmus, and photophobia. The ERG findings in the complete rod monochromat show a nonrecordable photopic response and a normal scotopic response.

Incomplete rod monochromatism is characterized by

a reduced number of functioning cones. There may be some sensation of color, but it is abnormal. Visual acuity is reduced to the 20/50 to 20/200 level, and there is mild photophobia and mild nystagmus. Thus patients' symptoms are very similar to those of patients with blue cone monochromatism. Inheritance patterns differ, as does one subjective test, but symptoms and electrophysiologic findings are very similar in these two conditions, and accurate diagnosis is difficult.[293]

Color Mechanism Abnormalities

Abnormality of the red color mechanism is a *protan color defect*. This causes a confusion between red and green colors. A complete defect (protanopia) reduces the visible spectrum in the longer wavelengths (vision normally mediated by red cones). Individuals with this defect are more visually handicapped than are those with color vision defects involving green- or blue-sensitive cones. Inheritance is X-linked recessive, with a 1% incidence rate for both the complete and incomplete varieties of protan defect.

Abnormality of the green color mechanism is a *deutan color defect*. This defect also causes a confusion between red and green colors; thus many investigators inappropriately link both the protan and deutan color vision defects to a similar color mechanism abnormality, referred to as the red/green color defect. The deutan defect is actually a separate color vision defect and affects only the green color mechanism. Unlike the patient with protanopia, the patient with deuteranopia perceives the full range of the visible spectrum. The inheritance pattern is also X-linked recessive. The complete deutan defect occurs in 1% of the population, whereas the incomplete deutan defect occurs more commonly, in 5% of the population.

Abnormality of the blue cone mechanism is a *tritan color defect*, causing a confusion between blue and yellow colors. Tritan defects are not generally simple congenital defects but are associated with other inherited abnormalities. Inherited tritan defects are rare, usually autosomal dominant, and often found in conjunction with an autosomal-dominant optic atrophy. These defects, both incomplete and complete, are most often acquired, as the blue mechanism seems particularly sensitive to the toxic effects of drugs and other pathologic conditions.[293,296,298]

COLOR VISION TESTS

This section presents several of the more popular tests used to evaluate color vision.[256]

Pseudoisochromatic (Color) Plates

Color plates are probably the most popular color vision tests available. Color plates are inexpensive, easy to administer, and require little special equipment. They provide qualitative information about the patient's color perception and are usually used as screening devices. A patient with a mild color vision defect may not be detected with the use of color plates. Unfortunately, color plates are only about 90% accurate and are prone to fading; normal individuals can appear to be color defective if faded plates are used.[190]

Detection of color perception abnormality by using the color plates is based on the inability of those with color defects to distinguish shades of color produced by varying mixtures of the primary colors. Those with defects have ranges of color confusion that are exploited by the plates. Because of his or her inability to distinguish these colors, the patient sees a different number or symbol on the plate than would a normal subject. Interpretation of test results is simple and provides a useful indication of whether an abnormality is present. The plates are less useful for diagnosis of a specific abnormality.

Arrangement Tests

Several types of arrangement tests are available for the diagnosis of color vision defects. These tests require the patient to arrange colored caps into a graded color order. The arrangement of caps reveals the ability of the patient to perceive a subtle color gradation. Again, the results are qualitative. Arrangement tests require a minimal level of cognitive functioning and are not suitable for very young children. Patients with poor visual acuity (about 20/100 or worse) may have difficulty seeing the caps and will perform poorly on the tests, although their color vision may be normal. All arrangement tests should be performed under the manufacturers' lighting specifications. Poor lighting may cause errors in the test results. Soiled caps can also produce errors. Care should be taken to prevent patients from touching the colored portion of the caps.

The Farnsworth-Munsell D-15 panel is an arrangement test that is simple to administer and that can be used for children about 5 years of age and older. It can be administered quickly and provides easy differentiation between protan, deutan, and tritan defects. The test consists of 15 movable caps of different saturated colors and one stationary reference cap. The patient is required to arrange the caps in proper color order. The way the patient arranges the caps determines normality or a specific color defect. The D-15 panel will not detect subtle defects because of the full saturation of the colors.[101]

The desaturated 15 panel, designed by Lanthony, uses desaturated colors and is an excellent test for detecting subtle color vision defects. Both the D-15 panel and the desaturated panel are easy to administer, produce reliable results, and are scored in a similar fashion. On the underside of each cap is a number corresponding to its appropriate place in proper color order. The score sheet places the numbers in consecutive, circular order. The cap order determined by the patient is recorded in a "connect-the-dots" manner. If the patient puts the number 15 cap next to the number 1 cap, the scorer would connect cap 1 and cap 15 with a line. These lines, if they cross from one side of the circle to the other, represent an abnormal color vision axis along which there is confusion (see Figures 101 through 104).

The most popular extended arrangement test is the Farnsworth-Munsell 100-hue test. The test consists of 85 hues divided into four boxes with 21 or 22 caps per box. At both ends of the box are reference caps. The

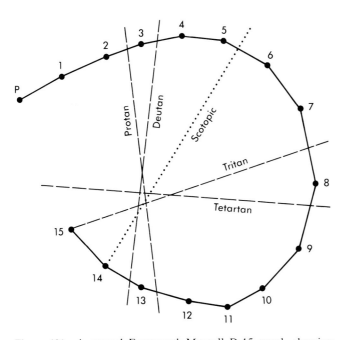

Figure 101. A normal Farnsworth-Munsell D-15 panel, showing no axis of confusion.

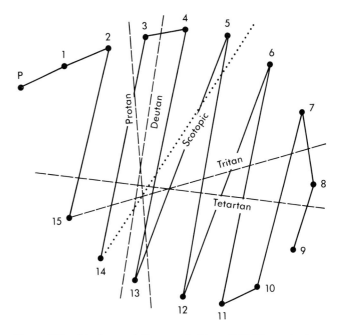

Figure 103. An abnormal Farnsworth-Munsell D-15 panel, showing a deutan axis of confusion.

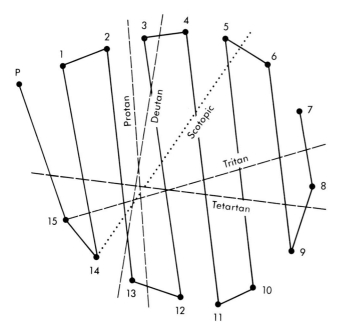

Figure 102. An abnormal Farnsworth-Munsell D-15 panel, showing a protan axis of confusion.

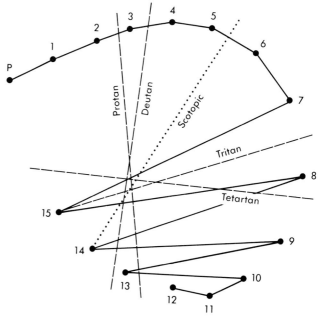

Figure 104. An abnormal Farnsworth-Munsell D-15 panel, showing a tritan axis of confusion.

patient is requested to arrange the colored caps in color order between the two reference caps. The colored caps are of equal lightness and are approximately equal in hue distance from one another. The caps compose a natural hue circle that represents a modified version of the full color spectrum.

The test was originally designed to screen individuals for possible employment in the textile industry, but over the years it has become known as an effective tool for diagnosing color vision defects. A score of fewer than 100 errors is generally considered normal; however, the age of the patient should be considered when evaluating the results. A 12-year-old child would need a score of greater than 200 to be clearly abnormal. A 25-year-old adult, however, would be considered abnormal with a score just over 100. An elderly adult may need a score as high as 300 to be considered abnormal. Scores in both eyes should be similar.[160]

Scores well above 100 can demonstrate a nonspecific abnormality, where no axis is seen; or reveal a specific defect (see Figures 105 through 108). Differ-

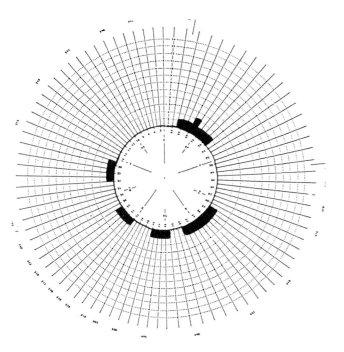

Figure 105. Normal results on the Farnsworth-Munsell 100-hue test.

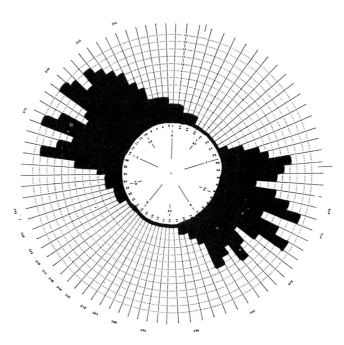

Figure 107. An abnormal Farnsworth-Munsell 100-hue test, showing a deutan axis of confusion.

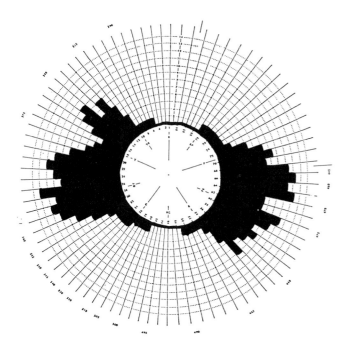

Figure 106. An abnormal Farnsworth-Munsell 100-hue test, showing a protan axis of confusion.

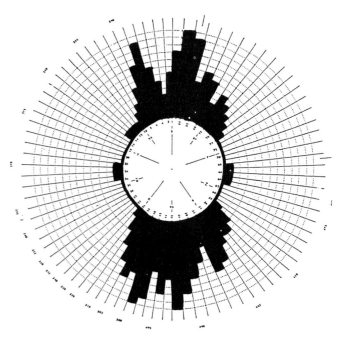

Figure 108. An abnormal Farnsworth-Munsell 100-hue test, showing a tritan axis of confusion.

entiation between protan and deutan defects can be difficult, and additional tests may be necessary to support the diagnosis. As with the D-15 panel, each cap has a number on its underside indicating its proper position, but the scoring technique is not the same. The number represents the ideal relationship of that cap to the others within the box. The score for each cap is the absolute difference between the cap and the two that surround it. If the caps are in proper order, the absolute score for the cap is two. Thus, a score of two represents no deviation, and a score greater than two represents a deviation. The score sheet is a circle with the numbers within it. For every number there is a level of deviation away from two. The score for each number is plotted along the circle, and then the dots are connected. The area with the greatest level of deviation represents the area of confusion, which corresponds to the type of color perception abnormality present.[31,101,102]

Color Matching Tests (Anomaloscope)

The previously discussed color tests are qualitative in nature, so they cannot fully reveal the severity of a defect. However, the anomaloscope can provide such information. The most common instrument is the Nagel anomaloscope produced by Schmidt and Haensch, which detects red/green abnormalities. A mixture of two primary colors (red and green) is adjusted by the patient to match a test color (yellow). The Rayleigh equation states that a mixture of spectral red light and spectral green light will produce a sensation equivalent to a pure spectral yellow light; that is, (X) red + (Y) green = yellow. The coefficients of red (X) and green (Y) are the quantities of those colors used for the match. All normal subjects use approximately the same ratio of primary red and green to match a pure spectral yellow. The range of red/green color quantity to match yellow is very narrow, so detection of a patient with even a slight red/green defect is relatively easy. The patient with a protan defect will need more red to match yellow, and one with a deutan defect will need more green in the mixture. The normal range on the Nagel anomaloscope is a red/green mixture numerically represented between 37 and 45 (see Table 13).[322]

Differentiation between a patient with protanopia and one with deuteranopia can be difficult because both are able to match pure spectral yellow with pure green to pure red. An intensity series using the Nagel anomaloscope can help distinguish between the two abnormalities. A patient with deuteranopia matches the range of green through red with a similar yellow intensity (10 to 20 on the spectral yellow scale). However,

Table 13 NAGEL ANOMALOSCOPE READINGS* IN PATIENTS WITH COLOR DEFECTS

Anomaloscope readings showing the normal range and abnormal ranges for protan and deutan defects.[296]

NORMAL TRICHROMATIC VISION	PROTAN DEFECTS	DEUTAN DEFECTS
Range: 37 to 45	**Protanopia (Intensity Matching Abnormal,† Farnsworth-Munsell 100-Hue Protan Axis)** Range: 0 to 73	**Deuteranopia (Intensity Matching Normal,† Farnsworth-Munsell 100-Hue Deutan Axis)** Range: 0 to 73
Probably Normal: Slightly Altered Equation Wide equation: 39 to 49 Less wide equation: 41 to 48 Wide equation shift to red end: 40 to 50 Wide equation shift to green end: 35 to 45 Wide equation shift to both ends: 35 to 50	**Protanomalous Defect—Mild** Protanomalous defect: narrow equation: 45 to 50 Protanomalous defect: wide equation: 41 to 55 Slight protanomalous defect: equation: 42 to 55 Slight protanomalous defect: wide equation: 41 to 57	**Deuteranomalous Defect—Mild** Deuteranomalous defect: mild: 20 to 30
	Protanomalous Defect—Moderate to Severe Protanomalous defect: mild to moderate: 40 to 57 Protanomalous defect: moderate: 50 to 73 Protanomalous defect: moderate to severe: 25 to 73	**Deuteranomalous Defect—Moderate** Deuteranomalous defect: mild to moderate (narrow equation): 10 to 20 Deuteranomalous defect: mild to moderate: 6 to 30 Deuteranomalous defect: moderate: 0 to 25 Deuteranomalous defect: moderate: 0 to 30

*These readings represent the relative red and green content of the mixture used to match yellow (0, pure green; 73, pure red).
†See Figure 109.
Patient data courtesy of Diedre Martin, Jules Stein Eye Institute, Los Angeles, Cal.

a patient with protanopia uses a high intensity of yellow (very bright) to match green and uses no yellow (appears black) when matching red because he or she cannot distinguish this portion of the color spectrum (see Figure 109).[31]

Test for Rod Monochromatism

Several color vision tests are available that are used to evaluate the possible achromatic patient (no cones). The Sloan achromatopsia test was devised to test patients suspected of having achromatopsia. The test is made up of 17 gray rectangles of graduated saturation level, from nearly white to nearly black. Each rectangle has a fixed color circle in the center. The test plate has a gray-colored center. The patient is asked to identify the rectangle with the matching outer rectangle and inner circle. For the normal individual the test plate is the only one with a perfect match. The achromatic patient however, can match all the test colors (red, orange, yellow, green, blue, and pink) with 1 of the 17 gray rectangles. If a patient matches all six test colors with the gray rectangles, a diagnosis of complete rod monochromatism can be entertained. However, if a patient can identify even one of the test colors, then complete rod monochromatism is ruled out.[335]

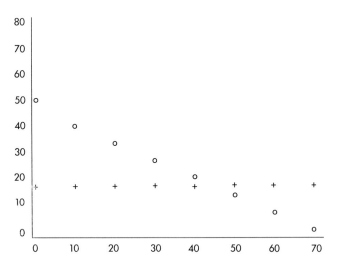

Figure 109. A graph of test yellow intensity against a red/green mixture, as read from the Nagel anomaloscope, using a yellow test target. The relative brightness of the yellow target is indicated on the ordinate. The red/green mixture, from pure green (0) to pure red (73), is indicated on the abscissa. Note that the patients with deuteranopia (+) consistently use a relatively dim yellow, between 10 and 20, regardless of the red/green combination. Patients with protanopia (○) change the luminosity level; pure spectral green is matched to a very bright yellow, whereas red is matched to nearly black.[298] (Patient data courtesy of Deidre Martin, Jules Stein Eye Institute, Los Angeles, Cal.)

Test for Blue Cone Monochromatism

A new color vision test to identify persons with X-linked blue cone monochromatism has been devised by Berson and colleagues.[25] The test comprises color plates with three blue/green arrows and one purple/blue arrow. The patient is asked if one of the four arrows appears to be different. The achromatic patient will see no difference. The patient with blue cone monochromatism, who has short wavelength–sensitive cones, will easily see the purple/blue arrow as different from the other three. The main disadvantage to both the Sloan achromatopsia test and the Berson arrow test is that evaluation of the incomplete rod monochromatic patient is unsatisfactory.

Successful Color Vision Testing

Proper assessment of color vision can be accomplished only if the tests are properly executed. A patient's eyes should never be dilated when tested. The natural coloration of the human lens may alter the person's color perception. This is particularly noticeable when the patient's eyes are dilated. The patient should always wear his or her best correction when tested so that refractive errors do not influence the outcome of the test. Each test should be given at the distance specified by the manufacturer and under the proper lighting conditions. Care must be taken to ensure that test objects are not soiled or faded.

Differentiating Severe Congenital Color Vision Defects

Inherited achromatopsia, or complete absence of color vision, is a very rare occurrence. Most patients with achromatopsia suffer from an acquired retinal disease, such as cone degeneration. In the event of a true congenital defect, three possible causes of profound loss of color perception must be considered: complete rod monochromatism, incomplete rod monochromatism, or blue cone monochromatism.

Complete rod monochromatism has very specific characteristics and can be easily diagnosed if proper tests are administered. This is not so with incomplete rod or blue cone monochromatism, both of which manifest similar signs and symptoms and often cannot be easily distinguished.

The complete rod monochromatic patient, also known as the typical achromatic patient, manifests total stationary loss of color perception, a visual acuity of 20/200, photophobia, and nystagmus. The nystagmus may be severe at a young age but may lessen by the second to third decade. Family history usually includes consanguinity, and the condition is inherited as an autosomal recessive trait. ERGs reveal nonrecordable or severely abnormal photopic responses but normal scotopic responses. Dark adaptometry may reveal an abnormal cone section, and visual fields often reveal a central scotoma.

Most color vision tests will reveal a severe abnormality. The D-15 panel may reveal no axis dominance or a scotopic axis. The complete rod monochromatic patient may make numerous errors on the 100-hue test without evidence of axis dominance, but this may result partly from their poor visual acuity.[46] The patient may also be able to match pure spectral green to pure spectral red with a yellow test object on the anomaloscope, producing a Rayleigh matching range of 0 to 73. Unfortunately, this pattern is commonly seen in persons with an end-stage cone dystrophy. The two tests that are diagnostically helpful are the Sloan achromatopsia test and the Berson arrow test.

The patient with complete rod monochromatism will be able to match the inner circle with the outer rectangle on all of the Sloan test plates and will not be able to differentiate any of the test arrows in the Berson test. Both of these tests are essential in diagnosing rod monochromatism. If the patient can see one of the colors on the Sloan test or differentiate the test arrow, the diagnosis of complete rod monochromatism is ruled out.

Incomplete rod monochromatism resembles a mild complete rod monochromatism. The incomplete rod monochromatic patient has a reduced visual acuity of 20/60 to 20/200 and reduced color perception but possesses some color sensation. Photophobia and nystagmus are also present, but may be milder than that seen in patients with complete rod monochromatism. The photopic ERG is abnormal but usually recordable, and the scotopic ERG is generally normal. There is generally a family history of consanguinity. Some studies have suggested that complete and incomplete rod monochromatism may be variations within the same pedigree, but the diagnoses in these cases may have been based on inappropriate testing procedures.[298]

Color vision tests suggest that, although both protan and deutan defects can be observed in incomplete rod monochromatic patients, both types of defects are not present in one individual. This finding suggests that the blue cone mechanism is functioning in all such patients.

Tests for screening red/green color defects are usually failed by patients with incomplete rod monochromatism, and the D-15 panel reveals either a protan or a scotopic axis. The Sloan achromatopsia test may reveal a large number of matched items; however, because all incomplete rod monochromatic patients are able to identify some colors, there will not be a 100% matching as seen in those with complete rod monochromatism.

The incomplete rod monochromatic patient is also able to identify the test arrow on the Berson test, thus making it a useful test for differentiating the complete from incomplete rod monochromat. Unfortunately, the Berson arrow test is not useful in differentiating those with incomplete rod monochromatism from those with X-linked blue cone monochromatism.

Color matching and spectral sensitivity are important diagnostic tools in the differentiation of incomplete rod monochromatism from blue cone monochromatism. Both processes present similar signs and symptoms as well as similar results on standard color vision tests.

In the protan type of incomplete rod monochromatism, there is evidence on color matching and spectral sensitivity of normally functioning middle wavelength–sensitive (green) cones and rod photopigment, with a spectral sensitivity characteristic of rhodopsin. The incomplete rod monochromatic patient with a deutan-type defect shows evidence on color matching and spectral sensitivity of normally functioning long wavelength–sensitive (red) cones and rod photopigment, with a spectral sensitivity characteristic of rhodopsin.[294]

This constellation of signs and symptoms is similar to that found in a patient with cone dystrophy. Careful ocular history will reveal progression of the disease in the latter patient; progression is absent in inherited achromatopsia.

The X-linked blue cone monochromatic patient also has reduced visual acuity and poor color perception. Pendular nystagmus and photophobia may also be present. The photopic ERG is reduced or nonrecordable, and the scotopic ERG is normal. Visual acuity is not generally reduced to the level of 20/200 because blue cones are present in the macula; however, the fovea is blue-cone free, which causes some acuity reduction.

Unfortunately, standard color vision tests may not be helpful in establishing a diagnosis of X-linked blue cone monochromatism. In many cases, the diagnosis of cone dystrophy or incomplete rod monochromatism may be made erroneously. Because the blue cones are functioning normally, most of the standard color vision tests reveal a red/green color defect. The Rayleigh matching range of such a patient is similar to that of a complete rod monochromatic patient. On the Sloan achromatopsia test, some colors (presumably blue and yellow) are identified, and on the Berson test, the X-linked blue monochromatic patient can identify the test arrow. The patient is dichromatic at mesopic and low photopic levels, revealing two active photopigments, the first being that of short wavelength–sensitive (blue) cones and the second being that of rhodopsin. The patient is monochromatic at photopic or scotopic levels of illumination, behaving in a manner similar to that of the complete rod monochromatic patient. Spectral sensitivity reveals responses similar to those found in short wavelength–sensitive (blue) cones, without evidence of middle or long wavelength–sensitive (green and red) cone response.[202,296]

Acquired Color Vision Abnormalities

Acquired color vision defects can be observed in approximately 5% of the total population and can be caused by factors such as age, systemic disease, chemical exposure (e.g., toxins or medications), head injury, and ocular disease.

Congenital color vision defects manifest with findings typical of the affected color mechanism. Acquired color vision defects, however, do not always follow set patterns, making diagnosis more difficult. In general, acquired defects reflect a progressive secondary problem associated with a primary causative agent, such as disease, trauma, or chemical exposure. Typical patterns may exist but are not always observable. The pattern seen may suggest a progression from normal color vision to anomalous trichromatic to dichromatic color vision. In extreme cases, the person may progress to monochromatic vision. Loss of visual acuity often accompanies such progression. In some abnormalities, widespread loss of color discrimination may occur before extensive loss of visual acuity occurs.

Some specific characteristics assist in the differentiation of congenital versus acquired color vision defects. Acquired color vision defects may possess one or more of the following characteristics: an unequal manifestation of color defect between the eyes; a color defect associated with another ocular disturbance, such as visual acuity loss, visual field loss, or abnormal ERG; a blue-yellow defect occurring as often as a red-green defect; males and females being equally affected; color perception improving with larger test targets; and a sudden onset or change in color perception.[293] Any of these characteristics should suggest an acquired process to the physician.

Color vision tests have been designed mainly to test congenital defects; however, acquired defects can also be adequately evaluated. The screening test commonly used for such evaluation is the Standard Pseudoisochromatic Plates, which features separate booklets for congenital and acquired color vision testing. For extensive testing, the Farnsworth-Munsell 100-hue test is the test of choice. As visual acuity declines, however, the results may become uninterpretable. In such cases, the D-15 panel, which does not rely on particularly good visual acuity, may provide superior information.[46]

DARK ADAPTOMETRY TESTS

Dark adaptometry is a test of the ability of the photoreceptors to increase their sensitivity in the dark and is indicated in patients complaining of nyctalopia. The test, generally performed with the Goldmann-Weekers dark adaptometer, involves initial dark adaptation for 2 minutes, followed by light adaptation for 5 minutes. The light adaptation segment of the test is essential; it causes a standard bleaching of the rod and cone pigments so that a standard dark adaptation curve can be obtained. After light adaptation is complete, the background light is extinguished and the patient is asked to identify the test target.

The test target consists of a very dim light or target that is adjusted in intensity by a technician until the patient states that the light is barely visible. Once the patient identifies the target, the technician turns the adaptometer off, then slowly increases its intensity until the patient can again see the target. This procedure is repeated throughout the examination. When the patient states that the light is visible, the technician marks the test strip. The vertical axis of the strip represents log units of light, and the horizontal axis represents time. Thus the patient's response represents the least intensity of light seen at any point in time after the background adaptation light is extinguished.

The dark adaptation curve has a characteristic shape in the normal individual (see Figure 110). The first 5 minutes are represented by a rapid increase in sensitivity, which is viewed as a steeply declining curve. This curve represents cone function. Initially, after bleaching, the cones can only see a very bright target light, but they quickly adapt (normally 5 minutes or less) to a normal cone threshold (the least amount of light at which cones function). The curve levels off for a few minutes, until the rod adaptation causes a further increase in sensitivity. This is the *rod/cone break*. After this point the rods are the cells responsible for further adaptation. The rods adapt to dark more slowly, and this is viewed as a gradually descending slope. The rods are approximately 80% to 90% dark-adapted after 30 minutes in the dark (the usual completion time for the test), and rods in the normal individual are 3 log units (1000 times) more sensitive to dim lights than are cones.

If the patient being tested complains of nyctalopia and there is abnormality of the rod system, the dark adaptation curve will appear abnormal. If only the rods are affected, the abnormality will occur only in the rod

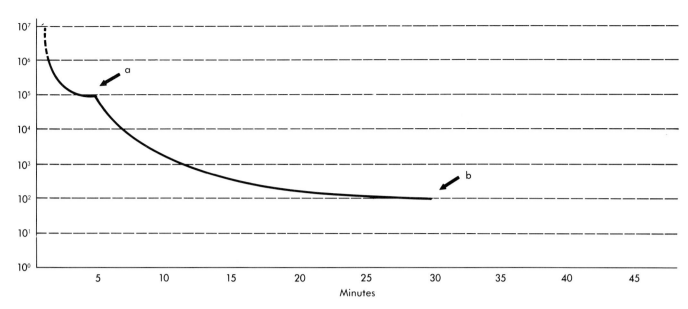

Figure 110. A normal dark adaptometry curve. **A,** A normal cone adaptation curve, with normal rod/cone break after 5 minutes of dark adaptation. **B,** A normal final rod threshold.

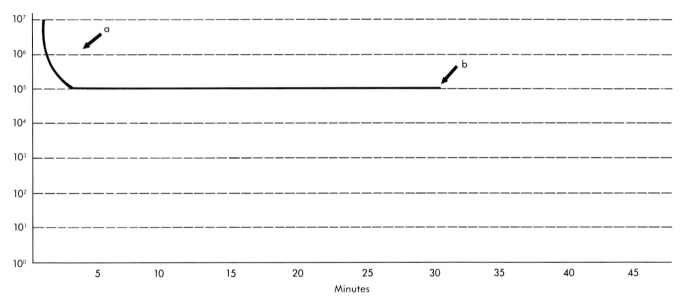

Figure 111. An abnormal rod dark adaptometry curve. **A,** A normal cone adaptation curve, without evidence of a rod/cone break. **B,** An abnormal final rod threshold, without evidence of an increased retinal sensitivity over time. Dark adaptometry curves displaying this pattern are typical of those associated with abnormality of the rod system, such as retinitis pigmentosa.

aptation segment and will result in an elevated final rod threshold. If the patient has some functioning rods, his or her final rod threshold will be located between the normal rod threshold and the normal cone threshold. However, if the patient has only normally functioning cones and a complete abnormality of the rod system, that patient's final rod threshold will be at the level of a normal cone threshold (see Figure 111). This indicates that no additional adaptation (increase in retinal sensitivity) occurred past the initial adaptation of the cones.

Dark adaptometry tests can also be revealing in patients who have abnormalities of the cone system. In the patient with rod monochromatism, the initial cone adaptation curve will be abnormal. The curve will not have the typical, rapidly declining slope that is observed in the normal patient, but will instead have a delayed, slowly declining slope. Additionally, there will be little or no evidence of a rod/cone break (see Figure 112).

Some patients (e.g., those with retinitis pigmentosa) have both a rod and cone system abnormality. In such

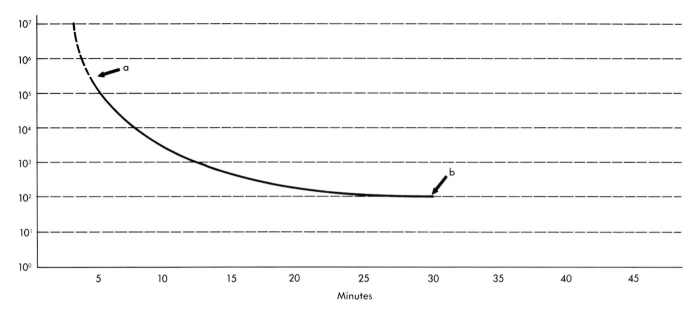

Figure 112. An abnormal cone dark adaptometry curve. **A,** An abnormal cone adaptation curve, without evidence of a rod/cone break. **B,** A normal final rod threshold. Dark adaptometry curves displaying this pattern are typical of those associated with abnormality of the cone system, such as those seen in complete rod monochromatism.

patients the cone adaptation curve and the rod adaptation curve will both be abnormal. This may be represented as an elevated final rod threshold combined with an abnormality in the cone adaptation curve. In severe cases there is no additional increase in retinal sensitivity beyond that which is initially observed. Thus the patient is unable to see lights dimmer than the brightest target light, and, in the most severe cases, the patient cannot see the brightest target light until after 5 minutes of dark adaptation.

In a few, very rare, retinal diseases the patient has the ability to adapt to dark, but the adaptation process is delayed and prolonged. The best known of these entities is Oguchi's disease. In these patients, the cone adaptation curve may be somewhat less steep, followed by a normal cone threshold, but with a delay of the rod/cone break. The patient at 30 minutes in the dark is still actively dark adapting, and the test should be continued. A final rod threshold in the normal range may not be observed until the patient has been in the dark anywhere from 1 to 3 hours. Any patient suspected of having Oguchi's disease should be tested beyond the standard 30 minutes. If the rod/cone break is delayed, the final rod threshold very likely will also be delayed (see Figure 113).

The dark adaptometry test is a subjective test, requiring cooperation from the patient and expert administration by the technician. The patient must be cooperative and capable of comprehension. Patients who are too young or developmentally delayed will not perform this test well, primarily because of its length. However, when establishing final rod threshold is necessary for diagnosis, such patients can be left in the dark or fitted with red goggles for 30 minutes and then tested for 5 to 10 minutes. Even very young children can often tolerate the test if it is sufficiently short. Patients who are not reliable at stating when they first see the test target provide unreliable data. The technician may not be able to obtain sufficient cooperation if a patient is malingering, but the variable responses will reveal this condition.

The light adaptation portion of the test must also be properly executed. If the patient does not open his or her eyes fully during this period, the photopigments may not become adequately bleached. If this occurs, the cone adaptation curve may not appear normal, but the final rod threshold will be accurate.

The area of the retina being tested plays a significant role in the normality of the dark adaptation curve. Initially, the macular area is tested for the cone adaptation segment. The patient is encouraged to fixate on the center portion of the back of the adaptometer bowl. After the rod/cone break, the patient is asked to fixate on the red light above the target in the bowl. This red fixation light allows testing of the most sensitive portion of the retina, the area with a high concentration of rods, located between 10 to 15 degrees from the center of the visual field. In newer models of the Goldmann-Weekers dark adaptometer, several additional fixation lights are positioned so that other areas of the retina can be tested.

The dark adaptation test evaluates the most sensitive

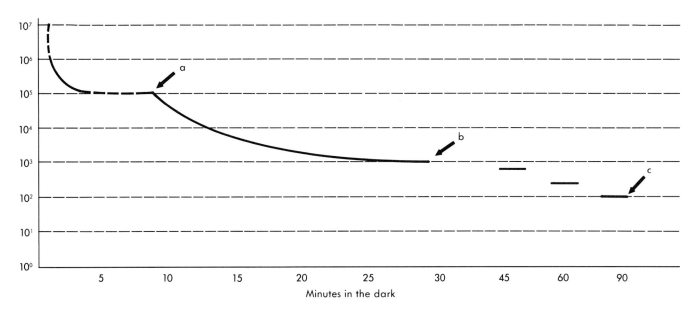

Figure 113. An abnormal rod dark adaptometry curve (delayed). **A,** A normal cone adaptation curve, with prolongation of the rod/cone break. **B,** An elevated final rod threshold after 30 minutes of dark adaptation. **C,** Continuation of dark adaptation shows a normal final rod threshold after 90 minutes. Dark adaptometry curves displaying this pattern are typical of those associated with abnormality in adaptation, such as those seen in Oguchi's disease.

patch of retina in the area tested. The test is reliable only in generalized retinal diseases. Focal retinal abnormality may cause very misleading test results varying from normal to grossly abnormal, depending on whether fixation is on a normal or an adjacent scotomatous area of retina.

For optimal results, the dark adaptometry curve is used as a psychophysical representation of retinal function along with the ERG, which provides objective findings of overall retinal function. Lastly, final rod threshold should always be obtained monocularly because both eyes may not function equivalently.[3,212]

MACULAR FUNCTION TESTS

Macular function can easily be assessed with five subjective tests: (1) visual acuity charts (Snellen type), (2) the Amsler grid, (3) contrast sensitivity, (4) the glare test, and (5) the macular stress test. Visual acuity charts and the Amsler grid are most commonly used in offices during routine screening of macular function, whereas the other tests are used primarily in research laboratories. Unfortunately, all subjective tests require patient cooperation for valid results to be obtained. Patients can report worse vision than they actually have (feigning blindness) or misunderstand the instructions and not respond accurately. Care must be taken when giving instructions, and appropriate tests must be administered to those with language or literacy barriers.

Visual Acuity Charts

The test most commonly administered for assessment of macular function is the Snellen-type visual acuity chart. This familiar test requires the patient to correctly identify letters of the alphabet or objects (similar to Allen cards) that are placed at a specified distance away from the patient. The chart contains letters of varying sizes corresponding to their true distance from the patient if all letters were subtending the same prescribed five degrees.

Visual acuity tests are performed without dilation and without prescription lenses in both near-vision and distance-vision testing. The patient's current prescription is then used for both near and distance testing. If the patient's vision does not improve with lenses, a pinhole is used. This helps determine if the problem is refractive in nature, or if it is caused by other abnormalities. Vision should be the same for near and distance testing. If these results are not comparable, a refractive problem should be suspected.

Snellen-type charts test two different visual thresholds, one being the visibility threshold and the other being the resolution threshold. The visibility threshold is based on the smallest object correctly identified, where the contrast between the background and the object are constant and only the size changes (e.g., 20/20 or 20/30). The resolution threshold is based on the actual shape of the object. Objects of similar shape can be easily confused, and actual resolution of the object must be made for recognition.

Several other visual acuity charts are commercially available and include the Landolt C test, the Sloan chart, and the Bausch and Lomb chart. Illiterate charts include the Snellen E chart, the Kindergarten chart, and Allen cards.[310]

Amsler Grid

The Amsler grid was designed to detect subtle macular area defects and metamorphopsia. Many macular problems cause metamorphopsia, but this may not be readily detected on Snellen-type charts. When held at 30 cm, the grid tests the central 10 degrees of the visual field, or the macular area. The test is performed with the patient wearing his or her best correction, eyes undilated, at the proper distance and always monocularly. The patient is asked to identify any holes or wavy lines that may be present. This is an excellent tool for identifying small scotomas in the central 10 degrees, which may not be found with other visual field tests. The tests are on regular sheets of paper, quite inexpensive, and easy to perform. Thus it is possible to send an Amsler grid home with a patient if a progressive process is suspected so that the patient can note any change.

LABORATORY TESTS
Contrast Sensitivity Test

Several tests of macular function are used primarily in the laboratory or research setting but are slowly being incorporated into the office. The contrast sensitivity test is very sensitive and provides information about retinal function that is not directly related to the visibility threshold or visual acuity. The test, made up of sinusoidal gratings of different contrast and spatial frequency, detects abnormalities in a patient's ability to perceive those gratings. The subjective response to the gratings may in fact provide significantly more information than do standard visual acuity charts. A patient who sees 20/20 on a Snellen chart may complain of seeing poorly (i.e., everything being in a fog), but that difficulty might not be confirmed unless a contrast sensitivity test is performed. This test is particularly useful in detecting optic nerve diseases where visual acuity has not been affected. Early changes in contrast sensitivity have been reported in glaucoma and several other retinal diseases. This test is simple to use, but it depends on patient cooperation and understanding. Improper results may be obtained if the patient does not have a clear understanding of what is expected. Error in results may also occur if proper lighting is not maintained, and many manufacturers actually provide a light meter to help ensure proper lighting conditions.

The test is performed much like the Snellen test. The patient looks at a series of gratings at various angles and reports the direction of the lines that have varying contrast and separation.

Glare Test

The glare test examines the level of visual disturbance attributable to glare. Glare is a common complaint from those with early cataracts, and, although the cataract itself may not warrant surgery, the effects of glare produced by the cataract may be quite debilitating. To evaluate this, the patient is asked to identify the opening in the Landolt C, as he or she would if being tested with a regular acuity chart. The C does not change in size but changes in contrast. The letter is on a white, opaque background, and a light is projected from behind the C from a slide projector. The light produced from the slide projector is also uniform. The only condition that varies is the contrast. If a patient with a cataract can correctly identify the opening of the C only under high contrast, the cataract is producing a sufficient amount of glare to be debilitating.

Macular Stress Test

The macular stress test is used in some clinics for evaluating macular function. The tester first bleaches the retina in the macular area by shining a light in the patient's eye for 10 seconds. The patient is then asked to read the acuity chart one line above their maximum acuity (i.e., 20/25 if they see 20/20). The time it takes for the patient to read three letters correctly is recorded. There should be very little time difference between the two eyes. Most normal individuals will read the line within the first 50 seconds after the light has been extinguished. However, in patients with macular abnormalities, the resolution time can be as long as 8 minutes.

The resolution is caused by a resynthesis of the visual pigments in the photoreceptors. Ocular abnormalities of the outer segments or the retinal pigment epithelium (in the macular area) may cause a prolongation of resolution. Patients with optic nerve disease and glaucoma function normally on this test. Thus the differentiation between macular and optic nerve diseases can be facilitated with the macular stress test.[147]

VISUAL FIELD TESTS

Peripheral vision is tested with visual field equipment that tests the functioning capacity of the peripheral retina. Although visual acuity is not directly tested with this equipment, sensitivity of peripheral areas can be evaluated. This evaluation is essential in diagnosing various retinal diseases.

The three types of visual field tests are the suprathreshold static, the below-threshold static, and the below-threshold kinetic fields.

1. The suprathreshold static field (i.e., the Field Master) uses a spot of one intensity and one size presented in an on/off fashion. This is a gross test of peripheral retinal function and can detect only widespread or absolute visual field defects. Subtle defects will be missed, not only because of the suprathreshold light source, but also because there are very few areas of the retina tested with this type of apparatus.
2. The below-threshold static field (i.e., the Octopus perimeter) also uses an on/off light stimulus. The advantage of this visual field test is its use of multiple test object sizes and multiple light intensities. Thus subtle defects or relative scotomas can be easily identified. This equipment is computerized, reducing the potential for error if an inexperienced technician is performing the test. The peripheral retina is systematically tested in that the distance between locations of the retina tested are predetermined by the computer program.
3. The below-threshold kinetic field (i.e., the Goldmann perimeter) also uses multiple test object sizes and light intensities. This visual field test is controlled by a technician, who presents a test object to the patient, bringing the object from the unseeing periphery to the seeing periphery. The patient responds by telling the technician when the object is seen. Isopters are recorded and determined by the test object seen. Very subtle defects can be detected by the well-trained technician. Unfortunately, erroneous findings often result if the technician is not well trained.

Visual field testing can be very useful in diagnosing retinal disease. Areas of nonfunctioning retina will appear as absolute scotomas, whereas the areas of retina that are functioning below normal will demonstrate a relative scotoma. Visual fields are very revealing in many disease processes, including retinal diseases, where the seeing and nonseeing retina can be mapped out. Thus progression can be observed as a decrease of functioning retinal area and expressed as reduced visual fields.[258]

REFERENCES

1. Ackerman J, Brody PE, Kanarek I, and Gottlieb F: Macular wrinkling and atypical retinitis pigmentosa in Laurence-Moon-Biedl-Bardet syndrome, Ann Ophthalmol 12:632, 1980.
2. Alfano JE: Ocular aspects of the maternal rubella syndrome, Trans Am Acad Ophthalmol Otolaryngol 70:235, 1966.
3. Alpern M: Rod vision. In Potts AM, editor: The assessment of visual function, St. Louis, 1972, The CV Mosby Co.
4. Amman F: Investigations cliniques et genetiques sur le syndrome de Bardet-Biedl en Suisse, J Genet Hum 18(suppl):1, 1970.
5. Appel I, and Barishak YR: Histopathological changes in siderosis bulbi, Ophthalmologica 176:205, 1978.
6. Arden GB, Friedmann A, and Kolb H: Anticipation of chloroquine retinopathy, Lancet 1:1164, 1962.
7. Ashton N: Central areolar choroidal sclerosis: a histo-pathological study, Br J Ophthalmol 37:140, 1953.
8. Auerbach E: Electroretinographical and psychophysical studies in achromats, Mod Probl Ophthalmol 13:169, 1974.
9. Auerbach E, Godel V, and Rowe H: An electrophysiological and psychophysical study of two forms of congenital night blindness, Invest Ophthalmol 8:332, 1969.
10. Auerbach E, and Merin S: Achromatopsia with amblyopia. I. A clinical and electroretinographical study of 39 cases, Doc Ophthalmol 37:79, 1974.
11. Avila MP, Weiter JJ, Jalkh AE, Trempe CL, Pruett RC, and Schepens CL: Natural history of choroidal neovascularization in degenerative myopia, Ophthalmology 91:1573, 1984.
12. Ayazi S, and Fagan R: Pattern dystrophy of the pigment epithelium, Retina 1:287, 1981.
13. Bachynski BN, Flynn JT, Rodrigues MM, Rosenthal S, Cullen R, and Curless RG: Hyperglycemic acidotic coma and death in Kearns-Sayre syndrome, Ophthalmology 93:391, 1986.
14. Bagolini B, and Ioli-Spada G: Bietti's tapetoretinal degeneration with marginal corneal dystrophy, Am J Ophthalmol 65:53, 1968.
15. Bassen FA, and Kornzweig AL: Malformation of the erythrocytes in a case of atypical retinitis pigmentosa, Blood 5:381, 1950.
16. Bateman JB, Riedner ED, Levin LS, and Maumenee IH: Heterogeneity of retinal degeneration and hearing impairment syndromes, Am J Ophthalmol 90:755, 1980.
17. Baum JL, Tannenbaum M, and Kolodny EH: Refsum's syndrome with corneal involvement, Am J Ophthalmol 60:699, 1965.
18. Belin MW, Baltch AL, and Hay PB: Secondary syphilitic uveitis, Am J Ophthalmol 92:210, 1981.
19. Benson WE: An introduction to color vision. In Duane T, editor: Clinical ophthalmology, vol 3, Philadelphia, 1986, Harper & Row, Publishers, Inc.
20. Berson EL, Gouras P, and Gunkel RD: Progressive cone-rod degeneration, Arch Ophthalmol 80:68, 1968.
21. Berson EL, Gouras P, and Gunkel RD: Progressive cone degeneration, dominantly inherited, Arch Ophthalmol 80:77, 1968.
22. Berson EL, Rosen JB, and Simonoff EA: Electroretinographic testing as an aid in detection of carriers of X-chromosome–linked retinitis pigmentosa, Am J Ophthalmol 87:460, 1979.
23. Berson EL, Rosner B, and Simonoff E: Risk factors for genetic typing and detection in retinitis pigmentosa, Am J Ophthalmol 89:763, 1980.
24. Berson EL, Sandberg MA, Maguire A, Bromley WC, and Roderick TH: Electroretinograms in carriers of blue cone monochromatism, Am J Ophthalmol 102:254, 1986.
25. Berson EL, Sandberg MA, Rosner B, Birch DG, and Hanson AH: Natural course of retinitis pigmentosa over a three-year interval, Am J Ophthalmol 99:240, 1985.
26. Berson EL, Sandberg MA, Rosner B, and Sullivan PL: Color plates to help identify patients with blue cone monochromatism, Am J Ophthalmol 95:741, 1983.
27. Berson EL, Shih VE, and Sullivan PL: Ocular findings in patients with gyrate atrophy on pyridoxine and low-protein, low-arginine diets, Ophthalmology 88:311, 1981.
28. Betten MG, Bilchik RC, and Smith ME: Pigmentary retinopathy and myotonic dystrophy, Am J Ophthalmol 72:720, 1971.
29. Bietti G: Ueber familiäres Vorkommen von "Retinitis punctata albescens" (verbunden mit "Dystrophia marginalis cristallinea corneae"), Glitzern des Glaskörpers und anderen degenerativen Augenveränderungen, Klin Monatsbl Augenheilkd 99:737, 1937.
30. Birch J, Chisholm IA, Kinnear P, Marré M, Pinckers AJLG, Pokorny J, Smith VC, and Verriest G: Acquired color vision defects. In Pokorny J, Smith VC, Verriest G, and Pinckers AJLG, editors: Congenital and acquired color vision defects, New York, 1979, Grune & Stratton, Inc.
31. Birch J, Chisholm IA, Kinnear P, Pinckers AJLG, Pokorny J, Smith VC, and Verriest G: Clinical testing methods. In Pokorny J, Smith VC, Verriest G, and Pinckers AJLG, editors: Congenital and acquired color vision defects, New York, 1979, Grune & Stratton, Inc.
32. Bird AC: X-linked retinitis pigmentosa, Br J Ophthalmol 59:177, 1975.
33. Bisland T: The Laurence-Moon-Biedl syndrome: report of a typical case with complete necropsy, Am J Ophthalmol 34:874, 1951.
34. Blach RK, Jay B, and Kolb H: Electrical activity of the eye in high myopia, Br J Ophthalmol 50:629, 1966.
35. Blackwell HR, and Blackwell OM: Blue mono-cone monochromacy. A new color vision defect, J Opt Soc Am 47:338, 1957.
36. Blair CJ: Geographic atrophy of the retinal pigment epithelium: a manifestation of senile macular degeneration, Arch Ophthalmol 93:19, 1975.
37. Blair NP, Albert DM, Liberfarb RM, and Hirose T: Hereditary progressive arthro-ophthalmopathy of Stickler, Am J Ophthalmol 88:876, 1979.
38. Blair NP, Goldberg MF, Fishman GA, and Salzano T: Autosomal dominant vitreoretinochoroidopathy (ADVIRC), Br J Ophthalmol 68:2, 1984.

39. Bloom LH, Swanson DE, and Bird AC: Adult vitelliform macular degeneration, Br J Ophthalmol 65:800, 1981.
40. Blumenkranz MS, Gass JDM, and Clarkson JG: Atypical serpiginous choroiditis, Arch Ophthalmol 100:1773, 1982.
41. Boldrey EE, Egbert P, Gass JDM, and Friberg T: The histopathology of familial exudative vitreoretinopathy: a report of two cases, Arch Ophthalmol 103:238, 1985.
42. Boniuk M, and Zimmerman LE: Ocular pathology in the rubella syndrome, Arch Ophthalmol 77:455, 1967.
43. Bowen P, Ferguson-Smith MA, Moiser D, Lee CSN, Butler HG: The Laurence-Moon syndrome: association with hypogonadotropic hypogonadism and sex-chromosome aneuploidy, Arch Intern Med 116:598, 1965.
44. Bridges CDB, and Alvarez RA: Selective loss of 11-cis vitamin A in an eye with hereditary chorioretinal degeneration similar to sector retinitis pigmentosa, Retina 2:256, 1982.
45. Brinkley JR, Jr, Dubois EL, and Ryan SJ: Long-term course of chloroquine retinopathy after cessation of medication, Am J Ophthalmol 88:1, 1979.
46. Brown L, Govan E, and Block MT: The effect of reduced visual acuity upon Farnsworth 100-hue test performance, Ophthalmic Physiol Opt 3:7, 1983.
47. Burian HM, and Burns CA: Ocular changes in myotonic dystrophy, Am J Ophthalmol 63:22, 1967.
48. Burns RP, Lovrien EW, and Cibis AB: Juvenile sex-linked retinoschisis: clinical and genetic studies, Trans Am Acad Ophthalmol Otolaryngol 75:1011, 1971.
49. Campo RV, and Aaberg TM: Ocular and systemic manifestations of the Bardet-Biedl syndrome, Am J Ophthalmol 94:750, 1982.
50. Canny CLB, and Oliver GL: Fluorescein angiographic findings in familial exudative vitreoretinopathy, Arch Ophthalmol 94:1114, 1976.
51. Carr RE: Central areolar choroidal dystrophy, Arch Ophthalmol 73:32, 1965.
52. Carr RE: Vitamin A therapy may reverse degenerative retinal syndrome, Clin Trends 8:8, 1970.
53. Carr RE: Congenital stationary nightblindness, Trans Am Ophthalmol Soc 72:448, 1974.
54. Carr RE, and Gouras P: Oguchi's disease, Arch Ophthalmol 73:646, 1965.
55. Carr RE, and Noble KG: Choroideremia, Ophthalmology 87:169, 1980.
56. Carr RE, and Ripps H: Rhodopsin kinetics and rod adaptation in Oguchi's disease, Invest Ophthalmol 6:426, 1967.
57. Carr RE, Ripps H, Siegel IM, and Weale RA: Rhodopsin and the electrical activity of the retina in congenital night blindness, Invest Ophthalmol 5:497, 1966.
58. Carr RE, Ripps H, Siegel IM, and Weale RA: Visual functions in congenital night blindness, Invest Ophthalmol 5:508, 1966.
59. Carr RE, and Siegel IM: The vitreo-tapeto-retinal degenerations, Arch Ophthalmol 84:436, 1970.
60. Carr RE, and Siegel IM: Unilateral retinitis pigmentosa, Arch Ophthalmol 90:21, 1973.
61. Carr RE, and Siegel IM: The retinal pigment epithelium in ocular albinism. In Zinn KM, and Marmor MF, editors: The retinal pigment epithelium, Cambridge, Mass., 1979, Harvard University Press.
62. Cavender JC, and Ai E: Hereditary macular dystrophies. In Duane TD, editor: Clinical ophthalmology, vol 3, Philadelphia, 1986, Harper & Row, Publishers, Inc.
63. Cherry PMH: Usher's syndrome, Ann Ophthalmol 5:743, 1973.
64. Chew EY, Deutman AF, and Cruysberg JRM: Macular changes in myotonic dystrophy. In Ryan SJ, Dawson AK, and Little HL, editors: Retinal diseases, Orlando, Fl., 1985, Grune & Stratton, Inc.
65. Chisholm IA, and Dudgeon J: Pigmented paravenous retinochoroidal atrophy: helicoid retino-choroidal atrophy, Br J Ophthalmol 57:584, 1973.
66. Chopdar A: Reticular dystrophy of retina, Br J Ophthalmol 60:342, 1976.
67. Cibis GW, Morey M, and Harris DJ: Dominantly inherited macular dystrophy with flecks (Stargardt), Arch Ophthalmol 98:1785, 1980.
68. Cibis PA, Yamashita T, and Rodriguez F: Clinical aspects of ocular siderosis and hemosiderosis, Arch Ophthalmol 62:180, 1959.
69. Clarkson JG, and Altman RD: Angioid streaks, Surv Ophthalmol 26:235, 1982.
70. Cogan DG, Kuwabara T, Kolodny E, and Driscoll S: Gangliosidoses and the fetal retina, Ophthalmology 91:508, 1984.
71. Condon GP, Brownstein S, Wang NS, Kearns AF, and Ewing CC: Congenital hereditary (juvenile X-linked) retinoschisis: histopathologic and ultrastructural findings in three eyes, Arch Ophthalmol 104:576, 1986.
72. Condon PI, and Serjeant GR: Ocular findings in elderly cases of homozygous sickle-cell disease in Jamaica, Br J Ophthalmol 60:361, 1976.
73. Connell MM, Poley BJ, and McFarlane JR: Chorioretinopathy associated with thioridazine therapy, Arch Ophthalmol 71:816, 1964.
74. Copenhaver RM, and Goodman G: The electroretinogram in infantile, late infantile, and juvenile amaurotic family idiocy, Arch Ophthalmol 63:559, 1960.
75. Coppeto J, and Ayazi S: Annular macular dystrophy, Am J Ophthalmol 93:279, 1982.
76. Cortin P, Archer D, Maumenee IH, Feiock K, and Speros P: A patterned macular dystrophy with yellow plaques and atrophic changes, Br J Ophthalmol 64:127, 1980.
77. Cox J: Colour vision defects acquired in diseases of the eye, Br J Physiol Optics 18:3, 1961.
78. Criswick VG, and Schepens CL: Familial exudative vitreoretinopathy, Am J Ophthalmol 68:578, 1969.
79. Cruess AF, Schachat AP, Nicholl J, and Augsburger JJ: Chloroquine retinopathy: is fluorescein angiography necessary? Ophthalmology 92:1127, 1985.
80. Daily MJ, and Mets MB: Fenestrated sheen macular dystrophy, Arch Ophthalmol 102:855, 1984.
81. Davidorf FH: Thioridazine pigmentary retinopathy, Arch Ophthalmol 90:251, 1973.
82. de Jong PTVM, de Jong JGY, de Jong-Ten Doeschate JMM, and Delleman JW: Olivopontocerebellar atrophy with visual disturbances: an ophthalmologic investigation into four generations, Ophthalmology 87:793, 1980.
83. de Jong PTVM, and Delleman JW: Pigment epithelial pattern dystrophy: four different manifestations in a family, Arch Ophthalmol 100:1416, 1982.
84. Deutman AF: Benign concentric annular macular dystrophy, Am J Ophthalmol 78:384, 1974.
85. Deutman AF, and Jansen LMAA: Dominantly inherited drusen of Bruch's membrane, Br J Ophthalmol 54:373, 1970.
86. Deutman AF, and Kovács B: Argon laser treatment in complications of angioid streaks, Am J Ophthalmol 88:12, 1979.
87. Deutman AF, Pinckers AJLG, and Aan de Kerk AL: Dominantly inherited cystoid macular edema, Am J Ophthalmol 82:540, 1976.

88. Deutman AF, Pinckers AJL, and Yuzawa M: Further findings in dominant cystoid macular dystrophy. In Henkind P, editor: Acta: XXIV international congress of ophthalmology, Philadelphia, 1983, JB Lippincott Co.
89. Deutman AF, Van Blommestein JDA, Henkes HE, Waardenburg PJ, and Solleveld-van Driest E: Butterfly-shaped pigment dystrophy of the fovea, Arch Ophthalmol 83:558, 1970.
90. Dhanda RP: Electroretinograms in myopic retinal degeneration, Jpn J Ophthalmol 10(suppl):325, 1966.
91. Dobbie JG, Fetkenhour CL, and Shoch D: Central areolar pigment epithelial (CAPE) dystrophy, Trans Am Ophthalmol Soc 73:141, 1975.
92. Douglas AA, Waheed I, and Wyse CT: Progressive bifocal chorio-retinal atrophy: a rare familial disease of the eyes, Br J Ophthalmol 52:742, 1968.
93. Duinkerke-Eerola KU, Cruysberg JRM, and Deutman AF: Atrophic maculopathy associated with hereditary ataxia, Am J Ophthalmol 90:597, 1980.
94. Eagle RC, Jr, Lucier AC, Bernardino VB, Jr, and Yanoff M: Retinal pigment epithelial abnormalities in fundus flavimaculatus: a light and electron microscopic study, Ophthalmology 87:1189, 1980.
95. Ellis DS, and Heckenlively JR: Retinitis punctata albescens: fundus appearance and functional abnormalities, Retina 3:27, 1983.
96. Epstein GA, and Rabb MF: Adult vitelliform macular degeneration: diagnosis and natural history, Br J Ophthalmol 64:733, 1980.
97. Epstein RL: Inborn metabolic disorders and the eye. In Peyman GA, Sanders DR, and Goldberg MF, editors: Principles and practice of ophthalmology, Philadelphia, 1980, WB Saunders Co.
98. Falls HF: Sex-linked ocular albinism displaying typical fundus changes in the female heterozygote, Am J Ophthalmol 34:41, 1951.
99. Farkas TG: Drusen of the retinal pigment epithelium, Surv Ophthalmol 16:75, 1971.
100. Farkas TG, Krill AE, Sylvester VM, and Archer D: Familial and secondary drusen: histologic and functional correlations, Trans Am Acad Ophthalmol Otolaryngol 75:333, 1971.
101. Farnsworth D: The Farnsworth-Munsell 100-hue and dichotomous tests for color vision, J Opt Soc Am 33:568, 1943.
102. Farnsworth D: The Farnsworth-Munsell 100-Hue test for the examination of color discrimination, manual, Baltimore, 1957, Munsell Color Company, Inc.
103. Favre M: À propos de deux cas de dégénérescence hyaloïdéo-rétinienne, Ophthalmologica 135:604, 1958.
104. Federman JL, Shields JA, and Tomer TL: Angioid streaks. II. Fluorescein angiographic features, Arch Ophthalmol 93:951, 1975.
105. Ferry AP, Llovera I, and Shafer DM: Central areolar choroidal dystrophy, Arch Ophthalmol 88:39, 1972.
106. Fetkenhour CL, Choromokos E, Weinstein J, and Shoch D: Cystoid macular edema in retinitis pigmentosa, Trans Am Acad Ophthalmol Otolaryngol 83:515, 1977.
107. Fetkenhour CL, Gurney N, Dobbie JG, and Choromokos E: Central areolar pigment epithelial dystrophy, Am J Ophthalmol 81:745, 1976.
108. Fishman G: Hereditary retinal and choroidal diseases: electroretinogram and electro-oculogram findings. In Peyman GA, Sanders DR, and Goldberg MF, editors: Principles and practice of ophthalmology, Philadelphia, 1980, WB Saunders Co.
109. Fishman GA: Fundus flavimaculatus: a clinical classification, Arch Ophthalmol 94:2061, 1976.
110. Fishman GA: Progressive human cone-rod dysfunction (dystrophy), Trans Am Acad Ophthalmol Otolaryngol 81:716, 1976.
111. Fishman GA: Retinitis pigmentosa: genetic percentages, Arch Ophthalmol 96:822, 1978.
112. Fishman GA: Electroretinography and inherited macular dystrophies, Retina 5:172, 1985.
113. Fishman GA, Buckman G, and Van Every T: Fundus flavimaculatus: a clinical classification, Doc Ophthalmol Proc Ser 13:213, 1977.
114. Fishman GA, Carrasco C, and Fishman M: The electro-oculogram in diffuse (familial) drusen, Arch Ophthalmol 94:231, 1976.
115. Fishman GA, Farber MD, and Derlacki DJ: X-linked retinitis pigmentosa: profile of clinical findings, Arch Ophthalmol 106:369, 1988.
116. Fishman GA, Fishman M, and Maggiano J: Macular lesions associated with retinitis pigmentosa, Arch Ophthalmol 95:798, 1977.
117. Fishman GA, Goldberg MF, and Trautmann JC: Dominantly inherited cystoid macular edema, Ann Ophthalmol 11:21, 1979.
118. Fishman GA, Jampol LM, and Goldberg MF: Diagnostic features of the Favre-Goldmann syndrome, Br J Ophthalmol 60:345, 1976.
119. Fishman GA, Rhee AJ, and Blair NP: Blood-retinal barrier function in patients with cone or cone-rod dystrophy, Arch Ophthalmol 104:545, 1986.
120. Fishman GA, Trimble S, Rabb MF, and Fishman M: Pseudovitelliform macular degeneration, Arch Ophthalmol 95:73, 1977.
121. Fishman GA, Weinberg AB, and McMahon TT: X-linked recessive retinitis pigmentosa: clinical characteristics of carriers, Arch Ophthalmol 104:1329, 1986.
122. Fishman GA, Woolf MB, Goldberg MF, and Busse B: Reticular tapeto-retinal dystrophy: as a possible late stage of Sjögren's reticular dystrophy, Br J Ophthalmol 60:35, 1976.
123. Fishman GA, Young RSL, Schall SP, and Vasquez VA: Electro-oculogram testing in fundus flavimaculatus, Arch Ophthalmol 97:1896, 1979.
124. Flanders M, Lapointe ML, Brownstein S, and Little JM: Keratoconus and Leber's congenital amaurosis: a clinicopathological correlation, Can J Ophthalmol 19:310, 1984.
125. Forsius HR, Eriksson AW, Suvanto EA, and Alanko HI: Pseudoinflammatory fundus dystrophy with autosomal recessive inheritance, Am J Ophthalmol 94:634, 1982.
126. Foxman SG, Heckenlively JR, Bateman JB, and Wirtschafter JD: Classification of congenital and early onset retinitis pigmentosa, Arch Ophthalmol 103:1502, 1985.
127. Foxman SG, Heckenlively JR, and Sinclair SH: Rubeola retinopathy and pigmented paravenous retinochoroidal atrophy, Am J Ophthalmol 99:605, 1985.
128. Franceschetti A, and François J: Fundus flavimaculatus, Arch Ophthalmol (Paris) 25:505, 1965.
129. François J, De Rouck A, Cambie E, and De Laey JJ: Visual functions in pericentral and central pigmentary retinopathy, Ophthalmologica 165:38, 1972.
130. François J, De Rouck A, and Golan A: ERG in sectorial pigmentary retinopathy, Doc Ophthalmol Proc Ser 13:239, 1977.
131. François J, and Verriest G: Rétinopathie pigmentaire unilatérale, Bull Soc Belge Ophtamol 99:479, 1951.

132. François J, Verriest G, and De Rouck A: A new pedigree of idiopathic congenital night-blindness: transmitted as a dominant hereditary trait, Am J Ophthalmol 59:621, 1965.
133. Frangieh GT, Green WR, and Fine SL: A histopathologic study of Best's macular dystrophy, Arch Ophthalmol 100:1115, 1982.
134. Frank HR, Landers MB III, Williams RJ, and Sidbury JB: A new dominant progressive foveal dystrophy, Am J Ophthalmol 78:903, 1974.
135. Fraser HB, and Wallace DC: Sorsby's familial pseudoinflammatory macular dystrophy, Am J Ophthalmol 71:1216, 1971.
136. Gass JDM: Photocoagulation of macular lesions, Trans Am Acad Ophthalmol Otolaryngol 75:580, 1971.
137. Gass JDM: Drusen and disciform detachment and degeneration, Trans Am Ophthalmol Soc 70:409, 1972.
138. Gass JDM: Drusen and disciform macular detachment and degeneration, Arch Ophthalmol 90:206, 1973.
139. Gass JDM: A clinicopathologic study of a peculiar foveomacular dystrophy, Trans Am Ophthalmol Soc 72:139, 1974.
140. Gass JDM: Stereoscopic atlas of macular diseases, diagnosis and treatment, ed 3, pp. 98-100, St. Louis, 1987, The CV Mosby Co.
141. Gass JDM: Stereoscopic atlas of macular diseases, diagnosis and treatment, ed 3, pp. 312-313, St. Louis, 1987, The CV Mosby Co.
142. Gass JDM: Stereoscopic atlas of macular diseases, diagnosis and treatment, ed 3, pp. 614-615, St. Louis, 1987, The CV Mosby Co.
143. Gass JDM, and Clarkson JG: Angioid streaks and disciform macular detachment in Paget's disease (osteitis deformans), Am J Ophthalmol 75:576, 1973.
144. Gelber PJ, and Shah A: Fluorescein study of albipunctate dystrophy: report of a case, Arch Ophthalmol 81:164, 1969.
145. Gills JP, Jr, and Paton D: Mottled fundus oculi in pseudoxanthoma elasticum: a report on two siblings, Arch Ophthalmol 73:792, 1965.
146. Giuffrè G, and Lodato G: Vitelliform dystrophy and pattern dystrophy of the retinal pigment epithelium: concomitant presence in a family, Br J Ophthalmol 70:526, 1986.
147. Glaser JS, Savino PJ, Sumers KD, McDonald SA, and Knighton RW: The photostress recovery test in the clinical assessment of visual function, Am J Ophthalmol 83:255, 1977.
148. Godtfredsen E, and Jensen SF: Dystrophia myotonica and retinal dystrophy, Acta Ophthalmol 47:565, 1969.
149. Goodman G, Ripps H, and Siegel IM: Cone dysfunction syndromes, Arch Ophthalmol 70:214, 1963.
150. Gouras P, Carr RE, and Gunkel RD: Retinitis pigmentosa in abetalipoproteinemia: effects of vitamin A, Invest Ophthalmol 10:784, 1971.
151. Gow J, and Oliver GL: Familial exudative vitreoretinopathy: an expanded view, Arch Ophthalmol 86:150, 1971.
152. Green WR: Pathology of the retina. In Frayer WG, editor: Lancaster course in ophthalmic histopathology, unit 9, Philadelphia, 1981, FA Davis Co.
153. Green WR, Friedman-Kien A, and Banfield WG: Angioid streaks in Ehlers-Danlos syndrome, Arch Ophthalmol 76:197, 1966.
154. Grizzard WS, Deutman AF, Nijhuis F, and Aan de Kerk A: Crystalline retinopathy, Am J Ophthalmol 86:81, 1978.
155. Grøndahl J: Autosomal recessive inheritance in "senile" retinitis pigmentosa, Acta Ophthalmol 65:231, 1987.
156. Gutman I, Walsh JB, and Henkind P: Vitelliform macular dystrophy and butterfly-shaped epithelial dystrophy: a continuum? Br J Ophthalmol 66:170, 1982.
157. Hadden OB, and Gass JDM: Fundus flavimaculatus and Stargardt's disease, Am J Ophthalmol 82:527, 1976.
158. Hamilton AM, and Bird AC: Geographical choroidopathy, Br J Ophthalmol 58:784, 1974.
159. Hampton GR, Kohen D, and Bird AC: Visual prognosis of disciform degeneration in myopia, Ophthalmology 90:923, 1983.
160. Han DP, and Thompson HS: Nomograms for the assessment of Farnsworth-Munsell 100-hue test scores, Am J Ophthalmol 95:622, 1983.
161. Hansen E, Bachen NI, and Flage T: Refsum's disease: eye manifestations in a patient treated with low phytol, low phytanic acid diet, Acta Ophthalmol 57:899, 1979.
162. Harris GS, and Yeung JWS: Maculopathy of sex-linked juvenile retinoschisis, Can J Ophthalmol 11:1, 1976.
163. Havener WH: Cerebellar-macular abiotrophy, Arch Ophthalmol 45:40, 1951.
164. Hayasaka S, and Okuyama S: Crystalline retinopathy, Retina 4:177, 1984.
165. Hayasaka S, Shiono T, Mizuno K, Sasayama C, Akiya S, Tanaka Y, Hayakawa M, Miyake Y, and Ohba N: Gyrate atrophy of the choroid and retina: 15 Japanese patients, Br J Ophthalmol 70:612, 1986.
166. Hayasaka S, Shoji K, Kanno CI, Oura F, and Mizuno K: Differential diagnosis of diffuse choroidal atrophies: diffuse choriocapillaris atrophy, choroideremia, and gyrate atrophy of the choroid and retina, Retina 5:30, 1985.
167. Hayes KC: Retinal degeneration in monkeys induced by deficiencies of vitamin E or A, Invest Ophthalmol 13:499, 1974.
168. Heckenlively JR: Preserved para-arteriole retinal pigment epithelium (PPRPE) in retinitis pigmentosa, Br J Ophthalmol 66:26, 1982.
169. Heckenlively JR, and Kokame GT: Pigmented paravenous retinochoroidal atrophy, Doc Ophthalmol Proc Ser 40:235, 1984.
170. Heckenlively JR, Martin D, and Levy J: Chloroquine retinopathy, Am J Ophthalmol 89:150, 1980.
171. Heckenlively JR, Martin DA, and Rosales TO: Telangiectasia and optic atrophy in cone-rod degenerations, Arch Ophthalmol 99:1983, 1981.
172. Heckenlively JR, Martin DA, and Rosenbaum AL: Loss of electroretinographic oscillatory potentials, optic atrophy, and dysplasia in congenital stationary night blindness, Am J Ophthalmol 96:526, 1983.
173. Heckenlively JR, and Weleber RG: X-linked recessive cone dystrophy with tapetal-like sheen: a newly recognized entity with Mizuo-Nakamura phenomenon, Arch Ophthalmol 104:1322, 1986.
174. Henkind P, Carr RE, and Siegel IM: Early chloroquine retinopathy: clinical and functional findings, Arch Ophthalmol 71:157, 1964.
175. Hertzberg R: Twenty-five-year follow-up of ocular defects in congenital rubella, Am J Ophthalmol 66:269, 1968.
176. Hill DA, Arbel KF, and Berson EL: Cone electroretinograms in congenital nyctalopia with myopia, Am J Ophthalmol 78:127, 1974.
177. Hirose T, Lee KY, and Schepens CL: Wagner's hereditary vitreoretinal degeneration and retinal detachment, Arch Ophthalmol 89:176, 1973.

178. Hirose T, Lee KY, and Schepens CL: Snowflake degeneration in hereditary vitreoretinal degeneration. Am J Ophthalmol 77:143, 1974.
179. Hirose T, and Miyake Y: Pigmentary paravenous chorioretinal degeneration: fundus appearance and retinal functions, Ann Ophthalmol 11:709, 1979.
180. Hirose T, Schepens CL, Brockhurst RJ, Wolf E, and Tolentino FI: Congenital retinoschisis with night blindness in two girls, Ann Ophthalmol 12:848, 1980.
181. Hirose T, and Wand O: Amaurosis congenita (Leber), Ann Ophthalmol 7:59, 1975.
182. Hirose T, Wolf E, and Hara A: Electrophysiological and psychophysical studies in congenital retinoschisis of X-linked recessive inheritance, Doc Ophthalmol Proc Ser 13:173, 1977.
183. Hirose T, Wolf E, and Schepens CL: Retinal functions in snowflake degeneration, Ann Ophthalmol 12:1135, 1980.
184. Hittner HM, Borda RP, and Justice J, Jr: X-linked recessive congenital stationary night blindness, myopia, and tilted discs, J Pediatr Ophthalmol Strabismus 18:15, 1981.
185. Hittner HM, Ferrell RF, Borda RP, and Justice J, Jr: Atypical vitelliform macular dystrophy in a 5-generation family, Br J Ophthalmol 68:199, 1984.
186. Hodes BL, Feiner LA, Sherman SH, and Cunningham D: Progression of pseudovitelliform macular dystrophy, Arch Ophthalmol 102:381, 1984.
187. Hoskin A, Sehmi K, and Bird AC: Sorsby's pseudoinflammatory macular dystrophy, Br J Ophthalmol 65:859, 1981.
188. Hotchkiss ML, and Fine SL: Pathologic myopia and choroidal neovascularization, Am J Ophthalmol 91:177, 1981.
189. Hsieh RC, Fine BS, and Lyons JS: Patterned dystrophies of the retinal pigment epithelium, Arch Ophthalmol 95:429, 1977.
190. Ichikawa H, Hukami K, Tanabe S, and Kawakami G: Standard pseudoisochromatic plates, manual, Tokyo, 1978.
191. Ide CH, and Wilson RJ: Juvenile retinoschisis, Br J Ophthalmol 57:560, 1973.
192. Jay M: The Eisdell pedigree: congenital stationary night blindness with myopia, Trans Ophthalmol Soc UK 103:221, 1983.
193. Kaiser-Kupfer MI, deMonasterio FM, Valle D, Walser M, and Brusilow S: Gyrate atrophy of the choroid and retina: improved visual function following reduction of plasma ornithine by diet, Science 210:1128, 1980.
194. Kandori F: Very rare case of congenital nonprogressive night blindness with fleck retina, Jpn J Clin Ophthalmol 13:384, 1959.
195. Kandori F, Setogawa T, and Tamai A: Electroretinographical studies on "fleck retina with congenital non-progressive night-blindness," Yonago Acta Med 10:98, 1966.
196. Kandori F, Tamai A, Kurimoto S, and Fukunaga K: Fleck retina, Am J Ophthalmol 73:673, 1972.
197. Kandori F, Tamai A, Watanabe T, and Kurimoto S: Unilateral pigmentary degeneration of the retina, Am J Ophthalmol 66:1091, 1968.
198. Kaufman SJ, Goldberg MF, Orth DH, Fishman GA, Tessler H, and Mizuno K: Autosomal dominant vitreoretinochoroidopathy, Arch Ophthalmol 100:272, 1982.
199. Kearns TP: External ophthalmoplegia, pigmentary degeneration of the retina, and cardiomyopathy: a newly recognized syndrome, Trans Am Ophthalmol Soc 63:559, 1965.
200. Kearns TP, and Sayre GP: Retinitis pigmentosa, external ophthalmoplegia, and complete heart block: unusual syndrome with histologic study in one of two cases, Arch Ophthalmol 60:280, 1958.
201. Kingham JD, Fenzl RE, Willerson D, and Aaberg TM: Reticular dystrophy of the retinal pigment epithelium: a clinical and electrophysiologic study of three generations, Arch Ophthalmol 96:1177, 1978.
202. Kinnear P, Marré M, Pokorny J, Smith VC, and Verriest G: Specialized methods of evaluating color vision defects. In Pokorny J, Smith VC, Verriest G, and Pinckers AJLG editors: Congenital and acquired color vision defects, New York, 1979, Grune & Stratton, Inc.
203. Klein RM, and Curtin BJ: Lacquer crack lesions in pathologic myopia, Am J Ophthalmol 79:386, 1975.
204. Klein R, Lewis RA, Meyers SM, and Myers FL: Subretinal neovascularization associated with fundus flavimaculatus, Arch Ophthalmol 96:2054, 1978.
205. Klien BA: Angioid streaks: a clinical and histopathologic study, Am J Ophthalmol 30:955, 1947.
206. Klien BA, and Krill AE: Fundus flavimaculatus: clinical, functional and histopathologic observations, Am J Ophthalmol 64:3, 1967.
207. Knave B: Electroretinography in eyes with retained intraocular metallic foreign bodies: a clinical study, Acta Ophthalmol [Suppl] 100:1, 1969.
208. Knobloch WH, and Layer JM: Clefting syndromes associated with retinal detachment, Am J Ophthalmol 73:517, 1972.
209. Kolb H, and Galloway NR: Three cases of unilateral pigmentary degeneration, Br J Ophthalmol 48:471, 1964.
210. Kornzweig AL, and Bassen FA: Retinitis pigmentosa, acanthrocytosis, and heredodegenerative neuromuscular disease, Arch Ophthalmol 58:183, 1957.
211. Kozy D, Doft BH, and Lipkowitz J: Nummular thioridazine retinopathy, Retina 4:253, 1984.
212. Krill AE: Clinical aspects of night vision. In Potts Am, editor: The assessment of visual function, St. Louis, 1972, The CV Mosby Co.
213. Krill AE, and Archer D: Classification of the choroidal atrophies, Am J Ophthalmol 72:562, 1971.
214. Krill AE, Archer D, and Martin D: Sector retinitis pigmentosa, Am J Ophthalmol 69:977, 1970.
215. Krill AE, Archer D, and Newell FW: Fluorescein angiography in retinitis pigmentosa, Am J Ophthalmol 69:826, 1970.
216. Krill AE, and Deutman AF: Dominant macular degenerations: the cone dystrophies, Am J Ophthalmol 73:352, 1972.
217. Krill AE, Deutman AF, and Fishmann M: The cone degenerations, Doc Ophthalmol 35:1, 1973.
218. Krill AE, and Fishman GA: Acquired color vision defects, Trans Am Acad Ophthalmol Otolaryngol 75:1095, 1971.
219. Krill AE, and Folk MR: Retinitis punctata albescens: a functional evaluation of an unusual case, Am J Ophthalmol 53:450, 1962.
220. Krill AE, and Klien BA: Flecked retina syndrome, Arch Ophthalmol 74:496, 1965.
221. Krill AE, Klien BA, and Archer DB: Precursors of angioid streaks, Am J Ophthalmol 76:875, 1973.
222. Krill AE, and Lee GB: The electroretinogram in albinos and carriers of the ocular albino trait, Arch Ophthalmol 69:32, 1963.
223. Krill AE, and Martin D: Photopic abnormalities in congenital stationary nightblindness, Invest Ophthalmol 10:625, 1971.

314. Ryan SJ, Jr, Knox DL, Green WR, and Konigsmark BW: Olivopontocerebellar degeneration: clinicopathologic correlation of the associated retinopathy, Arch Ophthalmol 93:169, 1975.
315. Sabates R, and Kolder HE: Peripapillary pigmentary retinochoroidal degeneration, Ann Ophthalmol 14:681, 1982.
316. Sandvig K: Central, areolar choroidal atrophy: a report on four cases, Acta Ophthalmol 37:325, 1959.
317. Sarks SH: Senile choroidal sclerosis, Br J Ophthalmol 57:98, 1973.
318. Sassani JW, Brucker AJ, Cobbs W, and Campbell C: Progressive chloroquine retinopathy, Ann Ophthalmol 15:19, 1983.
319. Schatz H, Maumenee AE, and Patz A: Geographic helicoid peripapillary choroidopathy: clinical presentation and fluorescein angiographic findings, Trans Am Acad Ophthalmol Otolaryngol 78:747, 1974.
320. Schlaegel TF, Jr, and Kao SF: A review (1970-1980) of 28 presumptive cases of syphilitic uveitis, Am J Ophthalmol 93:412, 1982.
321. Schlernitzauer DA, and Green WR: Peripheral retinal albinotic spots, Am J Ophthalmol 72:729, 1971.
322. Schmidt I: Some problems related to testing color vision with the Nagel anomaloscope, J Opt Soc Am 45:514, 1955.
323. Schocket SS, Lakhanpal V, and Varma SD: Siderosis from a retained intraocular stone, Retina 1:201, 1981.
324. Schubert G, and Bornschein H: Beitrag zur Analyse des menschlichen Elektroretinogramms, Ophthalmologica 123:396, 1952.
325. Shields JA, and Tso MOM: Congenital grouped pigmentation of the retina: histopathologic description and report of a case, Arch Ophthalmol 93:1153, 1975.
326. Siegel IM, Graham CH, Ripps H, and Hsia Y: Analysis of photopic and scotopic function in an incomplete achromat, J Opt Soc Am 56:699, 1966.
327. Sieving PA, Fishman GA, Alexander KR, and Goldberg MF: Early receptor potential measurements in human ocular siderosis, Arch Ophthalmol 101:1716, 1983.
328. Silva-Lopez F: Pigmentacion agrupada retiniana, Arch Soc Oftal Hispano-Am 8:448, 1948.
329. Singerman LJ, Berkow JW, and Patz A: Dominant slowly progressive macular dystrophy, Am J Ophthalmol 83:680, 1977.
330. Singerman LJ, and Hatem G: Laser treatment of choroidal neovascular membranes in angioid streaks, Retina 1:75, 1981.
331. Sjögren H: Dystrophia reticularis laminae pigmentosae retinae: an earlier not described hereditary eye disease, Acta Ophthalmol 28:279, 1950.
332. Skalka HW: Vitelliform macular lesions, Br J Ophthalmol 65:180, 1981.
333. Slagsvold JE: Fenestrated sheen macular dystrophy: a new autosomal dominant maculopathy, Acta Ophthalmol 59:683, 1981.
334. Slezak H, and Hommer K: Fundus pulverulentus, Albrecht v Graefes Arch Klin Exp Ophthalmol 178:177, 1969.
335. Sloan LL: Congenital achromatopsia: a report of 19 cases, J Opt Soc Am 44:117, 1954.
336. Sloan LL, and Feiock K: Acuity-luminance function in achromatopsia and in progressive cone degeneration: factors related to individual differences in tolerance to bright light, Invest Ophthalmol 11:862, 1972.
337. Slusher MM, and Hutton WE: Familial exudative vitreoretinopathy, Am J Ophthalmol 87:152, 1979.
338. Smith BF, Ripps H, and Goodman G: Retinitis punctata albescens: a functional and diagnostic evaluation, Arch Ophthalmol 61:93, 1959.
339. Smith JL, Gass JDM, and Justice J, Jr: Fluorescein fundus photography of angioid streaks, Br J Ophthalmol 48:517, 1964.
340. Smith VC, Pokorny J, Delleman JW, Cozijnsen M, Houtman WA, and Went LN: X-linked incomplete achromatopsia with more than one class of functional cones, Invest Ophthalmol Vis Sci 24:451, 1983.
341. Smith VC, Pokorny J, and Newell FW: Autosomal recessive incomplete achromatopsia with protan luminosity function, Ophthalmologica 177:197, 1978.
342. Smith VC, Pokorny J, and Newell FW: Autosomal recessive incomplete achromatopsia with deutan luminosity, Am J Ophthalmol 87:393, 1979.
343. Sogg RL, Steinman L, Rathjen B, Tharp BR, O'Brien JS, and Kenyon KR: Cherry-red spot-myoclonus syndrome, Ophthalmology 86:1861, 1979.
344. Sommer A, Tjakrasudjatma S, Djunaedi E, and Green WR: Vitamin A–responsive panocular xerophthalmia in a healthy adult, Arch Ophthalmol 96:1630, 1978.
345. Sorr EM, and Goldberg RE: Vitelliform dystrophy in a 64-year-old man, Am J Ophthalmol 82:256, 1976.
346. Sorsby A, and Crick RP: Central areolar choroidal sclerosis, Br J Ophthalmol 37:129, 1953.
347. Sorsby A, Joll-Mason ME, and Gardener N: A fundus dystrophy with unusual features, Br J Ophthalmol 33:67, 1949.
348. Sperling MA, Hiles DA, and Kennerdell JS: Electroretinographic responses following vitamin A therapy in α-beta-lipoproteinemia, Am J Ophthalmol 73:342, 1972.
349. Stickler JB, Belau PG, Farrell FJ, Jones JD, Rugh DG, Steinberg AG, and Ward LE: Hereditary progressive arthroophthalmopathy, Mayo Clin Proc 40:433, 1965.
350. Sukumlyn SW: Grouped pigmentation of the retina, Am J Ophthalmol 29:1458, 1946.
351. Swanson D, Rush P, and Bird AC: Visual loss from retinal oedema in autosomal dominant exudative vitreoretinopathy, Br J Ophthalmol 66:627, 1982.
352. Takki K: Differential diagnosis between the primary total choroidal vascular atrophies, Br J Ophthalmol 58:24, 1974.
353. Takki K: Gyrate atrophy of the choroid and retina associated with hyperornithinaemia, Br J Ophthalmol 58:3, 1974.
354. Takki K, and Simell O: Genetic aspects in gyrate atrophy of the choroid and retina with hyperornithinaemia, Br J Ophthalmol 58:907, 1974.
355. Tasman W, Augsburger JJ, Shields JA, Caputo A, and Annesley WH, Jr: Familial exudative vitreoretinopathy, Trans Am Ophthalmol Soc 79:211, 1981.
356. Teng KH: Further contributions to the fundus Xerophthalmicus, Ophthalmologica 150:219, 1965.
357. Toussaint D, and Danis P: An ocular pathologic study of Refsum's syndrome, Am J Ophthalmol 72:342, 1971.
358. Turut P, Puech B, François P, and Hache JC: "Fundus flavimaculatus" à hérédité dominante (a propos de deux families): considérations nostologiques sur la moladie de Stargardt, Bull Soc Ophtalmol Fr 75:309, 1975.
359. Van den Biesen PR, Deutman AF, and Pinckers AJLG: Evolution of benign concentric annular macular dystrophy, Am J Ophthalmol 100:73, 1985.
360. Veld M in 'T, and Oosterhuis JA: Adult-onset foveomacular pigment epithelial dystrophy, Doc Ophthalmol 52:419, 1982.
361. Verdaguer JT: Juvenile retinal detachment, Am J Ophthalmol 93:145, 1982.

362. Vine AK, and Schatz H: Adult-onset foveomacular pigment epithelial dystrophy, Am J Ophthalmol 89:680, 1980.
363. Von Sallmann L, Gelderman AH, and Laster L: Ocular histopathologic changes in a case of α-beta-lipoproteinemia (Bassen-Kornzweig syndrome), Doc Ophthalmol 26:451, 1969.
364. Wataga T: A histopathological study of retinitis punctata albescens, Jpn J Clin Ophthalmol 14:552, 1960.
365. Watzke RC, Folk JC, and Lang RM: Pattern dystrophy of the retinal pigment epithelium, Ophthalmology 89:1400, 1982.
366. Weekley RD, Potts AM, Reboton J, and May RH: Pigmentary retinopathy in patients receiving high doses of a new phenothiazine, Arch Ophthalmol 64:65, 1960.
367. Weiner LP, Konigsmark BW, Stoll J, Jr, and Magladery JW: Hereditary olivopontocerebellar atrophy with retinal degeneration: report of a family through six generations, Arch Neurol 16:364, 1967.
368. Weingeist TA, Kobrin JL, and Watzke RC: Histopathology of Best's macular dystrophy, Arch Ophthalmol 100:1108, 1982.
369. Weise EE, and Yannuzzi LA: Ring maculopathies mimicking chloroquine retinopathy, Am J Ophthalmol 78:204, 1974.
370. Weiss H, Annesley WH, Jr, Shields JA, Tomer T, and Christopherson K: The clinical course of serpiginous choroidopathy, Am J Ophthalmol 87:133, 1979.
371. Weiter J, and Fine BS: A histologic study of regional choroidal dystrophy, Am J Ophthalmol 83:741, 1977.
372. Welch RB: Bietti's tapetoretinal degeneration with marginal corneal dystrophy: crystalline retinopathy, Trans Am Ophthalmol Soc 75:164, 1977.
373. Weleber RG, and Kennaway NG: Clinical trial of vitamin B_6 for gyrate atrophy of the choroid and retina, Ophthalmology 88:316, 1981.
374. Weleber RG, Kennaway NG, and Buist NRM: Gyrate atrophy of the choroid and retina: approaches to therapy, Int Ophthalmol 4:23, 1981.
375. Weleber RG, and Tongue AC: Congenital stationary night blindness presenting as Leber's congenital amaurosis, Arch Ophthalmol 105:360, 1987.
376. Weleber RG, Tongue AC, Kennaway NG, Budden SS, and Buist NRM: Ophthalmic manifestations of infantile phytanic acid storage disease, Arch Ophthalmol 102:1317, 1984.
377. Winn S, Tasman W, Spaeth G, McDonald PR, and Justice J, Jr: Oguchi's disease in Negroes, Arch Ophthalmol 81:501, 1969.
378. Wiznia RA, Perina B, and Noble KG: Vitelliform macular dystrophy of late onset, Br J Ophthalmol 65:866, 1981.
379. Wojno T, and Meredith TA: Unusual findings in serpiginous choroiditis, Am J Ophthalmol 94:650, 1982.
380. Wolff SM: The ocular manifestations of congenital rubella, Trans Am Ophthalmol Soc 70:577, 1972.
381. Yamanaka M: Histologic study of Oguchi's disease: its relationship to pigmentary degeneration of the retina, Am J Ophthalmol 68:19, 1969.
382. Yanoff M, Rahn EK, and Zimmerman LE: Histopathology of juvenile retinoschisis, Arch Ophthalmol 79:49, 1968.
383. Young RSL, Krefman RA, and Fishman GA: Visual improvements with red-tinted glasses in a patient with cone dystrophy, Arch Ophthalmol 100:268, 1982.
384. Yuzawa M, Mae Y, and Matsui M: Bietti's crystalline retinopathy, Ophthalmic Paediatr Genet 7:9, 1985.

SUGGESTED READINGS

The following reference books provide additional information about the diseases and laboratory procedures discussed in this manual.

Diseases of the Retina and Choroid

Bloom MA, and Garcia CA: Manual of retinal and choroidal dystrophies, New York, 1982, Appleton-Century-Crofts.

Deutman AF: The hereditary dystrophies of the posterior pole of the eye, Assen, The Netherlands, 1971, Van Gorcum and Co.

Duke-Elder S: System of ophthalmology, vol 10, Diseases of the retina, St. Louis, 1967, The CV Mosby Co.

Franceschetti A, François J, and Babel J: Chorioretinal heredodegeneration, Springfield, Ill, 1974, Charles C Thomas, Publisher.

Gass JDM: Stereoscopic atlas of macular diseases: diagnosis and treatment, ed 3, St. Louis, 1987, The CV Mosby Co.

Harley RD: Pediatric ophthalmology, Philadelphia, 1983, WB Saunders Co.

Heckenlively JR: Retinitis pigmentosa, Philadelphia, 1988, JB Lippincott Co.

Krill, AE: Hereditary retinal and choroidal diseases, vol 2, New York, 1977, Harper & Row, Publishers, Inc.

Newsome DA, editor: Retinal dystrophies and degenerations, New York, 1988, Raven Press.

Ryan SJ, editor: Retina, St. Louis, 1989, The CV Mosby Co.

Yanoff M, and Fine BS: Ocular pathology, a text and atlas, New York, 1982, Harper & Row, Publishers, Inc.

Clinical Electrophysiology

Babel J, Stangos N, Korol S, and Spiritus M: Ocular electrophysiology: a clinical and experimental study of electroretinogram, electro-oculogram, visual evoked response, Stuttgart, Germany, 1977, Georg Thieme.

Carr RE, and Siegel IM: Visual electrodiagnostic testing: a practical guide for the clinician, Baltimore, 1982, Williams & Wilkins.

Galloway NR: Ophthalmic electrodiagnosis. Major problems in ophthalmology, vol 1, London, 1981, Lloyd-Luke Medical Books, Ltd.

Krill AE: Hereditary retinal and choroidal diseases, vol 2, New York, 1977, Harper & Row, Publishers, Inc.

Color Vision

Pokorny J, Smith VC, Verriest G, and Pinckers AJLG: Congenital and aquired color vision defects, New York, 1979, Grune & Stratton, Inc.

INDEX

A

Abetalipoproteinemia; *see* Bassen-Kornzweig syndrome
Achromatism; *see* Rod monochromatism
Achromatopsia; *see also* Rod monochromatism
    diagnosing, 260-261
    and ERG, 250
    Sloan test for, 260
Acquired color vision defects, 255, 262
Acuity, visual, explanation of, 13
Adaptometry, dark, explanation of, 13
Adult disease, 2
Adult-onset foveomacular vitelliform dystrophy of Gass, 60, 61t, **68-69***
Age of onset and disease classification, 2
Alagile's syndrome, 118t
Albers-Schönberg disease, 119t, 151t
Albinism, 100, 101, 102t-103t, **104-105**
    flowchart for, 101
    with hemorrhaging diathesis, 102t
    ocular, 103t
    oculocutaneous, 102t
    true, 100
Albinism-oligophrenia-microphthalmia, 102t
Albinoidism, 100, 103t
Albinotic spots, congenital grouped, 100, **106-107**
Albipunctate degeneration
    progressive, 114t
    stationary; *see* Fundus albipunctatus
Allen cards, 266
Alport's syndrome, 115t, 118t, 151t
Alström syndrome, 118t, 151t
Amaurosis congenita; *see* Amaurosis, congenital, Leber's
Amaurosis, congenital, Leber's, 119t, 121t, 122, **146-147**
    ERG and, 252
Amaurotic idiocy; *see* Neuronal ceroidlipofuscinosis
Amblyopia ex anopsia and VEP, 253
Amsler grid, 266
Anatomic basis of disease classification, 7-9

**t;* Indicates table mention; disease summaries are indicated by boldface type.

Anatomic localization, 7
Angiography, fluorescein, explanation of, 14
Angioid streaks, 47, **48-51**
Annular macular dystrophy, concentric, benign, 83, **88-89**, 167t
Anomaloscope, 259-260
Anomalous trichromatism, 189t
Apert's syndrome, 103t
Aplasia, retinal, 120t
    hereditary; *see* Leber's congenital amaurosis
Areolar choroidal dystrophy, central, 18, 19t, **34-37**
Areolar form of senile macular degeneration, 167t
Areolar pigment epithelial dystrophy, central, 83, **84-85**
Arrangement tests of color vision, 256-259
Arteriohepatic dysplasia, 118t
Arthroophthalmopathy
    hereditary, with Weill-Marchesani-like habitus, 209t
    progressive, 120t
    Stickler's 208, 209t, **216-219**
Ataxia, Friedreich's, 119t, 151t
Atrophy
    central choroidal vascular; *see* Central areolar choroidal dystrophy
    choriocapillaris, diffuse, 18, 19t, **32-33**, 122t
    chorioretinal; *see* Choroidal atrophies
    choroidal, 10t, 17-18, 19t, 22-43
        flowchart for, 20, 21
        serpiginous, helicoidal, or geographic, 18, 19t, **40-41**
    gyrate, 18, 19t, **26-29**, 122t
    muscular, progressive, neuritic, 118t
    olivopontocerebellar; *see* Olivopontocerebellar retinal degeneration
    paravenous chorioretinal, 120t
    progressive bifocal chorioretinal; *see* Progressive bifocal choroidal dystrophy
    retinochoroidal; *see* Chorioretinal atrophy(ies)
    vascular, diffuse total choroidal

Atrophy—cont'd
    vascular, diffuse total choroidal—cont'd
        of autosomal inheritance; *see* Gyrate atrophy
        of X-linked inheritance; *see* Choroideremia
Atypical monochromatism, 189t
Autosomal dominant dystrophy of retinal pigment epithelium of O'Donnell, Schatz, Reid, and Green, 61t
Autosomal dominant inheritance, 3
    pedigree chart for, 6
Autosomal dominant ocular albinism with deafness and freckles, 103t
Autosomal dominant oculocutaneous albinoidism, 103t
Autosomal dominant vitreoretinochoroidopathy, 118t, 208, 209t, 226-227
Autosomal inheritance, diffuse total choroidal vascular atrophy of; *see* Gyrate atrophy
Autosomal recessive inheritance, 3
    pedigree chart for, 7
Autosomal recessive ocular albinism, 103t
a-wave, 245
    enlarged, 247

B

Bard syndrome, 103t
Bardet-Biedl syndrome, 118t, 121t, 150, **154-155**, 167t
Bassen-Kornzweig syndrome, 118t, 121t, 150, **162-163**
Batten's disease, 118t
Batten-Vogt syndrome, 167t
Bausch and Lomb chart, 266
Bear track–grouped pigmentation, 100, **108-109**
Below-threshold kinetic fields, 267
Below-threshold static fields, 267
Benedikt and Werner, reticular dystrophy of, 61t
Benign concentric annular macular dystrophy, 83, **88-89**, 167t
Bergsma-Kaiser-Kupfer syndrome, 103t

Berkow, Patz, and Singerman, dominant slowly progressive macular dystrophy of, 60, 61t, **72-73**
Best's disease, 75, **76-81**
　ERG and EOG in, 251
Biedl-Bardet syndrome; *see* Bardet-Biedl syndrome
Bietti, crystalline retinopathy of, 18, **42-43,** 115t, 119t, 121t
Bifocal chorioretinal dystrophy, progressive, 18, 19t, **30-31**
Biphasic ERG, 246
Blindness, night; *see* Nyctalopia
Block-Sulzberger syndrome, 119t
Blue cone monochromatism, 188, 189t, **194-195**
　diagnosis of, 261-262
　test for, 260
Blue monocone monochromatism, 255
Bright-flash ERG, 248
Bruch's membrane, 8
　abnormalities of, 10t, 45-57
　disorders of, 10t, 47, 48-57
Bull's-eye maculopathy, 166t-167t
　of Deutman; *see* Benign concentric annular macular dystrophy
Butterfly-shaped dystrophy, 60, 61t, **62-63**
b-wave, 245
　reduction or loss of, 247
Byers, and Marmor, pattern dystrophy of retinal pigment epithelium of, 60, 61t, **70-71**

C

CAPE dystrophy; *see* Central areolar pigment epithelial dystrophy
Carotinemia, familial, 118t
Central areolar choroidal dystrophy, 18, 19t, **34-37,** 83
Central areolar pigment epithelial dystrophy, 83, **84-85**
Central cone monochromatism, 189t
Central retina, 7-8
Central retinitis pigmentosa, 120, 121t, **134-137**
Cerebrohepatorenal syndrome, 118t
Ceroidlipofuscinosis, neuronal, 118t, 167t
Charcot-Marie-Tooth disease, 118t
Chédiak-Higashi syndrome, 103t
Chloroquine retinopathy, 120t, **236-237**
Chloroquine toxicity, 167t
Choriocapillaris, 8
　diffuse atrophy of, 18, 19t, **32-33,** 122t
Chorioretinal atrophy(ies); *see also* Choroidal atrophies
　paravenous, 120t
　pigmented paravenous, 121t, 122, **148-149**
Chorioretinal degeneration, progressive, bifocal, **30-31;** *see also* Choroideremia

Chorioretinitis, luetic, congenital, **230-231**
Choroid, 8
　retina and vitreous, disorders of, 10-11
Choroidal atrophies, 10t, 17-18, 19t, 22-43
　flowchart of, 20, 21
　serpiginous, helicoidal, or geographic, 18, 19t, **40-41**
Choroidal detachment, 120t
Choroidal dystrophy
　central areolar, 18, 19t, **34-37;** *see also* Central areolar pigment epithelial dystrophy
　peripapillary, 18, 19t, **38-39**
Choroidal elastosis; *see* Angioid streaks
"Choroidal flush," 8
Choroidal sclerosis
　circinate, 18, 19t
　diffuse; *see* Diffuse choriocapillaris atrophy
　general; *see* Diffuse choriocapillaris atrophy
　peripapillary, 122t
Choroidal vascular atrophy
　of autosomal inheritance, diffuse total; *see* Gyrate atrophy
　of X-linked inheritance, diffuse total; *see* Choroideremia
Choroidal vessels, abnormalities of, 10t, 17-43
Choroideremia, 18, 19t, **22-25,** 122t
　and ERG, 250
Choroiditis
　guttate; *see* Dominant drusen (familial)
　Holthouse-Batten superficial; *see* Dominant drusen (familial)
　Hutchinson-Tay; *see* Dominant drusen (familial)
Circinate choroidal sclerosis, 18, 19t
Cockayne's syndrome, 118t, 151t
Cohen syndrome, 167t
Color matching tests, 259-260
Color mechanism, abnormalities of, 256
Color plates, 256
Color vision
　abnormalities of, 255
　defects of, 255-256
　　congenital, 255
　　differentiating, 260-262
　　stationary; *see* Cone disorders, stationary
　explanation of, 13
　and testing, 255-256
　testing of, successful, 260
　tests of, 256-262
Complete rod monochromatism, 255
　diagnosis of, 260-261
Concentric annular macular dystrophy, benign, 83, **88-89,** 167t
Cone degenerations
　and cone-rod degenerations, 10t, 111, 166-173
　and ERG, 250

Cone disorders, stationary, 11t, 188-195
　flowchart of, 188
　listing of, 189t
Cone dystrophy, 166, 166t, **168-169**
　late-onset, with Mizuo phenomenon, 166, **170-171,** 176
　X-linked recessive, with tapetal-like sheen; *see* Late-onset cone dystrophy with Mizuo phenomenon
Cone monochromatism, 189t
　blue; *see* Blue cone monochromatism
Cone system disorders, 11t, 188-195
Cone-rod degeneration, 166, **172-173**
　cone and, 10t, 111, 166-173
Congenital amaurosis, Leber's, 119t, 121t, 122, **146-147**
Congenital color vision defects, 255
　severe, differentiating, 260-262
Congenital cystic detachment; *see* X-linked juvenile retinoschisis
Congenital disease, 2
Congenital grouped albinotic spots, 100, **106-107**
Congenital hypopigmentation; *see* Albinism
Congenital luetic chorioretinitis, **230-231**
Congenital pigmentary anomalies, 10t, 100, 101, 102-109
Congenital retinoschisis; *see* X-linked juvenile retinoschisis
Congenital rubella retinitis, **232-233**
Congenital stationary nyctalopia, 176-187
　and ERG, 249
　with normal fundus, 176, 176t, **177-178**
Congenital vascular veils; *see* X-linked juvenile retinoschisis
Contrast sensitivity test, 266
Corneal dystrophy, marginal, tapetoretinal degeneration with; *see* Crystalline retinopathy of Bietti
Counseling, genetic, 3-4
Criswick-Schepens syndrome; *see* Familial exudative vitreoretinopathy
Cross-McKusick syndrome, 102t
Crystalline retinopathy of Bietti, 18, **42-43,** 115t, 119t, 121t
CSND; *see* Congenital stationary nyctalopia
Curve, dark adaptation, 262-263, 264, 265
Cystic detachment, congenital; *see* X-linked juvenile retinoschisis
Cystinosis, 119t
Cystoid macular dystrophy, dominant, 199, **200-201**

D

Dark adaptation curve, 262-263, 264, 265
Dark adaptometer, Goldmann-Weekers, 262

Dark adaptometry
  explanation of, 13
  tests of, 262-265
Deafness
  labyrinthine, pigmentary retinopathy with; *see* Usher's syndrome
  retinal degeneration and, disorders associated with, 151t
Deficiency, phytanic acid oxidase; *see* Refsum's disease
Degeneration
  albipunctate
    progressive, 114t
    stationary; *see* Fundus albipunctatus
  chorioretinal, progressive; *see* Choroideremia
  cone; *see* Cone dystrophy
  cone-rod, 10t, 111, 166-171, **172-173**
  honeycomb, Doyne's; *see* Dominant drusen (familial)
  hyaloideotapetoretinal; *see* Goldmann-Favre vitreoretinal dystrophy
  macular
    Holthouse-Batten; *see* Dominant drusen (familial)
    juvenile; *see* Stargardt's disease
    senile, areolar form of, 167t
  pallidal, and retinitis pigmentosa, 119t
  paravenous; *see* Pigmented paravenous chorioretinal atrophy
  reticular, 120t
  retinal
    and deafness, disorders associated with, 151t
    and EOG, 251
    olivopontocerebellar, 119t, 150, **164-165**, 167t
    rod-cone, and ERG, 250
    tapetoretinal; *see also* Retinitis pigmentosa
      and ERG, 250
      with marginal corneal dystrophy; *see* Crystalline retinopathy of Bietti
    vitreoretinal
      Favre's microfibrillar; *see* Goldmann-Favre vitreoretinal dystrophy
      snowflake, 120t, 208, 209t, 220-221
Degenerative myopia, 47, **56-57**, 122t
Detachment
  choroidal, 120t
  cystic, congenital; *see* X-linked juvenile retinoschisis
  retinal, 120t
Deutan color defect, 256
  and Nagel anomaloscope, 259t
Deuteranomaly, 189t
Deuteranopia, 189t, 256
Deutman, bull's-eye maculopathy of; *see* Benign concentric annular macular dystrophy
Diagnosis, differential, explanation of, 14
Diastrophic variant, 209t

Diathesis, hemorrhaging, albinism with, 102t
Dichromatism, 189t, 255
Differential diagnoses, explanation of, 14
Diffuse choriocapillaris atrophy, 18, 19t, **32-33**, 122t
Diffuse choroidal sclerosis; *see* Diffuse choriocapillaris atrophy
Diffuse total choroidal vascular atrophy
  of autosomal inheritance; *see* Gyrate atrophy
  of X-linked inheritance; *see* Choroideremia
Disease
  Albers-Schönberg, 119t, 151t
  Batten's, 118t
  Best's, 75, **76-81**
    ERG and EOG in, 251
  Charcot-Marie-Tooth, 118t
  classification of, 2
    anatomic basis of, 7-9
  flecked retina, 10t, 111, 112, 113, 114t-115t, 116-117
    flowchart for, 113
  Goldman-Favre, 119t
  Hooft, 119t
  inner retinal, 11t, 199-205
  Oguchi's, 176, 176t, **180-183**
  Paget's, 120t
    juvenile, 119t
  Pelizaeus-Merzbacher, 120t
  Refsum's, 120t, 121t, 150, 151t, **160-161**
  retinal
    other causes of, 229-241
    and pattern VER, 254
    review of, 15-241
  sea-blue histiocyte, 167t
  Stargardt's, 83, **92-95**, 114t, 119t, 166t
    dominant; *see* Dominant progressive foveal dystrophy
  Steinert's, 119t, 121t; *see also* Myotonic dystrophy of Steinert
  Tay-Sachs, 199, **204-205**
  Turner's, 120t
  Wagner's; *see* Wagner's vitreoretinal dystrophy
Disease summaries, format for, 12-14
Dominant cystoid macular dystrophy, 199, **200-201**
Dominant drusen (familial), 47, **54-55**, 114t
Dominant progressive foveal dystrophy, 83, **96-97**
  of Lefler, Wadsworth, and Sidbury; *see* Lefler-Wadsworth-Sidbury dystrophy
Dominant slowly progressive macular dystrophy of Singerman, Berkow, and Patz, 60, 61t, **72-73**
Dominant Stargardt's disease; *see* Dominant progressive foveal dystrophy

Donaldson-Fitzpatrick, 103t
Doyne's honeycomb degeneration; *see* Dominant drusen (familial)
Drusen
  dominant (familial), 47, **54-55**, 114t
  senile, 47
Dysgenesis neuroepithelialis retinae; *see* Leber's congenital amaurosis
Dysplasia
  arteriohepatic, 118t
  oculodentodigital, 119t
  renal, 120t
Dysplasia congenita, spondyloepiphyseal, 209t
Dysplasia spondyloepiphysiana congenita, 119t, 151t
Dystonic lipidosis; *see* Sea-blue histiocyte disease
Dystrophia reticularis laminae pigmentosae; *see* Reticular dystrophy of Sjögren
Dystrophy
  autosomal dominant, of retinal pigment epithelium of O'Donnell, Schatz, Reid, and Green, 61t
  butterfly-shaped, 60, 61t, **62-63**
  CAPE; *see* Dystrophy, central areolar pigment epithelial
  central areolar pigment epithelial, 83, **84-85**
  chorioretinal, progressive bifocal, **30-31**
  choroidal
    central areolar, 18, 19t, **34-37**
    peripapillary, 18, 19t, **38-39**
  cone; *see* Cone dystrophy
  cone-rod; *see* Cone-rod degeneration
  corneal, marginal, tapetoretinal degeneration with; *see* Crystalline retinopathy of Bietti
  epithelial, pigment, of Noble-Carr-Siegel, 83, **98-99**
  foveal, dominant progressive, 83, **96-97**
    of Lefler, Wadsworth, and Sidbury; *see* Lefler-Wadsworth-Sidbury dystrophy
  foveomacular pigment epithelial, adult-onset, 60, 61t, **68-69**
  foveomacular vitelliform, of Gass, adult-onset, 60, 61t, **68-69**
  ganglion cell, 199; *see also* Gangliosidosis
  Lefler-Wadsworth-Sidbury, 83, **90-91**
  macroreticular (spider dystrophy), 60, 61t, **66-67**
  macular; *see* Macular dystrophy
  myotonic, 119t, 121t
    of Steinert, 150, **158-159**
  pattern, of retinal pigment epithelium of Marmor and Byers, 60, 61t, **70-71**

Dystrophy—cont'd
　reticular
　　of Benedikt and Werner, 61t
　　of Sjögren, 60, 61t, **64-65,** 121t
　retinal
　　pigmentary sector; see Sector
　　　retinitis pigmentosa
　　primary; see Retinitis pigmentosa
　　rod-cone, 10t, 111, 118-149, 150-166, 166t
　　RPE; see Retinal pigment epithelium, dystrophies of
　　spider; see Macroreticular dystrophy (spider dystrophy)
　　tapetoretinal; see Choroideremia; Retinitis pigmentosa
　　vitelliform, ERG and EOG in, 251
　　vitreoretinal, 11t, 208, 209t, 210-227
　　　Goldmann-Favre, 121t, 208, 209t, **212-213**
　　　Wagner's, 120t, 208, 209t, **214-215**

E

Edema, macular, cystoid, dominant; see Dominant cystoid macular dystrophy
Elastosis, choroidal; see Angioid streaks
Electrooculogram, 250-251
　explanation of, 13
Electrophysiologic tests, review of, 245-254
Electroretinogram, 245-250
　explanation of, 13
EOG; see Electrooculogram
Epithelial dystrophy
　central areolar pigment, 83, **84-85**
　pigment, of Noble-Carr-Siegel, 83, **98-99**
Epithelium, retinal pigment; see Retinal pigment epithelium
ERG; see Electroretinogram
Evoked response, visual, explanation of, 14
External limiting membrane, 8
External ophthalmoplegia, progressive, with pigmentary retinopathy; see Kearns-Sayre syndrome
Exudative vitreoretinopathy, familial, 208, 209t, **222-225**

F

Familial carotinemia, 118t
Familial drusen, 47, **54-55,** 114t
Familial exudative vitreoretinopathy, 208, 209t, **222-225**
Familial foveal retinoschisis, 199, **202-203**
Familial idiocy, infantile; see Tay-Sachs disease
Familial pseudoinflammatory macular dystrophy of Sorsby, 47, **52-53**
Farnsworth-Munsell D-15 panel, 256-257

Farnsworth-Munsell 100-hue test, 257-259
Favre's microfibrillar vitreoretinal degeneration; see Goldmann-Favre vitreoretinal dystrophy
Fenestrated sheen macular dystrophy, 83, **86-87,** 167t
Fields, visual, explanation of, 13
Findings, key, explanation of, 12-13
Flash visual-evoked potential, 252
Flecked retina diseases, 10t, 111, 112, 113, 114t-115t, 116-117
　flowchart for, 113
Flecked retina of Kandori, 114t, 176, 176t, **186-187**
Flowchart
　for albinism, 101
　for choroidal atrophies, 20, 21
　for nystagmus, 190, 191
　for photophobia, 191
　for progressive nyctalopia, 123
　for stationary nyctalopia, 177
Fluorescein angiography, explanation of, 14
Flush, choroidal, 8
Flynn-Aird syndrome, 119t, 151t
Focal ERG, 249
Focal retinal pigment epithelial dystrophies, 10t, 83, 84-99
Fovea, butterfly-shaped pigment dystrophy of, 60, 61t, **62-63**
Foveal dystrophy, dominant progressive, 83, **96-97**
　of Lefler, Wadsworth, and Sidbury; see Lefler-Wadsworth-Sidbury dystrophy
Foveal retinoschisis, familial, 199, **202-203**
Foveomacular dystrophy of Gass; see Adult-onset foveomacular vitelliform dystrophy of Gass
Foveomacular pigment epithelial dystrophy, adult-onset; see Adult-onset foveomacular vitelliform dystrophy of Gass
Foveomacular vitelliform dystrophy of Gass, adult-onset, 60, 61t, **68-69**
Friedreich's ataxia, 119t, 151t
Fuch's gyrate atrophy; see Gyrate atrophy
Fucosidosis mucolipidoses, 167t
Fundus, normal
　congenital stationary night blindness with, 176, 176t, **178-179**
　photograph of, 7
Fundus albipunctatus, 114t, 176, 176t, **184-185**
Fundus flavimaculatus, 112, 114t, **116-117,** 119t
Fundus pulverulentus (Slezak and Hommer), 61t
Fundus xerophthalmicus; see Vitamin A deficiency retinopathy

G

Ganglion cell dystrophies, 199; see also Gangliosidosis
Ganglion cell layer, 8
Gangliosidosis, 199, **204-205**
Gargoylism, 119t
Generalized choroidal sclerosis; see Diffuse choriocapillaris atrophy
Generalized RPE dystrophy, 10t, 75, 76-81
Genetic counseling, 3-4
Geographic choroidal atrophy, 18, 19t, **40-41**
Glare test, 266
Goldmann-Favre disease, 119t
Goldmann-Favre vitreoretinal dystrophy, 121t, 208, 209t, **212-213**
Goldmann-Weekers dark adaptometer, 262
Green, O'Donnell, Schatz, and Reid, autosomal dominant dystrophy of retinal pigment epithelium of, 61t
Grid, Amsler, 266
Grönblad-Strandberg syndrome, 120t
Group, explanation of, 12
Guttate choroiditis; see Dominant drusen (familial)
Gyrate atrophy, 18, 19t, **26-29,** 122t

H

Hallervorden-Spatz syndrome, 115t, 119t, 167t
Hallgren's syndrome, 119t, 151t
Helicoidal choroidal atrophy, 18, 19t, **40-41**
Hemorrhaging diathesis, albinism with, 102t
Hereditary arthroophthalmopathy with Weill-Marchesani-like habitus, 209t
Hereditary retinal aplasia; see Leber's congenital amaurosis
Hereditary vitreoretinal dystrophy, Wagner's, 120t
Heredopathia atactica polyneuritiformis; see Refsum's disease
Heredoretinopathia congenitalis; see Leber's congenital amaurosis
Hermansky-Pudlak syndrome, 102t
Holthouse-Batten superficial choroiditis; see Dominant drusen (familial)
Homocystinuria, 119t
Honeycomb degeneration, Doyne's; see Dominant drusen (familial)
Hooft disease, 119t
Hunter's syndrome, 119t
Hurler syndrome, 119t, 151t
Hutchinson-Tay choroiditis; see Dominant drusen (familial)
Hyaloideotapetoretinal degeneration; see Goldmann-Favre vitreoretinal dystrophy

Hydroxychloroquine toxicity; *see* Chloroquine retinopathy
Hyperostosis corticalis deformans, 119t
Hyperoxaluria, primary, 115t
Hypopigmentation, congenital; *see* Albinism

I

Idiocy
    amaurotic; *see* Neuronal ceroidlipofuscinosis
    familial, infantile; *see* Tay-Sachs disease
Imidazole aminoaciduria, 119t
Incomplete rod monochromatism, 255-256
    diagnosis of, 261
Incomplete universal albinism, 102t
Incontinentia pigmenti, 119t
Infantile disease, 2
Infantile familial idiocy; *see* Tay-Sachs disease
Infantile phytanic acid storage, 119t
Inheritance
    autosomal, diffuse total choroidal vascular atrophy of; *see* Gyrate atrophy
    explanation of, 13
    patterns of, 3
        and disease classification, 2
        pedigree charts for, 6, 7
    X-linked, diffuse total choroidal vascular atrophy of; *see* Choroideremia
Inner nuclear layer, 8
Inner plexiform layer, 8
Inner retina, 8
    abnormalities of, 11t, 197-205
    diseases of, 11t, 199-205
Internal limiting membrane, 9
Intraocular foreign bodies, metallic, **238-239**
Inverse retinitis pigmentosa, 120, 121t, **134-137**

J

Juvenile disease, 2
Juvenile macular degeneration; *see* Stargardt's disease
Juvenile Paget's disease, 119t
Juvenile retinoschisis, X-linked, 120t, 208, 209t, **210-211**

K

Kandori, flecked retina of, 114t, 176, 176t, **186-187**
Kartagener's syndrome, 119t
Kearns-Sayre syndrome, 119t, 150, **156-157**
Key findings, explanation of, 12-13
Key symptoms, explanation of, 12
Kindergarten chart, 266
Kjellin syndrome, 115t
Kniest syndrome, 209t

L

Laboratory studies, explanation of, 13
Laboratory tests of macular function, 266
Labyrinthine deafness, pigmentary retinopathy with; *see* Usher's syndrome
Landolt C test, 266
Late receptor potential, 246
Late-onset cone dystrophy with Mizuo phenomenon, 166, **170-171**, 176
Latency in ERG waveform, 245
Laurence-Moon syndrome, 119t, 150
Laurence-Moon-Bardet-Biedl syndrome; *see* Bardet-Biedl syndrome
Leber's congenital amaurosis, 119t, 121t, 122, **146-147**
    ERG and, 252
Lefler-Wadsworth-Sidbury dystrophy, 83, **90-91**
Lesion(s)
    of optic nerve or tract, and VEP, 252
    predominant, appearance of, and classification of disease, 2
Light-dark ratio of EOG, 251
Lignac-Fanconi syndrome, 119t
Limiting membrane
    external, 8
    internal, 9
Lipidosis, dystonic; *see* Sea-blue histiocyte disease
Localization, anatomic, 7
Luetic chorioretinitis, congenital, **230-231**

M

Macroreticular dystrophy (spider dystrophy), 60, 61t, **66-67**
Macula lutea, 7
Macular degeneration
    Holthouse-Batten; *see* Dominant drusen (familial)
    juvenile; *see* Stargardt's disease
    senile, areolar form of, 167t
Macular dystrophy
    concentric annular, benign, 83, **88-89**, 167t
    cystoid, dominant, 199, **200-201**
    familial pseudoinflammatory, of Sorsby, 47, **52-53**
    fenestrated sheen, 83, **86-87**, 167t
    North Carolina; *see* Lefler-Wadsworth-Sidbury dystrophy
    of Singerman, Berkow, and Patz, dominant slowly progressive, 60, 61t, **72-73**
    vitelliform; *see* Best's disease
Macular function tests, 265-266
Macular pattern RPE dystrophies, 10t, 60, 61t, 62-73
Macular stress test, 266
Maculopathy, bull's-eye, 166t-167t
    of Deutman; *see* Benign concentric annular macular dystrophy

Malatia levantinese; *see* Dominant drusen (familial)
Mannosidosis, 119t
Manual, organization of, 9-14
Marginal corneal dystrophy, tapetoretinal degeneration with; *see* Crystalline retinopathy of Bietti
Marinesco-Sjögren syndrome, 119t
Marmor and Byers, pattern dystrophy of retinal pigment epithelium of, 60, 61t, **70-71**
Marshall's syndrome, 151t
Melanosis vasculorum retinae; *see* Angioid streaks
Mellaril toxicity; *see* Phenothiazine retinopathy
Membrane
    Bruch's, 8
        abnormalities of, 10t, 45-57
        disorders of, 10t, 47, 48-57
    limiting
        external, 8
        internal, 9
Mesopic ERG, 246
Metallic intraocular foreign bodies, **238-239**
Metallosis, 120t
Metallosis bulbi, 120t, **238-239**
Methoxyflurane toxicity, secondary oxalosis caused by, 115t
Meyer-Schwickerath and Weyers syndrome, 119t
Microfibrillar vitreoretinal degeneration, Favre's; *see* Goldmann-Favre vitreoretinal dystrophy
Mizuo phenomenon, late-onset cone dystrophy with, 166, **170-171**, 176
Monochromatism, 189t
    blue cone, 188, 189t, **194-195**
        diagnosis of, 261-262
        test for, 260
    blue monocone, 255
    rod, 188, 189t, **192-193**
        atypical incomplete, 189t
        complete, 255
            diagnosis of, 260-261
        incomplete, 255-256
            diagnosis of, 261
        test for, 260
Monocone monochromatism, blue, 255
Mucopolysaccharidoses, 119t, 151t, 167t
Multiplex inheritance, 4
Muscular atrophy, neuritic, progressive, 118t
Myopia
    degenerative, 47, **56-57**, 122t
    high, 119t
    pathologic progressive; *see* Degenerative myopia
Myotonic atrophica; *see* Myotonic dystrophy, of Steinert
Myotonic dystrophica; *see* Myotonic dystrophy, of Steinert

Myotonic dystrophy, 119t, 121t
    of Steinert, 119t, 121t, 150, **158-159**

N

Nagel anomaloscope, 259, 260
Negative ERG, 247
Nerve, optic, lesions of, and VEP, 252
Nerve fiber layer, 8-9
Nettleship-Falls X-linked ocular albinism, 103t
Neuritic muscular atrophy, progressive, 118t
Neuritis, optic, and P100, 253
Neuronal ceroidlipofuscinosis, 118t, 167t
Night blindness; see Nyctalopia
Noble-Carr-Siegel, pigment epithelial dystrophy of, 83, **98-99**
North Carolina macular dystrophy; see Lefler-Wadsworth-Sidbury dystrophy
Nuclear layer, 8
Nyctalopia
    progressive, 121t-122t
        flowchart for, 123
    stationary, 176t
        congenital, 176-187
        and ERG, 249
        with normal fundus, 176, 176t, **178-179**
    flowchart for, 177
Nystagmus, flowchart for, 190, 191

O

O'Donnell, Schatz, Reid, and Green, autosomal dominant dystrophy of retinal pigment epithelium of, 61t
O'Donnell and Welch, fenestrated sheen macular dystrophy of; see Fenestrated sheen macular dystrophy
Occlusion, vascular, 120t
Ocular albinism, 103t
Oculocutaneous albinism, 102t
Oculodentodigital dysplasia, 119t
Oguchi's disease, 176, 176t, **180-183**
Olivopontocerebellar retinal degeneration, 119t, 150, **164-165**, 167t
Onset, explanation of, 13
Ophthalmoplegia, external, progressive, with pigmentary retinopathy; see Kearns-Sayre syndrome
Ophthalmoplegic dystonic lipidosis; see Sea-blue histiocyte disease
Optic nerve or tract, lesions of, and VEP, 252
Optic neuritis and P100, 253
Oscillatory potentials, 248
    of ERG waveform, 245
Osteopetrosis, 119t, 151t
Osteoporosis, 119t
Outer nuclear layer, 8
Outer plexiform layer, 8
Oxalosis, 115t

P

P100, 253
Paget's disease, 120t
    juvenile, 119t
Pallidal degeneration and retinitis pigmentosa, 119t
Para-arteriolar retinal pigment epithelium, preserved, retinitis pigmentosa with, 121t, 122, **142-143**
Paravenous chorioretinal atrophy, 120t
    pigmented, 121t, 122, **148-149**
Pathologic progressive myopia; see Dégenerative myopia
Pathology, explanation of, 14
Pattern dystrophy of retinal pigment epithelium of Marmor and Byers, 60, 61t, **70-71**
Pattern VER, 253, 254
Patz, Singerman, Berkow and, dominant slowly progressive macular dystrophy of, 60, 61t, **72-73**
Peak delay in ERG waveform, 245
Pedigree charts, 4, 5, 6, 7
Pelizaeus-Merzbacher disease, 120t
Pericentral retinitis pigmentosa, 121t, 122, **138-141**
Peripapillary choroidal dystrophy, 18, 19t, **38-39**
Peripapillary choroidal sclerosis, 122t
Peripheral retina, 8
Phenomenon, Mizuo, late-onset cone dystrophy with, 166, **170-171**, 176
Phenothiazine retinopathy, 120t, **234-235**
Photophobia, flowchart for, 191
Photopic ERG, 246
Photoreceptor layer, 8
Photoreceptor–retinal pigment epithelium complex, abnormalities of, 10t-11t, 111-173
Photoreceptors, abnormalities of, 11t, 175-195
Phytanic acid oxidase deficiency; see Refsum's disease
Phytanic acid storage, infantile, 119t
Pierre Marie syndrome, 120t
Pigment epithelial dystrophy
    central areolar; see Central areolar choroidal dystrophy
    foveomacular, adult-onset; see Adult-onset foveomacular vitelliform dystrophy of Gass
    of Noble-Carr-Siegel, 83, **98-99**
Pigment epithelium, retinal; see Retinal pigment epithelium
Pigmentary anomalies, congenital, 10t, 100, 101, 102-109
Pigmentary retinal dystrophy, sector; see Sector retinitis pigmentosa
Pigmentary retinopathy, 120t
    bear track; see Bear track–grouped pigmentation
    causes of, 118t-120t
    with labyrinthine deafness; see Usher's syndrome
    progressive external ophthalmoplegia with; see Kearns-Sayre syndrome
    uniocular; see Unilateral retinitis pigmentosa
Pigmentation, bear track–grouped, 100, **108-109**
Pigmented paravenous chorioretinal atrophy, 121t, 122, **148-149**
PII, 246
PIII; see Late receptor potential
Plexiform layer, 8
Polar bear tracks; see Congenital grouped albinotic spots
Posterior pole disease, classification of, 2
PPRPE; see Retinitis pigmentosa, with preserved para-arteriolar retinal pigment epithelium
Preserved para-arteriolar retinal pigment epithelium, retinitis pigmentosa with, 121t, 122, **142-143**
Primary hyperoxaluria, 115t
Primary retinal dystrophy; see Retinitis pigmentosa
Prognosis, explanation of, 13
Progression
    and disease classification, 2
    explanation of, 13
Progressive albipunctate degeneration, 114t
Progressive arthroophthalmopathy, 120t
Progressive bifocal chorioretinal dystrophy, 18, 19t, **30-31**
Progressive choroidal degeneration; see Choroideremia
Progressive external ophthalmoplegia with pigmentary retinopathy; see Kearns-Sayre syndrome
Progressive foveal dystrophy, dominant, 83, **96-97**
    of Lefler, Wadsworth, and Sidbury; see Lefler-Wadsworth-Sidbury dystrophy
Progressive myopia, pathologic; see Degenerative myopia
Progressive neuritic muscular atrophy, 118t
Progressive nyctalopia, 121t-122t
    flowchart for, 123
Protan color defect, 256
    and Nagel anomaloscope, 259t
Protanomaly, 189t
Protanopia, 189t, 256
Pseudoinflammatory macular dystrophy of Sorsby, familial, 47, **52-53**
Pseudoisochromatic (color) plates, 256

Pseudoxanthoma elasticum, 120t
Psychophysical tests, review of, 255-267
Punctate oculocutaneous albinoidism, 103t

R

Rayleigh equation, 259
Receptor potential, late, 246
Recessive cone dystrophy, X-linked, with tapetal-like sheen; *see* Late-onset cone dystrophy with Mizuo phenomenon
References, explanation of, 14
Refraction, explanation of, 13
Refsum's disease, 120t, 121t, 150, 151t, **160-161**
Reid, Green, O'Donnell, and Schatz, autosomal dominant dystrophy of retinal pigment epithelium of, 61t
Renal dysplasia, 120t
Response, evoked, visual, explanation of, 14
Reticular degeneration, 120t
Reticular dystrophy
  of Benedikt and Werner, 61t
  of Sjögren, 60, 61t, **64-65,** 121t
Retina
  aplasia of, 120t
    hereditary; *see* Leber's congenital amaurosis
  central, 7-8
  choroid, and vitreous, disorders of, 10-11
  degeneration of
    and deafness, disorders associated with, 151t
    and EOG, 251
    olivopontocerebellar, 119t, 150, **164-165,** 167t
  detachment of, 120t
  diseases of
    flecked, 10t, 111, 112, 114t-115t, 116-117
      flowchart of, 113
    other causes of, 229-241
    and pattern VER, 254
  dystrophy of
    pigmentary, sector; *see* Sector retinitis pigmentosa
    primary; *see* Retinitis pigmentosa
  flecked, of Kandori, 114t, 176, 176t, **186-187**
  inner, 8
    abnormalities of, 11t, 197-205
    diseases of, 11t, 199-205
  peripheral, 8
Retinal pigment epithelium, 8
  abnormalities of, 10t, 59-109
  dystrophies of
    autosomal dominant, of O'Donnell, Schatz, Reid, and Green, 61t
    focal, 10t, 83, 84-99
    generalized, 10t, 75, 76-81

Retinal pigment epithelium—cont'd
  dystrophies of—cont'd
    pattern
      macular, 10t, 60, 61t, 62-73
        of Marmor and Byers, 60, 61t, **70-71**
      retinitis pigmentosa with preserved para-arteriolar, 121t, 122, **142-143**
      spots of, congenital grouped albinotic; *see* Congenital grouped albinoid spots
Retinal pigment epithelium–photoreceptor complex, abnormalities of, 10t-11t, 111-173
Retinal toxicity, 248
Retinitis, rubella, congenital, 232-233
Retinitis pigmentosa, 10t, 111, 118-149, 121t, **124-127**
  central, 120, 120t, 121t, **134-137**
  and ERG, 250
  inverse, 120, 120t, **134-137**
  pallidal degeneration and, 119t
  pericentral, 121t, 122, **138-141**
  with preserved para-arteriolar retinal pigment epithelium, 121t, 122, **142-143**
  sector, 120, 121t, **130-131**
  senile, 122
  sine pigmento, 120, 121t, **128-129**
  syndromes associated with, 10t, 111, 150-166
  unilateral, 120, 121t, **132-133**
  uniocular; *see* Retinitis pigmentosa, unilateral
Retinitis punctata albescens, 114t, 121t, 122, **144-145**
Retinochoroidal atrophy, pigmented paravenous; *see* Pigmented paravenous chorioretinal atrophy
Retinochoroiditis radiata; *see* Pigmented paravenous chorioretinal atrophy
Retinopathy
  chloroquine, 120t, **236-237**
  crystalline, of Bietti, 18, **42-43,** 115t, 119t, 121t
  phenothiazine, 120t, **234-235**
  pigmentary; *see* Pigmentary retinopathy
  tamoxifen, 115t
  vitamin A, 115t
  vitamin A deficiency, **240-241**
Retinoschisis
  foveal, familial, 199, **202-203**
  juvenile, X-linked, 120t, 208, 209t, **210-211**
Rod and cone ERGs, 246
Rod monochromatism, 188, 189t, **192-193**
  complete, 255
  diagnosis of, 260-261
  and ERG, 250

Rod monochromatism—cont'd
  incomplete, 255-256
    diagnosis of, 261
  test for, 260
Rod system disorders, 11t, 176-187
Rod/cone break, 262
Rod-cone degeneration and ERG, 250
Rod-cone dystrophies, 10t, 111, 118-149, 150-166, 166t
RPE; *see* Retinal pigment epithelium
Rubella retinitis, congenital, 120t, **232-233**

S

Saldino-Mainzer syndrome, 120t
Sanfilippo's syndrome, 119t
Schatz, Reid, Green, and O'Donnell, autosomal dominant dystrophy of retinal pigment epithelium of, 61t
Scheie's syndrome, 119t
Sclerosis, choroidal
  central areolar; *see* Central areolar choroidal dystrophy
  circinate, 18, 19t
  diffuse; *see* Diffuse choriocapillaris atrophy
  generalized; *see* Diffuse choriocapillaris atrophy
  peripapillary, 122t
Scotopic ERG, 246
Sea-blue histiocyte disease, 167t
Secondary oxalosis caused by methoxyflurane toxicity, 115t
Sector retinitis pigmentosa, 120, 121t, **130-131**
Senile disease, 2
Senile drusen, 47
Senile macular degeneration, areolar form of, 167t
Senile retinitis pigmentosa, 122
Senior-Loken syndrome, 120t
Serpiginous choroidal atrophy, 18, 19t, **40-41**
Sex-linked recessive inheritance, 3
  pedigree chart for, 6
Sheen macular dystrophy, fenestrated, 83, **86-87,** 167t
Sheen, tapetal-like, X-linked recessive cone dystrophy with; *see* Late-onset cone dystrophy with Mizuo phenomenon
Sidbury, Lefler, and Wadsworth, foveal dystrophy of; *see* Lefler-Wadsworth-Sidbury dystrophy
Simplex inheritance, 4
Singerman, Berkow, and Patz, dominant slowly progressive macular dystrophy of, 60, 61t, **72-73**
Sjögren, reticular dystrophy of, 60, 61t, **64-65,** 121t
Sjögren-Larsson syndrome, 167t

Slezak and Hommer's fundus pulverulentus, 61t
Sloan achromatopsia test, 260
Sloan chart, 266
Snellen E chart, 266
Snellen visual acuity chart, 265
Snowflake vitreoretinal degeneration, 120t, 208, 209t, **220-221**
Sorsby, familial pseudoinflammatory macular dystrophy of, 47, **52-53**
Spider dystrophy; *see* Macroreticular dystrophy
Spondyloepiphyseal dysplasia congenita, 209t
Spots, albinotic, congenital grouped, 100, **106-107**
Standard Pseudoisochromatic Plates, 262
Stargardt's disease, 83, **92-95,** 114t, 119t, 166t
  dominant; *see* Dominant progressive foveal dystrophy
Stationary albipunctate degeneration; *see* Fundus albipunctatus
Stationary cone disorders, 11t, 188-195
  flowchart of, 188
  listing of, 189t
Stationary nyctalopia, 176t
  congenital, 176-187
    and ERG, 249
    with normal fundus, 176, 176t, **178-179**
  flowchart for, 177
Steinert, myotonic dystrophy of, 150, **158-159**
Steinert's disease, 119t, 121t
Stickler's arthroophthalmopathy, 120t, 208, 209t, **216-219**
Streaks, angioid, 47, **48-51**
Stress test, macular, 266
Superficial choroiditis, Holthouse-Batten; *see* Dominant drusen (familial)
Suprathreshold static fields, 267
Symptoms
  and disease classification, 2
  key, explanation of, 12
Syndrome
  Alagile's, 118t
  Alport's, 115t, 118t, 151t
  Alström, 118t, 151t
  Apert's, 103t
  Bard, 103t
  Bardet-Biedl, 118t, 121t, 150, **154-155,** 167t
  Bassen-Kornzweig, 118t, 121t, 150, **162-163**
  Batten-Vogt, 167t
  Bergsma-Kaiser-Kupfer, 103t
  Block-Sulzberger, 119t
  cerebrohepatorenal, 118t
  Chédiak-Higashi, 103t
  Cockayne's, 118t, 151t
  Cohen, 167t

Syndrome—cont'd
  Criswick-Schepens; *see* Familial exudative vitreoretinopathy
  Cross-McKusick, 102t
  Donaldson-Fitzpatrick, 103t
  flecked retina; *see* Flecked retina diseases
  Flynn-Aird, 119t, 151t
  Grönblad-Strandberg, 120t
  Hallervorden-Spatz, 115t, 119t, 167t
  Hallgren's, 119t, 151t
  Hermansky-Pudlak, 102t
  Hunter's, 119t
  Hurler, 119t, 151t
  Kartagener's, 119t
  Kearns-Sayre, 119t, 150, **156-157**
  Kjellin, 115t
  Kniest, 209t
  Laurence-Moon, 119t, 150
  Laurence-Moon-Bardet-Biedl; *see* Bardet-Biedl syndrome
  Lignac-Fanconi, 119t
  Marinesco-Sjögren, 119t
  Marshall's, 151t
  Meyer-Schwickerath and Weyers, 119t
  Pierre Marie, 120t
  RP-associated, 10t, 111, 150-166
  Saldino-Mainzer, 120t
  Sanfilippo's, 119t
  Scheie's, 119t
  Sjögren-Larsson, 167t
  Stickler's; *see* Stickler's arthroophthalmopathy
  Usher's, 120t, 121t, 150, 151t, **152-153**
  Uyemura's; *see* Vitamin A deficiency retinopathy
  Waardenburg, 120t, 151t
  Waardenburg-like, 103t
  Zellweger, 118t
Synonyms, explanation of, 14
Syphilis, 120t, **230-231**

T

Tamoxifen retinopathy, 115t, 120t
Tapetoretinal degeneration
  and ERG, 250
  with marginal corneal dystrophy; *see* Crystalline retinopathy of Bietti
Tapetoretinal dystrophy; *see* Choroideremia; Retinitis pigmentosa
Tay-Sachs disease, 199, **204-205**
Testing, color vision and, 255-256
Test(s)
  arrangement, of color vision, 256-259
  for blue cone monochromatism, 260
  of color vision, 256-262
  contrast sensitivity, 266
  dark adaptometry, 262-265
  electrophysiologic, review of, 245-254
  Farnsworth-Munsell 100-hue, 257-259
  glare, 266
  laboratory, of macular function, 266

Test(s)—cont'd
  Landolt C, 266
  macular function, 265-266
  macular stress, 266
  psychophysical, review of, 255-267
  for rod monochromatism, 260
  Sloan achromatopsia, 260
  visual fields, 266-267
Thioridazine retinopathy; *see* Phenothiazine retinopathy
Topographic distribution and classification of disease, 2
Toxoplasmosis, 120t
Treatment, explanation of, 14
Trichromatic vision and Nagel anomaloscope, 259t
Trichromatism, 255
  anomalous, 189t
Tritan color defect, 256
Tritanomaly, 189t
Tritanopia, 189t
Turner's disease, 120t
Tyrosinase-negative oculocutaneous albinism, 102t
Tyrosinase-positive oculocutaneous albinism, 102t

U

Unilateral retinitis pigmentosa, 120, 121t, **132-133**
Uniocular pigmentary retinopathy; *see* Unilateral retinitis pigmentosa
Uniocular retinitis pigmentosa; *see* Unilateral retinitis pigmentosa
Universal albinism, incomplete, 102t
Usher's syndrome, 120t, 121t, 150, 151t, **152-153**
  Merin classification of, 119t
Uyemura's syndrome; *see* Vitamin A deficiency retinopathy

V

Vascular atrophy
  diffuse total choroidal
    of autosomal inheritance; *see* Gyrate atrophy
    of X-linked inheritance; *see* Choroideremia
Vascular occlusion, 120t
Vascular veils, congenital; *see* X-linked juvenile retinoschisis
VEP; *see* Visual-evoked potential
VER; *see* Visual evoked response
Vessels, choroidal, abnormalities of, 10t, 17-43
Vision, color; *see* Color vision
Visual acuity charts, 265-266
Visual acuity, explanation of, 13
Visual-evoked potential, flash, 252
Visual evoked response
  explanation of, 14
  flash, 252
  in optic atrophy, 252
  pattern, 253, 254

Visual evoked response—cont'd
    waveform for, 252
Visual fields, explanation of, 13
Visual fields test, 266-267
Vitamin A deficiency retinopathy,
    240-241
Vitamin A retinopathy, 115t
Vitelliform dystrophy
    ERG and EOG in, 251
    foveomacular, adult-onset, of Gass,
        60, 61t, **68-69**
Vitelliform macular dystrophy; see Best's
    disease
Vitreoretinal abnormalities, 11t, 207-227
Vitreoretinal degeneration
    Favre's microfibrillar; see
        Goldmann-Favre vitreoretinal
        dystrophy
    snowflake, 120t, 208, 209t, **220-221**
Vitreoretinal dystrophies, 11t, 208, 209t,
    210-227
    Goldmann-Favre, 121t, 208, 209t,
        212-213
    Wagner's, 120t, 208, 209t, **214-215**

Vitreoretinochoroidopathy, autosomal
    dominant, 118t, 208, 209t,
    226-227
Vitreoretinopathy, exudative, familial,
    208, 209t, **222-225**
Vitreous, choroid, and retina, disorders
    of, 10-11

W

Waardenburg syndrome, 120t, 151t
Waardenburg-like syndrome, 103t
Wadsworth, Sidbury, and Lefler, foveal
    dystrophy of; see
    Lefler-Wadsworth-Sidbury
    dystrophy
Wagner's vitreoretinal dystrophy, 120t,
    208, 209t, **214-215**
Waveform
    ERG, 245
        slowing of, 247
    VER, 252
Weill-Marchesani-like habitus, hereditary
    arthroophthalmopathy with,
    209t

Welch, O'Donnell and, fenestrated sheen
    macular dystrophy of; see
    Fenestrated sheen macular
    dystrophy
Werner, Benedikt and, reticular
    dystrophy of, 61t

X

X-linked inheritance, diffuse total
    choroidal vascular atrophy of;
    see Choroideremia
X-linked juvenile retinoschisis, 120t,
    208, 209t, **210-211**
X-linked recessive cone dystrophy with
    tapetal-like sheen; see
    Late-onset cone dystrophy with
    Mizuo phenomenon

Y

Yellow-mutant oculocutaneous albinism,
    102t

Z

Zellweger syndrome, 118t